RHEUMATOLOGICAL PHYSIOTHERAPY

CAROL DAVID MCSP
Therapies Audit and Research Co-ordinator
Midstaffordshire General Hospitals

JILL LLOYD BA MCSP
Lecturer in Physiotherapy
Department of Health Studies
Brunel University
Middlesex

 Mosby

London Philadelphia St Louis Sydney Tokyo

Publisher	**Jill Northcott**
Development Editor	**Gillian Harris**
Project Manager	**Louise Patchett**
Production	**Susan Walby**
Design	**Greg Smith**
Layout	**James Evoy**
Index	**Ann Marangos**
Cover Design	**Greg Smith**
Illustration Manager	**Danny Pyne**
Illustrator	**Deborah Gyan**

Copyright © 1999 Mosby International Limited

Published in 1998 by Mosby, an imprint of Mosby International Limited

ISBN 0 7234 2594 9

Printed by Printer Trento s.r.l., Trento, Italy

Set in: Scala: Fontworks. Interstate: Font Bureau. (Supplied by Fontworks UK)

For full details of all Mosby titles, please write to Mosby International Publishers Limited, Lynton House, 7-12 Tavistock Square, London WC1H 9LB, UK.

A CIP catalogue record for this book is available from the British Library.

It was a tremendous honour and challenge to be approached by Mosby to revise *Cash's Textbook of Orthopaedics and Rheumatology*. This task was especially daunting, given that Cash's was an established textbook which had been of assistance to many physiotherapists and students over the years, and we approached the project with some trepidation. In her introduction to the second edition, Marian Tidswell acknowledged the unenviable responsibility of the editor in deciding what should be included and what omitted in the light of progress in a constantly developing and evolving professional field. This latest edition goes beyond revision of the original text, and covers entirely new ground in several respects.

It would be more accurate to say that the book has been rewritten rather than revised; the format, structure and content have been completely reworked, with new chapters and authors. In common with previous editions, the chapters have been contributed by a multidisciplinary team of authors, who either practice within the NHS or teach physiotherapy and occupational therapy students. The decision to split the book into two volumes, Orthopaedics and Rheumatology, was natural given the considerable progress that has been made in both specialties in recent years. This has provided the opportunity to expand on the rheumatology topics covered in previous editions, and to introduce new chapters such as The Hand, The Foot and Joint Protection/Splinting.

This book also represents something of a departure in the way that it was edited, being a team effort by the committee of the Rheumatic Care Association of Chartered Physiotherapists. We owe a huge debt of thanks to Catherine Buckley, Cathy Cameron, Sue Hesketh, Phillippa Moreno, Suzanne Wells, and the many doctors, nurses, radiographers, lecturers and other work colleagues for their constructive comments on the manuscript. In addition Anne Chadwick, Nikki Chettle, Krysia Dziedzic, Liz Hall, Jackie Waterfield and Kay West not only reviewed the drafts but contributed chapters as well. We would also like to thank Nora Price for her support and encouragement.

In this book the reader will find a depth of information which will facilitate and encourage their reasoning process, and the material will be also be useful for other disciplines working in rheumatology. Multi-faceted rheumatological problems require multidisciplinary team solutions, and the reader is encouraged to consider not only their own intervention but also ways in which other members of the team can contribute to the patient's care. Pointers for possible management have been included, but the rest is up to the reader's ingenuity. This approach is geared to the needs of the honours-level undergraduate, and an atmosphere within the profession that demands the integration of research evidence into practice, rather than unquestioning acceptance of treatment formulae.

In concluding, we would like to acknowledge the enormous debt that we owe to those authors and editors who have gone before us, and hope that this book stimulates a new generation of readers to take this fascinating specialty forward.

Carol David
Jill Lloyd

Anne Chadwick MCSP
Lecturer/Practitioner in Rheumatology Physiotherapy,
Cannock Chase Hospital and Keele University.

Nikki Chettle MCSP
Senior Physiotherapist, Sandwell District Hospital.

Carol David MCSP **-Editor**
Therapies Audit and Research Co-ordinator, Mid
Staffordshire General Hospitals NHS Trust.

Krysia Dziedzic PhD MCSP
West Midlands Regional Clinical Physiotherapy Trials
Co-ordinator, Department of Physiotherapy, Keele
University.

Christine Fenelon MCSP
Senior Physiotherapist, Warrington Hospitals NHS
Trust.

Liz Hall MCSP
Senior Physiotherapist, Musgrove Park Hospital.

Dr Andrew Hassell MD MRCP
Consultant Rheumatologist, Staffordshire
Rheumatology Centre, Haywood Hospital.

Dianne Lloyd
Head Occupational Therapist, Royal Shrewsbury
Hospitals NHS Trust.

Jill Lloyd BA, MCSP **-Editor**
Lecturer, Department of Health Studies, Brunel
University.

Michael Monoghan
Senior Lecturer in Podiatry, Durham School of
Podiatric Medicine.

Professor David Pratt BSc MSc PhD MInstP CPhys MIPEM
Head of Department, Bioengineering Research Centre,
Dept of Rheumatology and Rehabilitation Medicine,
Derbyshire Royal Infirmary NHS Trust.

Sue Rimmer
Senior I Occupational Therapist, Chesterfield and
North Derbyshire Royal Hospital NHS Trust.

Dr Michael Shadforth MB FRCS
Consultant Rheumatologist, Staffordshire
Rheumatology Centre, Haywood Hospital.

Jane Stewart MSc SRCh
Research Associate, Postgraduate Institute for
Medicine and Dentistry, Newcastle University.

Mary Wade MSc DipCOT
Senior Lecturer in Occupational Therapy, School of
Health and Social Sciences, Coventry University.

Jackie Waterfield MSc Grad Dip Phys MCSP
Lecturer, Department of Physiotherapy Studies, Keele
University.

Kay West MCSP
Senior Physiotherapist, South Cleveland Hospital,
Middlesbrough.

Arthritis Care
18 Stephenson Way, London NW1 2HD

Arthritis Research Campaign
Copeman House, St Mary's Court, St Mary's Gate,
Chesterfield S41 7TD
(for patient information leaflets and more detailed
information for health professionals)

British Health Professionals in Rheumatology
41 Eagle St, London WC1R 4AR
(multidisciplinary group for all health professionals
interested in rheumatology)

Behçet's Syndrome Society
Mrs G Seaman, 3 Church Close, Lambourn, Hungerford
RG17 8PU

British Sjogren's Syndrome Association
Ms M Ford, 20 Kingston Way, Nailsea, Bristol BS19 2RA

Childrens Chronic Arthritis Association
47 Battenhall Ave, Worcester WR5 2HN

Dermatomyositis/Polymyositis Support Group
146 Newtown Rd, Woolston, Southampton SO19 9HR

Fibromyalgia UK
PO Box 206, Stourbridge DY9 8YL

Haemophilia Society
123 Westminster Bridge Rd, London SE1 7HR

Hypermobility Association
45A Anerley Rd, Crystal Palace, London SE19 2AS

Kawasaki Syndrome Support Group
National Co-ordinator, Ms S Davidson, 13 Norwood
Grove, Potters Green, Coventry CV2 2FR

Lady Hoare Trust for Physically Disabled Children
87 Worship St, London EC2A 2BE
(can be approached for financial support)

Lupus UK
1 Eastern Rd, Romford RM1 3NH

National AIDS Helpline
0800-567123

National Ankylosing Spondylitis Society
PO Box 179, Mayfield, East Sussex TN20 6ZL
(publish a very useful and informative newsletter)

National Association for the Relief of Paget's Disease
1 Church Rd, Eccles, Manchester M30 0DL

National Back Pain Association
16 Elmtree Rd, Teddington TW11 8ST

National Osteoporosis Society
PO Box 10, Radstock, Bath BA3 3YB

Psoriatic Arthropathy Alliance
PO Box 11, St. Albans AL2 3JQ

Raynauds and Scleroderma Association
Mrs A Mawdsley, 112 Crewe Rd, Alsager ST7 2JA

Repetitive Strain Injury Association
Chapel House, 152-156 High St, Yiewsley,
West Drayton UB7 7BD

Sarcoidosis and Interstitial Lung Association
Chest Clinic Office, Dulwich Hospital, East Dulwich
Grove, London SE22 8PT

Scleroderma Society
Mrs P Webster, 61 Sandpit Lane, St Albans AL1 4EY

Wegener's Granulomatosis Support Group
Mr T Clay, 30 Main St, Halton Village, Runcorn
WA7 2AN

USEFUL JOURNALS
Annals of the Rheumatic Diseases
Arthritis Care and Research
British Journal of Rheumatology

The following figures are courtesy of JH Klippel, P Dieppe, eds: *Rheumatology 1e* & *2e*, Mosby International, London, 1994 &1998 respectively:
7.1, 7.3, 7.4 a,b, 7.5, 7.6, 8.2 (John L Sherman, Washington Imaging Center, Washington DC), 8.6, 9.3, 10.1, 10.4, 12.1, 13.1, 13.3, 14.2, 15.1, 15.3 a,b, 15.4, 15.5, 15.6 a,b (Dr J Webb), 15.7.

Figure 7.2 is adapted from JH Klippel, P Dieppe, eds: *Rheumatology 1e*, Mosby International, London, 1994.

Table 4.2 is reproduced from Sim J, Waterfield J, *Validity, reliability and responsiveness*. In: Physiotherapy, Theory and Practice. Vol. 13(1), 1997. Reprinted by permission of Psychology Press Limited, Hove, UK.

Gratified thanks to the following individuals and organisations for their permission to reproduce/adapt materials:

Bioengineering Research Centre, Derbyshire Royal Infirmary NHS Trust, Derby (5.2)
ORLAU Publishing Ltd (5.3)
Evelyn M Phypers and Ann Jones (9.3)
T Butler (9.4)
Mark Elsmore (10.2)
ACR and Professor Carol Black (Table 13.1)

Every effort has been made to obtain permissions for copyright material in this book. Where this has not been possible, please contact the publisher, who will ensure that full acknowledgement is made in future editions.

SECTION 1

GENERAL TOPICS

rheumatology (roo·mat·ol·o·je). Branch
medicine which is concerned with the
diagnosis and treatment of rheumatic
disorders.

1

E Hall

MULTIDISCIPLINARY TEAM AND PATIENT EDUCATION

CHAPTER OUTLINE

- The team
- Teamwork in rheumatology
- Patient education in rheumatology
- What influences patient education?
- Patient partners

INTRODUCTION

This chapter aims to cover teamwork and patient education, two areas that seem at first to be unrelated. However, good teamwork is vital for good patient education, and a well-educated patient can become a valuable member of the team. Factors for successful teams are outlined in the first section, followed by a discussion of different types, advantages and disadvantages of patient education in the second.

THE TEAM

WHAT IS A TEAM?

A team is a group in which individuals share a common aim and in which the jobs and skills of each member fit in with those of the others (Adair, 1985). There are several key features in an effective team (Embling, 1995); these include shared goals, interdependence, co-operation, co-ordination of activities, task specialisation, division of effort and mutual respect.

Teams have characteristics and complexities which enable the team to be operationally effective. Some of the more common features of teams include communication, cohesiveness, morale, standards and structure (Adair, 1985).

Communication

Communication within a team must be multidirectional, which requires time for individual and group discussions and briefings. This ensures that the goals and objectives of the team remain clear and each member has an opportunity to have a voice. It is essential to hear and understand fellow team members' points of view, and the language used is clear to all team members. It is easy for a multidisciplinary team (MDT) to develop a hierarchical structure where information is passed up and down the disciplines, for example from the doctor to the therapists and nurses and back again. However, true team-working should be more interactive, with an exchange of ideas, opinions and information across professional boundaries. This interaction can be achieved through multidisciplinary meetings and ward rounds, case conferences, multidisciplinary audit and research projects, joint assessments and multidisciplinary notes.

Cohesiveness

An effective team has a cohesiveness or togetherness amongst its members, developed by sharing common aims and goals. Other factors contributing to cohesiveness include good leadership, working in the same place, effective communication, small team size and compatible personality types within the team.

Morale

Morale and atmosphere greatly influence the team's effectiveness. When morale is high efficiency increases and team members are more co-operative, enhancing development by improving team dynamics, creativity and outcomes.

Standards

The maintenance of standards, both personal and professional, is important to any team. Individual members who fail to achieve or maintain these often unwritten standards can reduce the efficiency of the team.

Structure

Structure is a necessary component of all teams and can be both formal and informal.

Formal

The formal structure is visible and easily documented; it represents the overall objectives of the team as well as those of individual members. The task or goal is broken down into its component parts and each team member is responsible for a specific component.

Informal

The informal structure is what actually happens behind the scenes, how the work gets done. Though individual team members have specific tasks, there is a certain amount of crossover of activities on a day to day basis. This involves a degree of flexibility and good communication to ensure that individuals do not lose sight of their tasks and the team remains focused on its objective.

Staff perceptions of how they fit into a team are important, especially team co-operation which can be broken down by interpersonal jealousies, crossing of professional boundaries and not fully understanding and respecting the skills of fellow team members. People may feel that they are being professionally threatened or compromised and that their own capacities and skills are not being fully used (Strasser et al., 1994). Regular meetings and communication help to avoid this situation.

WHAT IS TEAMWORK?

The Concise Oxford Dictionary defines teamwork as 'a combined effort or organised co-operation'. The individual efforts of team members merge into a single co-ordinated result, and the whole is more than the sum of its individual parts (Blake & Mouton, 1964). Effective teamwork can only be achieved when individuals apply their skills collaboratively rather than sequentially. Problems arise because of a lack of understanding of what true multidisciplinary teamwork involves. To many, the term MDT simply implies that different health care professionals treat the same patient, whereas a true MDT has a more structured form and involves collaboration, consensual decision-making and joint planning of patient care (Embling, 1995) leading to effective interdisciplinary management (McHugh et al. 1996).

The team approach also ensures that goals are reached in the most efficient way with minimal duplication of skills and documentation, and that the most suitably qualified member of the team deals with the problem in hand. Advice and information given to the patient should be reinforced, so that conflicting messages are not received which may lead to confusion and poor treatment compliance.

TEAMWORK IN RHEUMATOLOGY

Multidisciplinary teamwork in rheumatology is of major importance. The main objectives are to:
• Improve patient care.
• Deliver effective patient education.
• Increase interprofessional communication.
• Develop clinical audit and outcomes.

It has been shown that the team approach in the management of rheumatological conditions, especially rheumatoid arthritis (RA), leads to an improvement in the patient's health, functional ability and psychosocial well-being (Ahlmen et al., 1988). Health education using a team approach reduces health care costs whilst providing sustained benefits in health status (Lorig et al., 1993, Cronan et al., 1997) and multidisciplinary care helps to maintain functional ability (Hakala et al., 1994).

The increasing emphasis on professional accountability, evidence based medicine and audit, together with the need for a cost-effective and efficient service, must be considered when developing a MDT to provide a comprehensive service for the rheumatology patient.

Vliet Vlieland et al. (1996) studied the effectiveness of in-patient MDT care compared with routine out-patient treatment for RA. The study showed that a short period of in-patient care, despite the relatively increased costs, had a direct beneficial effect on disease activity and emotional status which was maintained for at least one year and was more effective than standard out-patient care. Many rheumatology patients will require ongoing care for the rest of their lives and as each new person is diagnosed, the numbers of patients requiring input from the medical profession increases, putting more strain on an already busy service. An effective and efficient team should be able to continue providing the comprehensive care despite these strains.

WHO MAKES UP THE TEAM?

The team comprises of many differing professionals. Rheumatological conditions are usually progressive and involve more than one system in the body. The team involved with any one patient may grow and alter as a variety of specialist skills may be required at different times throughout the disease course.

The patient is the most important member of the team. Patients know what problems they are having and how these problems are affecting their lives. Actively involving the patients in their care ensures that the team will be able to provide short- and long-term treatment plans that will be relevant to the patients' needs and personal beliefs. The integration of patients into the care team in this way has been shown to improve outcomes and compliance to the treatment plans suggested (Donovan, 1991).

THE MULTIDISCIPLINARY TEAM IN RHEUMATOLOGY

The core team consists of:
• Patients and Carers.
• General Practitioner.
• Rheumatologist.
• Physiotherapist.
• Occupational Therapist.
• Nursing Staff.

Other disciplines that may be involved at differing times include:
• Orthopaedic Consultants.
• Chiropodists.
• Orthotists/Appliance Officer.
• Dermatologists.
• Social Workers.
• Dieticians.
• Clinical Psychologists.
• Pharmacists.

The majority of the rheumatological MDTs are hospital based, which gives patients easy access to a variety of rheumatology specialists. However, some patients are never referred to a consultant but have their care co-ordinated by the General Practitioner (GP). The role of the Primary Care team and community centred care is increasing, especially since the introduction of GP fundholding practices. Nurses and physiotherapists work increasingly in GP practices, providing therapy and drug monitoring services locally to the patient. Good liaison between hospital-based and community-based staff allows a smooth transition of the patient's care from hospital to community following discharge. Schofield *et al.* (1990) commented that there is a danger that community care may merely consist of the transfer of patients from wards or out-patient clinics to the community while their care continues to be provided by hospital-based services. True community care involves care by professional staff based in the community and by the community itself.

Traditionally the co-ordination of the team, especially one which is hospital based, has been the domain of the doctor. However, it may be preferable to have another health professional fulfilling this role, in a position to provide a close link between the hospital and the community (Maycock, 1991). Each individual team member should know which health professional to refer to and the correct timing of such a referral. For example, early referral to an orthopaedic surgeon may enable more minor corrective surgery to be performed rather than a salvage procedure when all else has failed.

Although the relationship between the health professional team and the patient is important, a team may also include non health professionals such as employers, social services, voluntary organisations and even town planners and architects. Improving non health related matters as well as those directly related to health is important to attain the overall aim of an increased sense of well-being and functional ability for the patients (Vinicor, 1995). Physiotherapists working with patients with multisystem disorders may also require the skills and knowledge of other specialised staff within the physiotherapy network. This achieves the best possible outcome for the patient as well as enhancing and disseminating specialist knowledge among fellow physiotherapists.

In conclusion, teamworking is important in the management of rheumatological conditions. Improved patient care and reduced health care costs are the main outcomes of an efficient and effective MDT. Effective teams develop when each member contributes to the common aim and is committed to building the team. Creating an effective team does not occur overnight; it takes time, hard work, commitment and motivation to build and then to continue to develop. Teams have to evolve.

PATIENT EDUCATION IN RHEUMATOLOGY

Patient education is an important aspect in the overall management of rheumatology patients and its role should be complementary to any medical and therapeutic interventions.

To understand the importance of education it is necessary to appreciate the impact of a chronic disease such as arthritis on the lives of the patients, their families and friends, both physically and psychosocially.

Inflammatory and non-inflammatory arthritis can be unpredictable and disabling. However, the inflammatory arthritides cause more problems due to the systemic nature of the disease and the multiple joint involvement. This section will concentrate on the role of education in RA, the most common of the inflammatory joint diseases; however, many of the principles can be adopted in the management of other inflammatory and non-inflammatory arthritides.

WHY PATIENT EDUCATION?

The increasing prevalence of chronic disease creates a situation in which health or patient education has to focus not only on preventing illness but also on minimising its consequences and maximising the patient's capability for independent living. As arthritis has many physical, psychological and social implications, it is important to consider these prior to the development of any education programme aimed at improving functional and psychosocial well-being (Holman & Lorig, 1992).

Physical

The problems encountered are ones of increasing disability and pain, resulting in a variety of activity limitations in areas such as personal care, employment and leisure.

Psychological

Ahern *et al.* (1995) indicated that patients with RA were more preoccupied with their illness and its effects and readily admitted that psychological factors play a more important role than in osteoarthritis. The psychological factors of fear and anxiety due to the uncertainty and depression have all been recorded as prevalent emotions especially in the early stages of inflammatory arthritis (Frank & Maguire, 1988, Newman & Revenson 1993, DeVellis, 1993).

Depression is well recognised as a common psychological disturbance in any chronic condition. Wells *et al.* (1989) reported that depression could significantly increase disability, since patients are not in control of what is happening to them and feel unable to cope with the situation.

Social

Arthritis can affect relationships, and the patient's role within the family unit and society may be altered. Revenson & Majerovitz (1990) reported that family support and understanding is critical in enhancing well-being, healthy behaviours and compliance with treatment. However, social support may also have a negative effect if friends and carers are over-solicitous, unable to understand the patient's condition or unable to cope. Loss of employment, with its stigma and decreased financial resources, also has marked social and psychological implications.

The aims of an education programme are to enable patients to participate effectively in their own management, develop coping skills, make informed choices about their treatments and weigh up the consequences of their own actions or inactions. Patient education provides them with **choice** (Hill, 1995).

WHAT IS PATIENT EDUCATION?

The National Arthritis Advisory Board in the US recently developed standards for arthritis patient education (Burckhardt, 1994, Lorig & Visser, 1994). These standards include the following definition of patient education:

'Patient education is planned, organised learning experiences designed to facilitate voluntary adoption of behaviours or beliefs conducive to health. It is a set of planned educational activities that are separate from clinical patient care. The activities of a patient education programme must be designed to attain goals the patient has participated in formulating. The primary focus of these activities includes acquisition of information, skills, beliefs and attitudes which impact on health status, quality of life, and possibly health care utilisation.'

This definition emphasises the need not only to provide knowledge but also to change behaviour, which leads to improved health status, together with the importance of assessing the needs of the patients and tailoring the education to those needs (Taal *et al.*, 1996). Mazzuca (1982) stated that efforts to improve health by increasing patient knowledge alone were rarely successful. Behaviour-orientated programmes, taking the patients' individual environment and reactions into consideration, were consistently more effective and resulted in improved

outcomes and a greater sense of well-being. Hirano *et al.* (1994) concluded that the mechanisms that make patient education effective or the type of intervention or combination of interventions are still not known.

WHAT INFLUENCES PATIENT EDUCATION?

To enable patients to learn to manage their disease they may need to acquire new skills, and it is the role of health care professionals to collaborate with the patients to develop these skills, leading to effective self-management. Skills include those of a practical nature, i.e. pain relief, joint protection and exercise, and those that are non practical, i.e. problem-solving, decision-making and effective communication. To bring about behavioural change involves the enhancement of self-efficacy. This is self-confidence, patients' belief in themselves that they are able to perform new activities or tasks and cope with stressful or unknown situations.

Bandura (1986, 1992) discussed the social learning theory in which the author determined that human functioning is a result of the continuous interaction between biological, psychological, behavioural and environmental factors. Much of an individual's behaviour is motivated and regulated by internal standards and by self-evaluation of his or her own actions. Outcome expectations and self-efficacy expectations are very important mechanisms in the quest for behavioural change. A person's outcome expectation is that a particular behaviour will have a beneficial effect, whereas a self-efficacy expectation is the belief in the capability to perform that behaviour to achieve the desired outcome. Self-efficacy expectations affect behavioural choices in terms of the amount of effort the person will make to achieve a particular goal. In rheumatology patient education, where the aim is to provide the information and develop the skills necessary to achieve a greater degree of self-management, the influence of self-efficacy is high. In consequence, interventions to enhance self-management behaviour and health functioning should be aimed at strengthening self-efficacy expectations (Taal *et al.*, 1996).

What Influences Self-efficacy?

Self-efficacy expectations are derived from four principal sources of information: performance accomplishments, vicarious experience (modelling), verbal persuasion and physiological states. Performance accomplishment is the most influential source of efficacy information because people have to achieve the desired behavioural change by personally mastering new skills and not just watching others perform them (vicarious experience) or listening to people telling them what they should be doing (verbal persuasion). Learning to change reactions to certain physiological signals is also important. For example, the ability to distinguish pain following exercise from that of arthritis can make the difference between the sense of achievement of having been able to do certain exercises, and the negative thought that the arthritis has been made worse by the exercises.

Other Considerations

Patient education can be described as a means of enabling patients to cope better despite constraints placed on their lifestyle by arthritis. All patients are firstly individuals and secondly have arthritis and it is essential to provide advice and information that is specific to their individual needs. Exploring all avenues, not just the medical care system, is paramount to the achievement of physical and psychosocial well-being (Daltroy & Liang, 1991). Do not assume that what we as professionals think they *ought* to know is always what they *want* to know!

Personal beliefs

These beliefs determine what is acceptable and reasonable to apply to one's everyday life (Donovan, 1991) and lead patients to use certain recommended behaviours and reject others. Donovan *et al.* (1989) also stated that the patients should not be treated as a 'blank sheet of paper' assuming that any prior knowledge they have is incorrect or irrelevant. Individuals react to and cope with their arthritis very differently; it is important to acknowledge these differences and then decide how much, and in what format, information should be given to enable an individual to gain maximum benefit.

Information sources

The majority of patients want to gain as much information as possible about their particular condition and will use a variety of sources including books, family and friends, television and other patients. This information will be very varied; much of it will be relevant and helpful and unlikely to be harmful—however, this may not always be the case. It is therefore important to establish patients' own ideas about their arthritis and its management at an early stage in order to reinforce useful behaviours and to modify or eliminate negative ones.

Family influences

The influence and role of the family should never be underestimated (Revenson & Majerovitz, 1990). It is within this social setting that the patients have to live and function, and ignoring advice from well meaning family members may cause unwanted tensions within the family group. Some patients therefore may choose to take their advice and not to listen to the health professional. Involvement of family members in any management programme may help to overcome this situation.

NEGATIVE ASPECTS OF EDUCATION

Ewles & Simnett (1995) identified some of the pitfalls of promoting health by education:

- Patients don't always think the experts (i.e. health professionals) know best, as they can be proved wrong or change their minds.
- Patients may feel guilty because they are unable to do as they are being told or they may get angry at being told what to do.
- The behaviour of the individual may not be the cause of ill health.
- Individuals may not have the freedom of choice, even if it could lead to a physically and emotionally healthier lifestyle.

Tucker & Kirwan (1991) suggested that some patients, with recent onset of a chronic disease such as arthritis, have increased levels of depression and fear following education. This is especially true if the information given is irrelevant to their needs and does not relate to their personal beliefs.

TYPES OF PROGRAMMES

There are many different ways of providing information, changing behaviours and teaching self-help strategies. The majority of education programmes cover the following topics:

- Effects of arthritis: usual signs and symptoms, reasons for flare-ups and fatigue, effects on the body.
- Management: drug therapy and pain control, physical therapy, occupational therapy etc., doctor/patient communication, splinting.
- Self- management: self-help measures, home treatments and exercise, joint protection and the use of aids, relaxation, diet.
- The role of other members of the MDT: footwear and chiropody/podiatry.
- Common emotional feelings, sexual aspects.
- Self-help groups and hospital helplines; benefits and allowances.

The topics included must be identified as being important to the patients for the programme to be effective (Hill, 1990). It must be remembered that life as well as arthritis is not static, therefore education is always ongoing and must cater for the needs of the patients at varying stages of their disease. Hall & Ferguson (1992) investigated the need for patient education, and identified that only 50% of the patients questioned actually wanted a formal education programme. The other 50% wanted written information only or did not feel that they wanted any further information at all. It must not be assumed that all patients want to be involved in formal education programmes.

The most common patient education programme is that designed for small groups. The programme has a set timetable with different topics covered at each session. The programme is usually co-ordinated by one member of the MDT, calling on other members of the team to talk about their areas of expertise. The sessions, though structured, should be interactive with time for patient involvement and not just a formal teaching session.

This format can be used for out-patients and in-patients. A typical programme for out-patients would consist of weekly sessions of 1–2 hours each, over about 6 weeks. By the end of the course it would be hoped that all the original objectives had been achieved. Pimm *et al.* (1992) reported significant improvements in patients' knowledge gain, self-management skills and perceived control of their arthritis following such a programme, despite lack of change in functional ability, pain or emotional state.

1

For in-patients, the format is usually a rolling programme of about 2 weeks, with a different topic each day, ensuring that most patients cover all the topics at some stage during their stay in hospital. In situations where there may be only one or two patients on the ward, a less structured one-to-one approach is recommended.

Benefits of a group format are that patients have an opportunity to get to know other people with the same condition therefore they don't feel so isolated. It is also an opportunity to 'compare notes', a chance to exchange thoughts and ideas as well as offering support and advice. However, there are times when the patients may want to discuss any personal and sometimes delicate problems which they would not wish to discuss in a group setting and the opportunity to discuss these matters needs to be made available.

Co-ordinating and leading patient education programmes is not just the domain of health care professionals. The Arthritis Self-Management Programme (ASMP) developed in the US by Kate Lorig is being promoted and run in the UK by Arthritis Care. The programme aims to teach people the necessary skills to manage their arthritis and to regain control of their lives (Garner, 1996). The format is 6 weekly sessions facilitated by a pair of lay-leaders who have arthritis and have been specially trained to run the course. There is also input from professionals for some of the sessions. Topics covered are very similar to those covered in health professional-run programmes.

The course is very interactive, especially as there is not the health professional–patient scenario. Participants are encouraged to exchange thoughts and ideas, set goals and keep to contracts to enable them to achieve these goals. Short-term goal setting is encouraged so that patients take small achievable steps towards their ultimate goal. This helps to maintain a positive approach with fewer setbacks, and builds up self-efficacy (Bandura, 1977). The sessions also create a forum for discussing any related issues, i.e. fatigue, depression, coping strategies and relationships.

The results of a study by Lorig et al. (1993) showed that ASMP achieved a reduction in pain and depression and increased physical activity even though disability was unchanged. These benefits were sustained for at least 4 years after completing the course, were complementary to conventional therapy and reduced health care costs. The authors concluded that the study supported the use of taught behaviours, not primarily to improve health status but to promote the development of perceived self-efficacy.

Therefore, the teaching of knowledge and the learning of skills via patient education programmes can achieve similar results whether the courses are lay-person or professional led (Cohen et al., 1986). However, professionally taught groups show greater changes in knowledge, whereas lay-leader groups show greater changes in relaxation and a tendency towards less disability (Lorig et al., 1986).

Other methods of providing arthritis information include the use of written literature, audio-visual and computer based education packages. These have been proved to be useful tools and can be used as an adjunct to more conventional education programmes or on their own. Wetstone et al. (1985) evaluated a computer based programme and concluded that the patients gained significant improvements in knowledge, outlook on life and self-help behaviours as well as enjoying the style of presentation.

Professional-led patient education programmes can be costly in terms of professional time, and it has been postulated that self-instruction could provide similar benefits. Maggs et al. (1996) investigated the benefits of education by an instruction booklet alone versus information provided by a health professional. The results indicated that the knowledge gain was similar in both groups and that neither group improved health status or disability levels. With all the preceding information on the benefits of patient education groups it could be concluded that the use of information booklets has an important role in reinforcing verbal information.

An excellent source of further information on the topic of patient education is that by Hill (1997). This provides an overview of patient education for practising clinicians.

PATIENT PARTNERS

So far in this chapter, 'education' has implied the communication of knowledge from the health professional to the patient. In recent years, a new initiative has developed in which patients with arthritis are involved as educators in the training of health professionals (Gruppen et al., 1996). This scheme, known as patient partners, involves the training of patients in anatomy and joint examination. The patients then teach these skills to health professionals and students, enabling the students to practise identification of pathological features, and enabling the patient to correct them on their examination technique if it is uncomfortable. Although the concept originated in the US, several patient partners have now been trained and are working in the UK.

CONCLUSION

Patient education is an integral part of the management of rheumatological conditions. Education should enable patients to have a greater understanding of their disease, teach them how to manage their disease and gain greater control over their lives by building on their levels of perceived self-efficacy. Effective patient education involves the provision of information and advice that is relevant to the individual needs of the patient at that time. As patients' requirements vary throughout the course of their disease, it is essential that this education is progressive and in a format which suits the individual patient.

REFERENCES

Adair J. Teams. In: Adair J (ed). *Effective team building*. Aldershot: Gower; 1985.

Ahern MJ, McFarlane AC, Leslie A, Eden J, Roberts-Thomson PJ. Illness behaviour in patients with arthritis. *Ann Rheum Dis* 1995, **54**:245-250.

Ahlmen M, Sullivan M, Bjelle A. Team versus non team outpatient care in rheumatoid arthritis. *Arth Rheum* 1988, **31**:471-479.

Bandura A. Self-efficacy: Toward a unifying theory of behavioral change. *Psychol Rev* 1977, **84**:191-215.

Bandura A. *Social foundations of thought and action: a social cognitive theory*. Englewood, NJ: Prentice-Hall; 1986.

Bandura A. Self-efficacy mechanism in phychobiologic functioning. In: *Self-efficacy: thought control of action*. Edited by Schwarzer R. Washington DC: Hemisphere Publishing Corporation; 1992.

Blake R, Mouton J. *The Management Grid*. Houston, Texas: The Gulf Publication Company; 1964.

Burckhardt CS. Arthritis and musculoskeletal patient education standards. *Arth Care Res* 1994, **7**:1-4.

Cohen JL, Sauter SV, DeVellis RF, DeVellis BM. Evaluation of arthritis self-management courses led by laypersons and by professionals. *Arth Rheum* 1986, **29**:388-393.

Cronan TA, Groessl E, Kaplan RM. The effects of social support and education interventions on health care costs. *Arth Care Res* 1997, **10**:99-110.

Daltroy LH, Liang MH. Advances in patient education in rheumatic diseases. *Ann Rheum Dis* 1991, **50**:415-417.

DeVellis B. Depression in rheumatological diseases. Baillières *Clin Rheumatol* 1993, **7**:241-257.

Donovan J, Blake DR, Fleming WG. The patient is not a blank sheet: lay beliefs and their relevance to patient education. *Br J Rheumatol* 1989, **28**:58-61.

Donovan J. Patient education and the consultation: the importance of lay beliefs. *Ann Rheum Dis* 1991, **50**:418-421.

Embling S. Exploring multidisciplinary teamwork. *Br J Ther Rehab* 1995, **2**:142-144.

Ewles L, Simnett I. *Promoting health – a practical guide, 3rd edition*. London: Scutari; 1995, p35.

Frank AO, Maguire GP. *Disabling diseases: physical, environmental and psychosocial management*. Oxford: Heinemann Medical Books; 1988.

Garner A. Arthritis action. *Here's Health* 1996, Dec.**16**:27-29.

Gruppen LD, Branch VK, Laing TJ. The use of trained patient educators with rheumatoid arthritis to teach medical students. *Arthritis Care Res* 1996, **9**: 302-308.

Hakala M, Nieminen P, Koivist O. More evidence from a community based series of better outcome in rheumatoid arthritis. Data on the effect of multidisciplinary care on the retention of functional ability. *J Rheumatol* 1994, **21**:1432-1437.

Hall EC, Ferguson B. Identifying the need for patient education in rheumatoid arthritis in N. Staffordshire. *Clin Rheumatol* 1992, **11**:296-297 (abstract).

Hill J. Patient education: what to teach patients with rheumatic disease. *J Roy Soc Health* 1990, **110**:204-207.

Hill J. Patient education in rheumatic disease. *Nursing Standard* 1995, **9**:25-28.

Hill J. A practical guide to patient education and information giving. Baillières *Clin Rheumatol* 1997, **11**:109-127.

Hirano PC, Laurent DD, Lorig K. Arthritis patient education studies 1987-1991: a review of the literature. *Patient Education and Counselling* 1994, **24**:9-54.

Holman H, Lorig K. Perceived self-efficacy in self-management of chronic disease. In: Schwarzer R (ed): *Self-efficacy: thought control of action*. Washington DC: Hemisphere Publishing Corporation; 1992.

Lorig K *et al*. A comparison of lay-taught and professional-taught arthritis self-management courses. *J Rheumatol* 1986, **13**:763-767.

Lorig KR, Mazonson PD, Holman HR. Evidence suggesting that health education for self-management in patients with chronic arthritis has sustained health benefits while reducing health care costs. *Arth Rheum* 1993, **36**:439-446.

Lorig K, Visser A. Arthritis patient education standards: a model for the future. *Patient Education and Counselling* 1994, **24**:3-7.

Maggs FM, Jubb RW, Kemm JR. Single-blind randomized controlled trial of an educational booklet for patients with chronic arthritis. *Br J Rheumatol* 1996, **35**:775-777.

Maycock JA. Role of health professionals in patient education. *Ann Rheum Dis* 1991, **50**:429-434.

Mazzuca MA. Does patient education in chronic disease have therapeutic potential? *J Chronic Dis* 1982, **35**:521-529.

McHugh M, West P, Assalty C *et al*. Establishing an interdisciplinary patient care team. Collaboration at the bedside and beyond. *J Nursing Administration* 1996, **26**:21-29.

Newman SP, Revenson TA. Coping with rheumatoid arthritis. Baillières *Clin Rheumatol* 1993, **7**:259-80

Pimm TJ, Amos M, Byron MA. Evaluation of an out-patient education programme for people with rheumatiod arthritis. *Br J Rheumatol* 1992, **31**:77 (abstract).

Revenson TA, Majerovitz DM. Spouses' support provision to chronically ill patients. *Journal of Social and Personal Relationships* 1990, **7**:575-586.

Schofield T, Haslar J, Barnes G. Implications for practice. In: Haslar J, Schofield T (eds). *Continuing Care: the management of chronic disease*. Oxford: Oxford University Press; 1990, pp 64-83.

Strasser DC, Falconer JA, Martino-Saltzman D. The rehabilitation team: Staff perceptions of the hospital environment, the interdisciplinary team and interprofessional relations. *Arch Phys Med Rehabilitation* 1994, **75**:177-182.

Taal E, Rasker JJ, Wiegman O. Patient education and self-management in the rheumatic diseases: A self-efficacy approach. *Arthritis Care Res* 1996, **9**: 229-237.

Tucker M, Kirwan JR. Does patient education in rheumatoid arthritis have therapeutic potential? *Ann Rheum Dis* 1991, **50**:422-428.

Vinicor F. Interdisciplinary and intersectoral approach: a challenge for integrated care. *Patient Education and Counselling* 1995, **26**:267-272.

Vliet Vlieland TPM, Zwinderman AH, Vandenbrouke JP *et al*. A randomized clinical trial of in-patient multidisciplinary treatment versus routine out-patient care in active rheumatoid arthritis. *Br J Rheumatol* 1996, **35**:475-482.

Wells KB, Stewart A, Hays RD *et al*. The functioning and well-being of depressed patients: results from Medical Outcome Study. *JAMA* 1989, **262**:914-919.

Wetstone SL, Sheehan TJ, Votaw RG, Peterson MG, Rothfield N. Evaluation of a computer based education lesson for patients with rheumatoid arthritis. *J Rheumatol* 1985, **12**: 907-912

2 M Shadforth
IMMUNOLOGY, INFLAMMATION AND THE ACUTE PHASE RESPONSE

CHAPTER OUTLINE

- **The immune system**
- **The cellular immune system**
- **The humoral immune system**
- **Inflammation and the acute phase response**

- **The acute phase response**
- **Clinical applications of immunology and inflammation**

INTRODUCTION

While there is no real need to know the underlying process of disease in clinical practice, such understanding does help to plan the investigations needed to identify a problem and the treatment required. It also helps to explain to a patient what is being planned and why particular steps are being taken. Therapists and nurses are not responsible for planning an investigative routine for diagnosis, but they are involved in treatment and counselling of patients, and an understanding of the disease process gives a depth of knowledge which improves confidence and the ability to communicate plans and reasons.

Knowledge of the disease process in the inflammatory arthropathies has expanded phenomenally in the past 25 years and continues to expand exponentially. Terminology can be off-putting and it is easy to be frightened away from any attempt to understand the science. This chapter attempts to banish the mystery embroiled in immunology and inflammation by bringing it into simple logic and language.

The natural processes involved in an immune response are all common sense and are exactly what any organisation would put in place for protection. Whether the organisation is a country, a large business consortium or a living body, recognition of friend or foe, communication within the organisation and sanctions to remove and destroy a threat are vital. An invader must be recognised, then forces mobilised to immobilise and neutralise the foe. Damage to self will be incurred in that phase, so that during and following the action, repairs are required. While undertaking an action it may be prudent to sacrifice friendly positions or forces in order to achieve an end—thus damage may be self-inflicted.

In a living organism the immune system recognises the external threat, identifies it and attempts to destroy it, calling upon inflammation in the process. Inflammation is involved both in the destructive and the repair phase. Links exist with other systems for assistance as required. For instance, blood clotting to limit loss, and pain to limit use of the affected part are obvious accessories while the defensive and repair processes are underway.

The difficulty in understanding these systems stems mainly from the complexities of the safety and backup mechanisms. It is important not to take orders from an enemy—one must recognise 'self'. If a system fails, another must be available. Different approaches are needed for differing threats and regulation of the intensity and scope of the action is needed. Regulation also must be able to call a halt to an action when the threat is overcome. It seems likely that most of the inflammatory arthropathies arise from failure of these mechanisms, or perhaps the ability of an invader to overcome them. The following sections examine the basic principles of immunity and inflammation and how to relate these to our clinical concepts and actions.

2

TERMINOLOGY

Antigen

An antigen is a substance which invokes a response from the immune system. Antigens are almost always proteins, and will normally be foreign to the individual since clearly it would be inappropriate to be attacking one's own proteins. A situation known as 'tolerance' is produced for the proteins which make up 'self', and proteins seen by the immune system during foetal development fall into this category. Protein antigens may exist as free protein which can be dissolved in plasma or tissue fluid, or they may be fixed protein making up part of a structure such as a cell wall.

Immunoglobulins

These are a group of proteins in the blood, classified by their size and properties as immunoglobulin A, D, E, G and M, with further sub-divisions within those groups. The precise functions of the different sub-groups are beyond the scope of this chapter, but all are produced by the immune system as defence. When alluding to the group as a whole we refer to the immunoglobulin (e.g. IgG) but if we are indicating a specific protein within the group we refer to it as an antibody. For instance, an IgM antibody means a specific antibody which is a member of the IgM immunoglobulin group.

Antibody

An antibody is a specific immunoglobulin, produced in response to a specific antigen. It has the ability to bind to the antigen, forming an 'immune complex', and in so doing it may disable harmful effects of the antigen. If the antigen is a protein on the surface of a cell, such as a bacterium, the antibody will begin to disable the cell and will invoke the cascade of events produced by immune complex binding.

Immune Complex

When an antibody binds to an antigen, it produces an immune complex. In binding, the antibody changes appearance at molecular level, and this change is recognised by other protein systems such that they too are changed. The main protein involved here is complement.

Complement

Complement is a series of proteins normally present in the circulation in inactive form. Complement proteins are numbered as C1, C2 and so on, with letters given to fragments of the proteins which are formed after activation, e.g. C3d. Activation takes the form of a cascade, though not strictly in chronological order since not all were identified in sequence and the numbering was bestowed as they were discovered. Complement can be activated by certain surface characteristics found on some infective agents but the most effective activator of complement is the immune complex. Upon activation each protein produces fragments, many with their own function either as a messenger or as part of the complement protein complex. They also give rise to activation of the next complement protein, generating the complement cascade. Once fully activated the complement protein complex is capable of destroying a cell by puncturing the cell membrane and causing lysis. Complement does not respect identity and will destroy any cell within reach, rather as dropping a bomb will kill friends as well as foes in the area. The effectiveness of activated complement persists for a very short time and thus only cells in the immediate area of activation are likely to suffer.

Auto-immunity

This is the term applied when self proteins come under attack. This could occur if a protein which was not seen by the immune system during development becomes apparent. One possible scenario is that while proteins on the surface of cells are visible during development those in the interior are not. Should internal proteins become exposed, with for instance radiation injury to cells, then auto-immunity could ensue. Substances known as haptens are foreign molecules which are not proteins but which can activate the system by binding to 'self' proteins and altering their appearance, again giving a form of auto-immunity. Some drug reactions are produced in this way.

Rheumatoid Factor

This is an example of auto-immunity and is an IgM antibody directed against IgG. Initially rheumatoid factor (RF) was identified in the blood of patients with rheumatoid arthritis (RA) using the Rose–Waaler test. In this test a rabbit injected with red blood cells from a sheep will respond by producing antibodies against sheep red blood cells. If serum from the rabbit is then mixed in laboratory conditions with sheep red blood cells the antibody contained in the rabbit's serum will bind to the red cells, coating them in immunoglobulin. In sufficient quantity this would cause the red cells to stick together, a process called agglutination, and with complement present the cells would be destroyed by lysis. In lower quantities the red cells are coated with IgG, but not sufficient to upset the cells. Mixing a suspension of these cells with human serum has no effect unless RF is present in the human serum. If RF is present it will bind to the IgG on the cell surface and will make cells agglutinate just as if they had been exposed to greater quantities of rabbit antibody initially. Again the process is sensitive to quantity, and the result is expressed as a titre, i.e. the highest dilution which would still produce agglutination. Thus a result from the Rose–Waaler test could be '+ve 1:128', meaning 1 part serum diluted with 127 parts saline would still give a positive result. This test was refined to the 'Latex Test', where the red blood cells were replaced with particles of latex which had been coated with human IgG and the result still expressed as a titre. It is still used as a diagnostic test for RA, but techniques have been refined further and it is now automated by a laboratory process known as nephelometry with a result expressed in international units. The underlying immunology remains unchanged!

It is tempting to think of RF as the cause of RA but there is no evidence that this is so. Some patients with RA have a negative test for RF but still have the disease. In some of these cases IgG or IgA RF is found, rather than IgM. Only IgM RF is identified by the standard laboratory test. In most cases, however, if IgM RF is absent then so are the others and RF is not therefore a likely cause of the condition. Although not the cause it must have some bearing on the pathological process and its existence goes part way in helping us understand the disease process, as well as being a diagnostic aid.

Cytokines

These are proteins with specific effects, usually as a messenger and often attracting specific cells into the area in which they are required. Many proteins with defined functions are involved in immune and inflammatory reactions and often their names indicate their function. Interleukin (IL) for instance is responsible primarily for communication between leukocytes. There are a number of identified ILs and other functions may also be involved. IL-1, IL-6 and IL-11 stimulate the 'acute phase response' protein production. Interferons (IFN) and tumour necrosis factor (TNF) are also cytokines. TNF alpha is felt to play a major role in the inflammation in RA.

Acute Phase Response

This is the term given to the body's reaction to an insult of any sort. The insult may be an invasion giving an immune response or it may be a physical or chemical injury. A surgical operation will produce an acute phase response, so will a heart attack and so will an infection. The main element of the acute phase response is the production of acute phase response proteins. These acute phase proteins are produced predominantly by the liver and all have functions within the inflammatory process. There may be relative differences in the exact protein response produced by different insults but this aspect is incompletely understood. Different acute phase proteins are produced at different times within the reaction and there is a logic to both the time of their production and their function. Acute phase proteins are discussed further in the section on inflammation.

THE IMMUNE SYSTEM

Traditionally the immune system is divided into the cellular immune system and the humoral immune system, the latter so called since it exists in a soluble form in one or more of the four humors of early medicine, namely blood, bile, phlegm and lymph. While the cellular system can function independently, its abilities are strictly limited. The humoral system is dependent upon aspects of the cellular system for its existence, being produced by immune cells, but has much wider ranging powers.

At the molecular level, proteins exhibit a surface pattern which takes account of shape, electrical potential and water affinity. This applies either in their soluble form, or when they exist as part of a cell membrane. The immune system will use this pattern to recognise an invader and to produce defences specifically against it. Most defence functions exist in a quiescent form the whole time. They are activated by the immune recognition process and they must then stand down when the invader is cleared.

HUMAN LEUKOCYTE ANTIGEN TYPING

It will be helpful to examine some aspects of human leukocyte antigen (HLA) typing before discussing the mechanisms of the immune system proper. HLA refers to specific proteins which exist on the cell membrane of our leukocytes. These proteins are dictated by the genetic coding on part of the 6th chromosome. Each of us has an individual pattern of protein expression which can, amongst other things, be used to identify 'self'.

A major use of HLA typing has been in transplant surgery. Graft rejection depends upon the host (the patient receiving a graft) recognising that the graft does not belong. Tissue typing attempts to match as much of the protein pattern as possible in the hope that the host will not recognise the graft as different. Matching tissue type, along with immune suppression, has led to very much more successful transplantation. In much medical research, classification uses letters and numbers to catalogue discoveries. HLA proteins were given A, B and D identifiers, and the D area has been subdivided into DP, DQ and DR. Routine tissue typing detects four main proteins, although others exist, so an individual might type as A3, A8, B6 and B27. In transplant surgery, the aim is to find an organ from a donor who has three or four proteins the same as the recipient. The greater the match, the lower the chance of rejection.

While transplant surgery has had major benefits from tissue typing, other factors around tissue type have produced gains in other areas of medicine. Links have been discovered between tissue types, many in the HLA-D area, and susceptibility to a number of diseases or complications. Within rheumatology the best known link is between HLA B27 and ankylosing spondylitis but there are also connections between other tissue types and disease outcome, and with drug reactions. These are links and not origins. Having B27 tissue type does not cause ankylosing spondylitis. In the general population 8% have B27, and most of those do not have ankylosing spondylitis. Conversely 97% of those with ankylosing spondylitis are B27 positive. It seems likely that the way individuals handle an immune response is influenced by their tissue type and thus the link. Much remains to be discovered in this area.

Nature did not evolve tissue typing in order to help us with transplant surgery, nor even in the diagnosis of ankylosing spondylitis. The natural reason for its existence links with the immune functions of the cells. This identification on leukocytes also ensures that instructions are taken only from valid 'self' cells. Within the immune system there is a need for communication. One type of cell recognises an invader and communicates that fact to another, which in turn reacts itself or perhaps instructs a third to produce antibodies in defence.

HLA molecules are involved in presenting foreign antigens to specific lymphocytes called T cells. Protein fragments from such antigens become bound to HLA molecules in 'antigen presenting cells' such as macrophages. The HLA molecule plus bound antigen form a recognisable complex which produces an appropriate response when presented to and recognised by T cells. These proceed to enable the appropriate defence reaction.

THE CELLULAR IMMUNE SYSTEM

The cells of the immune system are all found in peripheral blood as the leukocyte population. These cells can leave the circulation and enter tissues at sites of inflammation or injury. The prime players in cellular immunity are given below.

MONOCYTES (MACROPHAGES)

The same cell has two names, being a monocyte when found in peripheral blood and a macrophage when found in other body fluids and tissues. Their prime function is recognising foreign material, and turning from resting into activated macrophages when they do so. As well as identifying an intruder and alerting other immune cells to it, they have a major scavenging function in mopping up operations later in an immune action.

Macrophages are important for digesting foreign antigens, such as those from bacteria, into small protein fragments. These fragments are transported to the surface of the macrophage where they may be recognised by T

cells. The macrophage thus acts as an 'antigen presenting cell'. Recognition of foreign antigen will stimulate the T cells to multiply and to produce cytokines. The latter will stimulate reactions in other types of lymphocyte, such as B cells, and in other cells involved with inflammation such as fibroblasts and endothelial cells of the blood vessel walls (Figure 2.1).

LYMPHOCYTES

Initially subdivided into large and small lymphocytes, simply from their appearance down a microscope, but now with much more knowledge of their functions into:

B cells

So called since they were originally identified in chickens where they are derived from a structure known as the **b**ursa of Fabricius. In humans they derive from the bone marrow. These cells are responsible for producing antibodies when activated, and in that state they are known as plasma cells.

T cells

These derive their name from the organ of their origin— the **T**hymus. Initially they were subdivided by their immunological properties and were named by those functions giving names such as 'T helper cell'. Now specific antibodies, produced in the laboratory and directed against proteins in the T cell walls, are used to identify the subtypes.

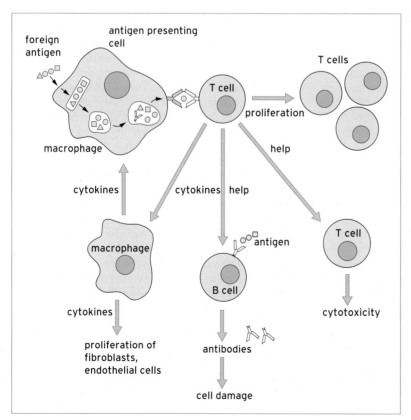

Figure 2.1 **Antigen presentation and immune cell communications leading to the immune response.**

One may come across cells with names such as CD4 or CD8, referring to the particular antibody which identifies the cell. CD4 positive T cells are T helper cells and CD8 positive T cells are cytotoxic T cells, so although names have varied the functions remain unchanged. T cells are thus divided into:

- T helper cells which promote activation of specific B cells.
- T suppressor cells which reduce activation of specific B cells.
- Cytotoxic T cells which destroy cells displaying specific antigens.

Natural Killer cells

Natural killer (NK) cells, also called null cells, have the ability to destroy other cells by surface contact, and are perhaps the only cells really deserving the title 'Cellular Immune System'. While initially classified with T cells, many immunologists now feel that NK cells should be classified separately. These cells are the mainstay of tumour immunity and are thought to police the body seeking and destroying malignancies. The cancer which kills you is the one you failed to kill! They also destroy other foreign cells and NK cells are those most responsible for transplant rejection. Some bacterial defence is largely dependent on the NK cell, tuberculosis being a prime example of this.

POLYMORPHONUCLEAR LEUKOCYTES

Also called neutrophils, or shortened to 'polymorphs', these are not strictly part of the cellular immune system since they are not involved in the instigation of the immune response. They are, however, very important in the inflammation which ensues and since this chapter covers inflammation they deserve a mention. It is difficult to separate precise roles of cells which are multi-functional, but the main purpose for the polymorph in this situation is the final destruction of cells and proteins identified as foreign. The polymorph achieves this by ingesting then digesting the material. Polymorphs are found in profusion when an inflammatory response is active. The predominant cells in fluid aspirated from an inflamed joint in RA are polymorphs. Polymorphs respond to the cytokines produced during the inflammatory process, and are essentially summoned to the site by chemical attraction. Enzymes released by polymorphs during the process seem likely to be responsible for much of the damage seen in a rheumatoid joint.

THE HUMORAL IMMUNE SYSTEM

Now that the inter-relationship of the cellular and the humoral immune system is better understood it is perhaps only history which maintains the terms. In practice the immune system functions as an entirety. The humoral system includes all the soluble factors involved. Immunoglobulins are generally considered as the mainstay but cytokines and other factors are important too. Neither these nor immunoglobulins would exist if the cellular immune system did not produce them.

Recognition of proteins immunologically relies on a number of properties. In much the same way as one looks for colour, size and shape when completing a jigsaw, so the immunoglobulins look for similar matches to attach to proteins. A protein is a string of amino-acids but it does not exist as a straight line. Because of attachments and electrical charges within the molecule, it acquires a three-dimensional shape and size, 'coloured' by static electrical charges and water affinities. The appearance is not unlike a length of multi-coloured knitting wool made into a ravel. One can imagine the vast number of variations in the surface pattern and colour which are possible. Perish the thought of completing a three-dimensional jigsaw made up from knitting wool!

The overall population of B cells is capable of producing so many different immunoglobulins that one will almost certainly match any given protein pattern. Each specific B cell will only produce one specific immunoglobulin, but somewhere in your circulation you have a B cell which will make a matching immunoglobulin for any foreign protein. The B cell itself does not recognise the need to produce immunoglobulin and it must be instructed to do so. Where a foreign protein invades the body it is recognised by an 'antigen presenting cell', usually a macrophage, which is activated in the process. This activated macrophage will proceed to meet with various lymphocytes as time passes and cells move around. Eventually it will meet with a T helper cell which recognises the appearance of the antigen it is presenting. The T helper cell is likewise triggered and goes on to meet with various B lymphocytes until, again, a match is found and that specific B lymphocyte is activated. The activated B lymphocyte is a plasma cell producing antibodies which match the size and shape, and often the electrical charge or water affinity, of the antigen in question. These antibodies are released into the circulation and will complex with the antigen when they meet. One plasma cell cannot make an impact, but a chain reaction ensues with more plasma cells produced and antibody levels increasing. Generally 10 days are required to build up effective levels of antibody against a new antigen, but a second meeting with the same antigen produces a more rapid response. This latter fact is the reason for acquired immunity, and we capitalise on this principle with immunisation. Where an invader is a complex of proteins, as in a bacterium, several proteins involved may act as antigens leading to more than one antibody being produced. Generally one particular antigen will be easier to recognise, immunologically speaking, and that will lead to more rapid antibody production than the others. This may lead to elimination of the invader before other antibody production has become established, but if not then, later antibodies represent an alternative method for producing the necessary result. When the threat has been overcome it is necessary to demobilise the troops. This is achieved by T suppressor cells which go on to deactivate plasma cells and antibody production. Deactivation is not total and detectable levels of specific antibody will remain in the circulation, usually for some years, after an immune response has finished.

To prevent an invader delivering false information, the immune cells will only communicate with other cells which are identifiable as allies. Each of these cells will only accept the instruction if the major histocompatibility complex (MHC) containing the HLA tissue type is recognised as belonging to 'self'. Cells come into physical contact and lock together, using specific cell binding areas called intercellular adhesion molecules (ICAMs) in order to exchange information needed for the immune response. This constitutes a safety mechanism, helping to ensure effective functioning of the systems. The MHC is also responsible for presenting the antigen to the T cell. As ever there can be situations which are unaccounted for and at present HIV seems to be able to mis-instruct the system, infecting the T cell which should be recognising it and defending against it and so reducing the availability of T helper cells in individuals suffering from AIDS. Given time natural selection would no doubt overcome that problem, unless modern medicine overcomes it first.

INFLAMMATION AND THE ACUTE PHASE RESPONSE

Treatments for rheumatological conditions frequently attempt to reduce inflammation, and we spuriously look upon inflammation as undesirable. However, we rely on inflammation to protect us and to heal damaged tissues. In many rheumatological conditions it is felt that the immune responses involved are prolonging inflammation inappropriately or that the limiting mechanisms have failed. In this event the inflammation is excessive and needs to be curtailed, but our approach needs to be balanced and it would be undesirable to abolish inflammation totally. In some situations the intention to limit it at all may be incorrect even though the patient's symptoms are improved by so doing. Sometimes the end justifies the means and it is appropriate to let nature take its course, despite a longer period of discomfort.

Inflammation may be induced by physical or chemical trauma, or by immune activation. Damaged tissues produce inflammation and in some instances inflammation damages tissue, producing a self-perpetuating situation unless some limiting processes are brought into play. When cells are damaged phospholipids, major constituents of cell membranes, are released. Cyclo-oxygenase, an enzyme, acts on phospholipids to produce prostaglandins. There are several types of prostaglandin and these are major mediators of inflammation. The main mode of action of most of the anti-inflammatory drugs used in rheumatology is to block the action of cyclo-oxygenase, reducing prostaglandins and thus inflammation (see Chapter 3). All inflammation is reduced by these agents, not just rheumatological inflammation, and unwanted effects such as increased gastric erosion and peptic ulceration ensue. Recently the identification of two types of cyclo-oxygenase has raised hopes of being able to be more specific in the blockade, perhaps reducing the unwanted effects of these agents. It is too early to say whether this is valid.

THE ACUTE PHASE RESPONSE

This occurs during inflammation and includes the production of specific proteins involved with inflammation and with specific functions to perform during the process. There are a number of 'acute phase proteins' and not all are mentioned here. Best known in rheumatology is C-reactive protein (CRP), the serum level of which is often used as a laboratory measure of inflammation. This protein appears able to function as a non-specific antibody. Since it is produced within 24 hours of an inflammatory insult, it can probably provide some of the function of specific antibodies while the production of these is awaited. The timing of acute phase protein production relates to their functions. The early CRP seems to encourage complement activation and thus increase the response. Alpha-1 anti-trypsin is another acute phase protein which is produced in increased quantities after 3 or 4 days. This is an anti-protease. Proteases are enzymes which destroy protein and in the early stage of inflammation they are released from cells involved in the inflammatory processes. Producing an anti-protease able to inactivate these enzymes at a stage when they may be damaging tissues which are healing seems sensible. Alpha-1 anti-trypsin has functions other than destroying enzymes and in RA it is found complexed with IgA. The presence of relatively high amounts of this complex seems to indicate more active disease, but as yet the significance is not understood. At a later stage again, the acute phase proteins produced have the ability to damp down the inflammatory response and clearly then have a limiting function. In the same way as the immune response is both self-perpetuating and self-limiting depending on the stage reached, so is the inflammatory response. These natural systems seem to display abundant common sense!

CLINICAL APPLICATIONS OF IMMUNOLOGY AND INFLAMMATION

An understanding of the processes involved in immunology and inflammation allows us to decide which laboratory investigations will be helpful in making a diagnosis, planning treatment and assessing the benefit of such treatment, and often in formulating a prognosis so that patients and their relatives can be counselled appropriately. Many of the investigations use immunological laboratory techniques to achieve the result. There is no need to understand the techniques used, nor is there a need for a full understanding of the meaning of many of the investigation results. It is helpful to be aware of the type of tests performed and the reasons for using them, and this section is a brief overview of that aspect.

From a physiotherapeutic viewpoint, choice of modalities of treatment may be influenced by knowledge of the underlying process. In some instances it may be appropriate to increase the blood supply to an affected area, increasing the inflammation and thus accelerating healing. Other situations may require reduction of inflammation to reduce pain, accepting that this may prolong the healing process but be more acceptable to the patient. In all healing situations physical routines to help regain functions which will have been reduced or lost during the inflammatory process are likely to be appropriate.

ERYTHROCYTE SEDIMENTATION RATE

This is the oldest investigation used and simply measures how quickly red cells settle through blood which is left standing for 1 hour. While simple, the factors which dictate how quickly cells do settle seem to be extremely complex and all the mechanisms involved are not yet fully understood. Major factors are the protein content of the plasma and the protein which coats the surface of the red cells. The presence of acute phase proteins in the plasma makes cells settle more quickly and elevates the erythrocyte sedimentation rate (ESR). Immunoglobulins similarly elevate it, as do lower levels of albumin. The ESR proves to be an easy way of assessing the level of the inflammation present and is used as such. If it is high then inflammation is likely to be active, and treatments which reduce it have probably reduced inflammation. Many other factors influence the ESR and it is quite non-specific. An elevated ESR can occur in conditions where inflammation is not involved. It is easy to forget that and assume the ESR reflects only inflammation. Not only can it reflect conditions other than inflammation, but it also gives no guarantee that any inflammation it is reflecting is due to the condition being investigated. Other passing problems in a patient can give a raised ESR and the results must be interpreted with caution and in the light of the clinical findings.

The level of ESR does vary between individuals. On the whole a value under 20 mm/hour can be considered normal, but having said that a patient who would normally have an ESR of 3 mm/hour would be revealing a problem with a value of 17 mm/hour. Unfortunately, patients do not present to doctors before they become unwell. We do not therefore know the usual level of an individual's ESR and results must be interpreted in the light of other clinical findings. Levels above 30 mm/hour should be considered as indicating a problem which may need further elucidation and levels over 60 mm/hour need further investigation to identify the reason unless that is already apparent. Older individuals tend to run higher levels and patients with long-standing inflammation, such as with RA, will often be relatively well despite an ESR between 30 and 60 mm/hour.

C-REACTIVE PROTEIN

Measured by immunological methods this investigation has become the most widely accepted method of assessing the degree of inflammation. It is a more difficult and more costly test but it is not affected by the non-inflammatory factors which may influence the ESR. Again the assumption that treatment which reduces the C-reactive protein (CRP) has improved the condition is tempting. As a rule this is

true, but again there is no guarantee that the inflammation being measured has arisen from the condition being treated and results must be interpreted with knowledge of clinical findings. Generally levels of ESR and CRP will run in parallel and when they do not, most rheumatologists feel that further investigations to explain the discrepancy are warranted. The collagenoses, particularly systemic lupus erythematosus (SLE), are liable to give an ESR result which is disproportionately high when compared with the CRP. The main advantage of CRP over ESR is that it specifically reflects inflammation almost all of the time.

A perfectly healthy individual should have an undetectable level of CRP in the serum. Laboratories will usually report this as 'less than 6', since very low levels cannot be quantified. As with the ESR different individuals vary in their expression of these factors and one cannot necessarily say that one patient with a level of 40 mg/l is more ill than another with a level of 30 mg/l. Where the level changes in the same individual it does indicate improvement or deterioration and effective treatment will reduce the CRP. This is often a very volatile and rapidly responsive test and it can change markedly within 24 hours. Very aggressive inflammation can produce values above 400 mg/l but in the inflammatory arthropathies levels between 20 and 200 mg/l are expected. Well-controlled patients can have undetectable levels, and that is a treatment ideal.

RHEUMATOID FACTOR

Most laboratories now report rheumatoid factor (RF) as international units (iu) but one may come across some which still report a 'Latex test titre' and older reports may be found which refer to the 'Rose–Waaler'. All these refer to the same finding and elevated levels indicate that RF is present in the serum. While this is evidence towards a diagnosis of RA it is not diagnostic and any chronic inflammatory condition may give a positive test. Equally, it is quite possible to have a negative result in patients with RA. Treatments can improve the disease activity without altering the level of RF and this test is not used to reflect the benefit of therapy but rather as an aid to diagnosis. It does influence prognosis to an extent and generally higher levels are indicative of more progressive disease, particularly in males.

A positive result is accepted at above 80 iu or for the Latex test a higher titre than 1:40. All results, but particularly borderline positive results, need to be interpreted in the light of clinical findings.

ANTI-NUCLEAR ANTIBODIES

Anti-nuclear antibody (ANA) is also referred to as anti-nuclear factor (ANF). This test relies on immunological laboratory methods and looks for the presence in the serum of antibodies against nuclear proteins. It is performed by exposing cells to serum from the patient, then to labelled antibodies against immunoglobulin. The cells are then examined microscopically and a pattern is observed if the test is positive. Results are expressed as a titre in the same way as the Latex or Rose–Waaler tests mentioned earlier, and the type of pattern observed is also reported. The pattern will be described as homogenous, speckled or nucleolar and this gives some guidance as to which particular ANA are present. This investigation superseded a method of identifying patients with SLE by looking in specially prepared blood for cells known as LE cells, and it is now superseded itself by methods which will identify specific ANA. It is still used routinely as a screening test for ANA but where a significant positive result is obtained the more specific tests will be performed. A positive ANA raises the possibility of the diagnosis being one of the collagenoses, or connective tissue diseases, but it is a relatively common finding in RA too.

Titres of less than 1:80 are not highly significant but may aid a diagnosis along with other findings.

SPECIFIC ANTI-NUCLEAR AND CYTOPLASMIC ANTIBODIES

A full classification of these is well beyond the scope of this chapter and they are mentioned now so that you will be aware of some of the terms. The presence of some, but not all, may be suspected from finding a positive Extractable Nuclear Antibodies (ENA). They will generally help formulate the diagnosis, or sometimes warn of possible complications in the condition being treated. Significantly positive DNA binding is relatively diagnostic for SLE. Positive antibodies against extractable nuclear antigens include a number of specific factors (e.g. RNP, Ro, La, Scl70) and these help in diagnosis and prognosis in collagenoses. Cytoplasmic antibodies such as Anti-Neutrophil Cytoplasmic Antibodies (ANCAs) are found in vasculitis and anti-cardiolipin antibodies indicate possible complications with the presence of lupus anti-coagulant.

Even Professors of Immunology admit to not understanding the full implications of all of these auto-antibodies and one need not lose sleep if this final paragraph appears daunting! The author hopes that it will indicate that much in Immunology is yet to be discovered and understood, but as the frontiers move forward so will the treatment and advice we can offer our patients improve.

ACKNOWLEDGEMENT

The author would like to thank Dr DL Mattey for Figure 2.1, and help with proof reading.

GENERAL READING

Isenberg DA. *Mechanisms of Autoimmunity*. Topical Reviews – Reports on Rheumatic Diseases (Series 2) Sept. 1992 No. 22. Arthritis and Rheumatism Council.

Playfair JL. *Immunology at a glance*. Oxford: Blackwell; 1996.

Roitt IM. *Essential immunology, 7th edition*. Oxford: Blackwell Scientific; 1991.

Roitt I, Brostoff J, Male D. *Immunology, 4th edition*. London: Mosby; 1996.

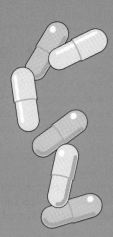

3

A Hassell

DRUG MANAGEMENT OF RHEUMATIC DISORDERS

CHAPTER OUTLINE

- **Non-steroidal anti-inflammatory drugs**
- **Slow acting anti-rheumatic drugs**
- **Newer anti-rheumatic agents**

- **Steroids**
- **Drugs used in the treatment of gout**
- **Agents used in the treatment/ prevention of osteoporosis**

INTRODUCTION

The aim of this chapter is to give some insight into the agents used in the management of rheumatic diseases (the main focus being on the inflammatory arthritides), their indications and limitations. In addition, a short description of some anti-rheumatic drugs under development will be given.

NON-STEROIDAL ANTI-INFLAMMATORY DRUGS

Non-steroidal anti-inflammatory drugs (NSAIDs) represent the usual mainstay of symptomatic treatment in patients with inflammatory arthritis. They will be dealt with in some detail as they will be the drugs most frequently encountered by physiotherapists. There are several different NSAIDs, all acting to decrease the cardinal symptoms and signs of inflammation—pain, stiffness, swelling and warmth.

THE RANGE OF NSAIDs

There are over 30 NSAIDs available for prescription. The drugs differ in terms of their chemical family (Table 3.1), their half life (the time taken for their plasma concentration to halve – this determines how frequently a drug must be taken), the nature of the preparation, the designated route

Chemical classification of non steroidal anti-inflammatory drugs	
Carboxylic acids:	aspirin, choline salicylate, diflunisal
Acetic acids:	diclofenac, indomethacin, tolmetin, *sulindac, etodolac
Propionic acids:	ibuprofen, naproxen, fenoprofen, tiaprofenic acid, ketoprofen, *fenbufen, flurbiprofen
Fenamic acids:	mefenamic acid
Enolic acids:	oxyphenbutazone, phenylbutazone, piroxicam, tenoxicam, azapropazone
Non-acidic compounds:	*nabumetone

*Prodrugs

Adapted from Brooks & Day, *N Engl J Med* 1991, 324:1716-1724.

Table 3.1 **Chemical classification of non steroidal anti-inflammatory drugs.**

of administration and whether they are a prodrug or not. Prodrugs are compounds which are themselves not active as anti-inflammatory agents but are metabolised in the body to the active anti-inflammatory compound.

Phenylbutazone is limited to hospital prescription for ankylosing spondylitis in the UK.

MECHANISMS OF ACTION

Prostaglandin synthesis is suppressed by NSAIDs (Figure 3.1)—at least partly by inhibiting the enzyme cyclo-oxygenase (COX). Prostaglandins produce many of the features of inflammation including warmth, erythema and oedema, and influence many of the cells and mediators involved in the immune response.

Recently there has been considerable interest in the discovery of different forms of COX, namely COX1 and COX2. COX1 has a 'housekeeping' role in the normal cell. It appears important in maintaining the integrity of gastric and duodenal mucosa, in regulating renal blood flow and in salt and water balance. COX2, by contrast, is associated with inflammation. There is thus the exciting prospect of developing agents which inhibit COX2 (and hence some of the manifestations of inflammation) while not affecting COX1 (and hence not causing some of the adverse effects of NSAIDs).

In addition to their effects on prostaglandin production, NSAIDs have effects on various other aspects of the inflammatory response, including leukotriene synthesis, superoxide production and cytokine production.

USES OF NSAIDs

Significant symptom relief is provided by NSAIDs, which is generally felt within days. In patients with spondyloarthropathies they may facilitate exercise. In rheumatoid arthritis (RA), while they provide symptomatic relief, there is no evidence that they have long-term beneficial effects on the outcome of the disease. The use of NSAIDs in osteoarthritis (OA) is open to debate. Because inflammation is often not a prominent feature of degenerative joint disease, and in view of the side effects of NSAIDs, there is a tendency to try and avoid NSAIDs in patients with this form of arthritis. Simple analgesics are generally sufficient, but in some cases NSAIDs are necessary for adequate symptom relief.

ADVERSE EFFECTS OF NSAIDs

Mild adverse effects with NSAIDs occur in approximately 10–15% of users. Serious side effects are rare, but because these agents are so widely prescribed a significant number of individuals are affected.

Gastrointestinal (GI)

The commonest adverse effects of NSAIDs are on the GI tract. In the upper GI tract they may be associated with erosions, with peptic ulceration (gastric or duodenal) and also with dyspepsia. Peptic ulceration may be complicated by perforation and bleeding. It has been estimated that 1 in 10,000 NSAID prescriptions issued to people over the age of 60 in the UK result in peptic ulcer complications. The risk of ulcer increases with higher NSAID doses. Generally, low dose ibuprofen is associated with the lowest risk of serious upper GI adverse effect. Diclofenac, naproxen and indomethacin are associated with intermediate risk of such adverse effects. Azapropazone is associated with the highest risk of serious upper GI side effects and also appears to carry higher risks of hepatic, renal and hypersensitivity reactions. Inflammation in the small and large intestine is also associated with NSAIDs.

Other drugs may be prescribed alongside NSAIDs to protect the gut. Misoprostol decreases the incidence of both gastric and duodenal ulcers in patients taking NSAIDs. Tablets have been produced which contain a NSAID component and a misoprostol component (e.g. arthrotec). However, misoprostol does not remove the risk of adverse effects but only decreases it. Moreover, misoprostol itself can cause diarrhoea and abdominal pain. Cimetidine and ranitidine decrease the incidence of duodenal but not gastric ulceration in individuals taking NSAIDs. Table 3.2 summarises the non-gastrointestinal side effects of NSAIDs.

SLOW ACTING ANTI-RHEUMATIC DRUGS (SAARDs)

A number of agents are used in an effort to control inflammatory arthritis, particularly RA. The terminology of these agents is confusing. They have been referred to as 'disease modifying anti-rheumatic drugs' (DMARDs), 'second-line agents' (to distinguish them from 'first-line' NSAIDs) and 'slow acting anti-rheumatic drugs' (SAARDs). For the purpose of this chapter they will be referred to as SAARDs (Table 3.3). These drugs come from very different chemical families but have a number of properties in common.

- Control of the symptoms and signs of RA—at least in the short- to medium-term. They have been shown to have a

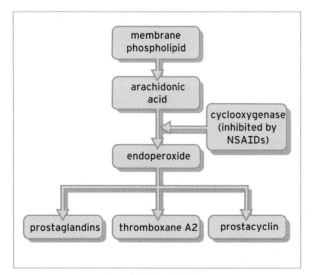

Figure 3.1 Non-steroidal anti-inflammatory drugs and prostaglandin synthesis.

beneficial effect on numbers of active joints, overall well being, function, and certain laboratory parameters of inflammation (e.g. the erythrocyte sedimentation rate (ESR)). Some effect in decreasing radiological progression has also been demonstrated.

• Delayed onset of action—typically it may take 2–4 months to see a response.

• Serious adverse effects—with the exception of the anti-malarials, haematological adverse effects occur with sufficient frequency to require regular blood test monitoring for individuals with inflammatory arthritis. The incidence of side effects (both major and minor) therefore limits their use.

• Mechanism of SAARDs' beneficial action—for the most part, this action in RA is not known.

Table 3.2 **Non-gastrointestinal side effects of non-steroidal anti-inflammatory drugs.**

Non-gastrointestinal side effects of non-steroidal anti-inflammatory drugs	
Renal	Nephropathy, impaired renal function Sodium retention – hypertension, oedema or heart failure Cystitis (particularly with tiaprofenic acid)
Skin	Rashes (particularly with fenbufen)
Hepatic	Transient rise in liver enzymes Hepatitis (rare)
Haematological	Iron deficiency anaemia (secondary to blood loss due to gastrointestinal erosion or ulceration), thrombocytopenia, neutropenia Aplastic anaemia (very rare except with phenylbutazone)
Respiratory	May precipitate asthma
Other	Headache and dizziness (particularly with indomethacin) Interact with numerous other commonly prescribed drugs including anticoagulants, anticonvulsants, diuretics

Slow acting anti-rheumatic drugs			
	Usual prescription regimen	Adverse effects	Comments
Chloroquine phosphate/ Hydroxychloroquine sulphate	Oral, daily	Minor: headaches, nausea Major: retinal toxicity (rare)	Sometimes used in combination with other slow acting anti-rheumatic drugs. Regular eye checks are recommended
Sulphasalazine	Oral, daily in divided doses	Minor: headaches, nausea, dizziness, skin rashes (can be major) Major: blood dyscrasias (abnormally low white cell-, red cell- or platelet-count), occasional liver abnormalities	Often used early in disease in the UK. Used in some combination regimes. Some efficacy in the seronegative spondyloarthropathies
D-Penicillamine	Daily dose on an empty stomach	Minor: nausea, abdominal pain, taste loss, mouth ulcers Major: blood dyscrasias (especially thrombocytopenia – low platelets); glomerulonephritis causing proteinuria; other autoimmune diseases – systemic lupus erythematosus, myositis, myasthenia gravis, bronchiolitis	

Table 3.3 **Slow acting anti-rheumatic drugs.**

	Usual prescription regimen	Adverse effects	Comments
Slow acting anti-rheumatic drugs (continued)			
Injectable gold (sodium aurothiomalate, aurothioglucose)	Intramuscular injection, initially 50 mg weekly, gradually decreasing to monthly. A 10 mg test dose is usually given first	Minor: rashes (can be major), itching, mouth ulcers (can be severe) Major: blood dyscrasias, glomerulonephritis with proteinuria, occasional pneumonitis or hepatitis	May slow radiological progression. Minor toxicity is often a problem – some rheumatologists are tending to use less gold and more methotrexate
Oral gold (auranofin)	Daily dose	Minor: diarrhoea, rash Major: proteinuria, thrombocytopenia	Major side effects much less common than with injectable gold but fewer patients respond
Methotrexate	Weekly dose, usually oral, sometimes intramuscular injection, sometimes subcutaneously (children)	Minor: nausea, vomiting, mouth ulcers (sometimes major). Folic acid may decrease the incidence of minor side effects Major: blood dyscrasias. Abnormal liver enzymes, fibrosis and cirrhosis Pneumonitis. Opportunistic infections	Methotrexate is a cytotoxic agent as well as having anti-inflammatory properties. It is used in the treatment of certain malignancies and severe psoriasis in a low dose regime. Effective in rheumatoid arthritis, psoriatic arthritis and myositis
Azathioprine	Daily in divided doses	Minor: nausea, vomiting, diarrhoea, rashes Major: blood dyscrasias, altered liver function. There may be an increased risk of subsequent lymphomas	Used in rheumatoid arthritis, and as a steroid sparing agent in other rheumatic conditions, including systemic lupus erythematosus and myositis
Cyclophosphamide	Daily oral, or inter-mittent 'pulse' regimes. Pulse regimens are given orally or intravenously, and may offer a better combination of efficacy and safety	Minor: nausea and vomiting. Alopecia Major: bone marrow suppression. Opportunistic infections. Later malignancies – lymphomas and bladder cancer. Haemorrhagic cystitis – may be partly prevented by a high fluid intake and taking the drug mesna at the same time. Infertility.	Potent highly toxic compound used in the treatment of tumours, lymphomas and leukaemias. In rheumatology, it is generally reserved for life threatening vasculitic conditions with major organ involvement (see Chapter 14). Also used for proliferative glomerulonephritis in systemic lupus erythematosus. Monitoring of blood tests is essential
Cyclosporin	Daily oral	Minor: nausea, headache, hirsutism, tremor Major: renal impairment with elevation of creatinine. Hypertension, hyperuricaemia and hyperkalaemia. Hepatotoxicity	Established role in the prevention of transplant rejection. Effective in rheumatoid arthritis. Not particularly toxic to the bone marrow. It has been used in rheumatoid arthritis in combination with other slow acting anti-rheumatic drugs (notably methotrexate)

Table 3.3 (continued) **Slow acting anti-rheumatic drugs.**

Although SAARDs have been shown to be of benefit in the short- to medium- term, a clear positive effect on the long-term outcome of patients with RA (e.g. quality of life, ability to continue working) has been more difficult to demonstrate, partly because of the logistic difficulties in designing studies to answer questions of long-term outcome. Most rheumatologists now agree that SAARDs do offer a significant benefit to individuals with RA while accepting that there is scope for improvement in terms of efficacy. One other area of consensus regarding SAARDs is the concept of early intervention: a significant proportion of joint damage in RA occurs within the first 2 years of disease. Effective control of inflammation at this stage in the disease appears important in controlling the disease process.

NEWER ANTI-RHEUMATIC AGENTS

NEW IMMUNOSUPPRESSIVE DRUGS

A number of new agents are currently under evaluation or development, such as leflunomide and FK506, an agent with cyclosporin like properties. Clinical trials are currently underway assessing the efficacy of these drugs.

MONOCLONAL ANTIBODIES

The rapid development of the technology to produce mono-clonal antibodies (MAb) has led to considerable excitement within the field of rheumatology. The effective use of MAb in therapy requires three conditions to be fulfilled:

- It must be possible to produce antibodies with the exact specificity. The antigen for which the antibody is specific may be an inflammatory cell or molecule. Attachment of the MAb to the antigen may result in death or neutral-isation of that cell.
- As these antibodies are usually produced in mice, the risk is that the patient's own immune system will recognise the mouse antibody and neutralise it and/or that the mouse antibody will cause an allergic reaction. The aim is to produce a 'humanised' MAb that is not recognised as foreign.
- The target for the MAb must be appropriate, i.e. there must be some confidence that neutralising that target will result in a beneficial effect. It is far from easy to predict the effect of interfering with one component of a very complex immune system.

A number of different MAb have been tried in RA with some success, including MAb specific for certain cell surface markers (e.g. the CD4 molecule which is expressed by T helper cells) and, specific for the cytokine tumour necrosis factor (TNF), anti-TNF MAb. Although intraven-ous anti-TNF has resulted in rapid, sustained improve-ments in measures of inflammation and function, further work is underway to establish its safety, dosage, periodicity of treatment and indications for its use. It is possible that a cocktail of MAb will eventually be used in the manage-ment of RA, each MAb dealing with a different aspect of the immune response.

CHEMICAL CYTOKINE MODIFIERS

Over the past decade considerable progress has been made in the identification and characterisation of cytokines. The identification of 'pro-inflammatory' cytokines which appear central in the pathology of RA (e.g. TNF-alpha, interleukin (IL)-1) has led to research into the therapeutic potential of cytokine inhibitors. Similarly, the observation that certain cytokines, e.g. IL-10, exert an important immunoregulatory effect has provoked interest in the therapeutic use of these molecules. This area of research is still in its infancy but studies into IL-10, IFN-gamma, IL-1 receptor antagonist and IL-2 fusion toxin are underway.

ARACHIDONIC ACID METABOLITE MODIFIERS

There are a number of developments in the field of prostaglandin inhibition. One is the advent of specific COX2 inhibitors to minimise toxicity while retaining efficacy (see section on NSAIDs above). Another has been the development of agents which act both as COX inhibitors and cytokine inhibitors.

ORAL TOLERANCE

The concept of immunological tolerance is currently being explored in RA therapeutic studies. Tolerance is the failure of the body's immune system to react to a specific mole-cule which would normally be antigenic. For example, in animal studies, guinea pigs normally respond to the injec-tion of foreign protein with an allergic reaction. However, prior feeding of high doses of the protein prevents this allergic reaction on subsequent injection of the protein. This tolerance is specific for that protein – the animals have normal allergic response to other foreign proteins. In rheumatology, the concept would be to tolerise RA patients to the target antigens against which the autoimmune response is directed—articular cartilage is one possible target. Studies are currently underway using Type II colla-gen from chicken bones as the tolerising agent.

STEROIDS

Systemic steroids are very effective anti-inflammatory agents, are immunosuppressive in high doses, and offer significant symptomatic relief in a number of inflamm-atory rheumatic disorders. However, even quite low doses are associated with potentially serious side effects which may cause significant morbidity. Osteoporosis has been found with doses as low as 7.5 mg daily. Systemic steroids include cortisone, hydrocortisone (cortisol), prednisolone and methylprednisolone.

The adverse effects are numerous and are largely dose related (Table 3.4). Systemic steroids are difficult to stop once started. They may switch off the patient's own (endogenous) steroid production and withdrawal may result in a 'steroid crisis' with a failure of cortisol produc-tion resulting in hypotension, hypoglycaemia and electro-lyte imbalance. Withdrawal can also lead to a marked flare in symptoms of the inflammatory disease.

STEROID USE

Vasculitis

High doses used initially, together with cytotoxic agents.

Connective Tissue Disorders

Low and intermediate doses are used in serositis or myositis in systemic lupus erythematosus (SLE) patients.

Inflammatory Muscle Diseases

Medium high doses for dermatomyositis and polymyositis, often with a cytotoxic agent such as azathioprine or methotrexate.

Rheumatoid Arthritis

Rheumatologists have tried to avoid steroids in treating the joint inflammation seen in rheumatoid arthritis (RA) as, although their initial use can be associated with excellent control of the disease, increasing doses are often required and it becomes very difficult to decrease or stop the steroids. Meanwhile, patients are at risk of steroid side effects. More recently there has been some interest in the concept of low dose steroids for RA. Kirwan (1995) found that patients with early RA suffered less radiological joint damage in the hands if given prednisolone compared with placebo. However, there have been a number of methodological criticisms of this paper. Sometimes a pulse of steroid (IV or IM) is used to induce remission when SAARD treatment is initiated.

INTRA-ARTICULAR CORTICOSTEROIDS

Local intra-articular or peri-articular injections are commonly used in rheumatology, and carry a much lower risk of side effects than systemic steroids.

Absolute contraindications are few. The most important is the presence of intra-articular sepsis. Foci of infection elsewhere in the body, especially infected skin ulcers, are relative contraindications as sepsis may develop in the locally immunosuppressed injected joint.

Peri-articular injections are often used to accelerate recovery of soft tissue problems although evidence proving their efficacy is relatively sparse.

Adverse effects of corticosteroids	
Metabolic	Weight gain (metabolic and appetite stimulation) Central obesity 'Buffalo hump' Muscle wasting Salt and water retention - oedema, hypertension
Endocrine	Hyperglycaemia Osteoporosis Stunting of normal growth
Skin	Atrophy Purpura Acne
Vascular	Hyperlipidaemia Atheroma
Bone	Osteoporosis Avascular necrosis
Neuro/Psychiatric	Mood changes, rarely psychosis Cataracts. Glaucoma
Immunological	Infections (opportunistic if high dose regimens)

Table 3.4 **Adverse effects of corticosteroids.**

DRUGS USED IN THE TREATMENT OF GOUT

TREATMENT OF THE ACUTE ATTACK

NSAIDs

Often the more potent NSAIDs, e.g. indomethacin, are used.

Colchicine

Colchicine is effective but frequent occurrence of side effects such as nausea, vomiting and abdominal pain mean that it tends to be reserved for individuals in whom NSAIDs are contraindicated. Less commonly it can cause GI bleeding and renal damage and, rarely, blood dyscrasias.

Intra-articular Steroids

Intra-articular steroids are very effective at settling the acute synovitis.

PREVENTION OF GOUT

Several agents, such as allopurinol, probenecid and sulfinpyrazone, effectively lower the serum urate level, and hence can prevent attacks of gout in the long-term. If started, the patient is committed to lifelong therapy. The decision is based on frequency of attacks, the presence or absence of tophi, and the potential efficacy of other treatment modalities (e.g. diet). Hypouricaemic therapy should not be started during an acute attack of gout as this may prolong the attack and make it more severe. In addition, initiation of hypouricaemic therapy can itself precipitate an attack of gout. To prevent this it is usual to give NSAIDs (or occasionally low dose colchicine) to cover the period following starting treatment with the hypouricaemic agent.

Allopurinol

Allopurinol inhibits the formation of uric acid. Minor side effects with allopurinol include GI disturbance. It can also result in skin rashes. Occasionally it causes a severe allergic reaction requiring steroid therapy. Sensitivity to allopurinol appears to be increased when there is renal impairment, in which circumstances lower doses should be used.

Probenecid and Sulfinpyrazone

Probenecid and sulfinpyrazone increase the renal excretion of urate. Minor side effects which may occur with these agents include GI disturbances. Both agents can result in crystallisation of urate in the urine. This is avoided by ensuring a high fluid intake, particularly during the first weeks of therapy. Both agents can cause hypersensitivity reactions, occasionally blood disorders and hepatic disturbances.

AGENTS USED IN THE TREATMENT/ PREVENTION OF OSTEOPOROSIS

The management and prevention of osteoporosis is a complex area which is beyond the scope of this chapter. A very brief outline of some of the agents used will be given.

CALCIUM, VITAMIN D AND METABOLITES OF VITAMIN D

The successful prevention/treatment of osteoporosis requires an adequate supply of the 'building blocks' of bone—calcium. Calcium needs vary with age, being increased during puberty, pregnancy, lactation and in old age. It has been recommended that women with post-menopausal osteopaenia should take at least 1500 mg calcium daily. This may require calcium supplements in individuals whose diet is not adequate. Various calcium salts are available and there is evidence that different salts are absorbed to differing degrees, e.g. calcium citrate malate may be better absorbed than calcium carbonate.

Vitamin D is similarly important in the prevention of osteoporosis. Various studies have shown an improvement in bone density with vitamin D supplementation. The most impressive effect on fractures was perhaps the study by Chapuy et al. (1994) which showed that hip fractures were 43% lower in individuals given calcium and vitamin D3 compared with placebo. The study population comprised 3270 ambulatory women (mean age 84 years) in nursing homes.

Calcitriol (1,25-dihydroxycholecalciferol), the most potent form of vitamin D, has also been shown to have some effect on diminishing vertebral fractures in osteoporotic women (Chapuy et al., 1994).

HORMONE REPLACEMENT THERAPY

A major factor in post-menopausal osteoporosis is the loss of oestrogen production. Oestrogen hormone replacement therapy (HRT) taken from the peri-menopausal period onwards largely prevents this form of osteoporosis. Moreover, HRT taken at any stage after the menopause, even up to 20 years, offers a significant anti-osteoporotic effect. As well as its beneficial effect on bone, oestrogen HRT has a positive effect on the incidence and severity of ischaemic heart disease (Compston, 1992).

Adverse Effects of Hormone Replacement Therapy

The incidence of uterine carcinoma is increased if oestrogens alone are taken post-menopausally. If progestogens are also taken the increase in uterine cancer is avoided. However, progestogens may be associated with troublesome symptoms including the withdrawal bleed which occurs with cyclical regimens. Moreover progestogens may decrease some of the beneficial cardiac effects of HRT.

There is evidence that prolonged use of HRT may be associated with an increased incidence of breast cancer. Studies have differed in their reported incidence of breast cancer in HRT takers. A recent meta-analysis found that the relative risk of breast cancer was 1.35 for women who had used HRT for 5 years or longer. In North America and Europe the cumulative incidence of breast cancer between the ages of 50 and 70 in never users of HRT is about 45 per 1000 women. In women who began HRT at age 50 years this was estimated to increase to about 47 in those who took HRT for 5 years, 51 in those who took HRT for 10 years and 57 in those who took it for 15 years (Collaborative Group on Hormonal Factors in Breast Cancer, 1997).

The risk of venous thrombosis had until recently been thought not to be increased in women taking HRT (unlike the oral contraceptive pill). However, recent studies have shown a small increase in risk of venous thrombosis, from an incidence of approximately 11 per 100,000 to one of 27 per 100,000 women per year (Daly et al., 1996).

BISPHOSPHONATES

These drugs were originally used mainly for the treatment of Paget's disease of bone and for malignant hypercalcaemia. At smaller doses they have also been found to be effective in the treatment of osteoporosis. They act by inhibiting the resorption of bone by osteoclasts and so decreasing bone turnover.

Pamidronate

Pamidronate is available only as an intravenous preparation.

Etidronate and Alendronate

Etidronate and alendronate have been shown to increase bone density (particularly vertebral), to decrease the rate of vertebral fractures in individuals who have suffered previous vertebral fractures, and, in the case of alendronate, to have some effect on decreasing osteoporotic hip fractures.

The major adverse effect of etidronate is impairment of mineralisation (and hence osteomalacia) when given for prolonged periods of time. Hence, for osteoporosis etidronate is given daily for 2 weeks every 3 months only, and for Paget's disease it is usually given daily for periods of 6 months. The newer bisphosphonates like alendronate are not associated with demineralisation problems and are taken daily. A significant potential adverse effect with alendronate is oesophageal ulceration, hence it is to be taken with a large glass of water and the patient must remain upright afterwards.

Calcitonin

Calcitonin inhibits osteoclastic bone resorption and is used in the treatment of Paget's disease, hypercalcaemia of malignancy and osteoporosis. It has to be given by intramuscular or subcutaneous injection, although trials with an intranasal preparation are well underway. Calcitonin appears to have no major side effects but does cause nausea, anorexia and also facial flushing.

SUMMARY

This chapter has attempted to illustrate some of the pharmacological approaches to treating patients with the spectrum of disorders encountered in rheumatology, and is by no means exhaustive. This is very much an expanding area. New agents are currently under investigation and it is likely that there will be several new therapies within the next few years.

REFERENCES

Chapuy MC, Arlott ME, Delmas PD *et al*. Effect of calcium and cholecalciferol treatment for three years on hip fractures in elderly women. *BMJ* 1994, **308**:1081-1082.

Collaborative group on hormonal factors in breast cancer: Breast cancer and hormone replacement therapy: collaborative reanalysis of the data from 51 epidemiological studies of 52,705 women with breast cancer and 108,411 women without breast cancer. *Lancet* 1997, **350**:1047-1059.

Compston JE. HRT and osteoporosis. *Br Med Bull* 1992, **48**:309-344.

Daly E, Vessey MP, Hawkins MM *et al*. Risk of venous thromboembolism in users of hormone replacement therapy. *Lancet* 1996, **348**:977-980.

Kirwan JR. The effect of glucocorticoids on joint destruction in rheumatoid arthritis. *N Engl J Med* 1995, **333**:3142-3146.

GENERAL READING

Borigini MJ, Paulus HE. Rheumatoid arthritis. In: Weisman MH, Weinblatt ME, eds. *Treatment of the rheumatic diseases*. Philadelphia: WB Saunders; 1995:31-51.

Brooks PM, Day RO. Non steroidal anti-inflammatory drugs - differences and similarities. *N Engl J Med* 1991, **324**:1716-1725.

Choy EHS, Panayi GS, Kingsley GH. Therapeutic monoclonal antibodies. *Br J Rheumatol* 1995, **34**:707-715.

Committee on Safety of Medicines: relative safety of oral non-aspirin NSAIDs. *Curr Prob Pharmacovigilance* 1994, **20**:9-11.

Emmerson BT. Antihyperuricaemics. In: Klippel JH and Dieppe PA, eds. *Rheumatology*. London: Mosby; 1994:8.15.1-8.15.6.

Felson DT, Anderson JJ, Meenan RF. The comparative efficacy and toxicity of second-line drugs in rheumatoid arthritis. Results of two meta-analyses. *Arthritis Rheum* 1990, **33**:1449-1461.

Furst DE. Combination DMARD therapy: rational and limitations. *Rheumatol Eur* 1995, **24**:190-194.

Kalden JR, Manger B. New therapeutic approaches in autoimmune rheumatic diseases, with special emphasis on rheumatoid arthritis. *Br J Rheumatol* 1995, **34**:193-196.

Kirwan JR. Systemic corticosteroids in rheumatology. In: Klippel JH, Dieppe PA, eds. *Rheumatology*. London: Mosby; 1994:8.11.1-8.11.6.

Kreme KM. The changing face of therapy for rheumatoid arthritis. *Rheum Dis Clin North America* 1995, **21**:845-852.

Langman MJS, Weil J, Wainwright P *et al*. Risk of bleeding peptic ulcer associated with individual non steroidal anti-inflammatory drugs. *Lancet* 1994, **343**:1075-1078.

Morrison E, Capell H. Corticosteroids in the management of rheumatoid arthritis. *Br J Rheumatol* 1996, **35**:2-4.

Paulus HE, Furst DE, Drogmoole SH. *Drugs for rheumatic diseases*. New York: Churchill Livingstone; 1987.

Weinblatt ME. Methotrexate. In: Kelsey WN, Harris ED, Ruddy S, Sledge CB, eds. *Textbook of rheumatology*. Philadelphia: W B Saunders; 1993.

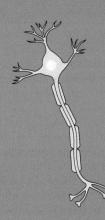

4

C David & J Waterfield

PAIN IN RHEUMATOLOGY

CHAPTER OUTLINE

- Pain mechanisms
- Peripheral pain mechanisms
- Clinical relevance

- Psychosocial factors
- Measurement

INTRODUCTION

Pain is an unpleasant sensory and emotional experience arising from actual or potential tissue damage, or described in terms of such damage (IASP, 1979). This definition encompasses the complexity of pain and identifies the uniqueness of the experience to the individual. This chapter aims to give an overview of mechanisms at work in the appreciation of pain, and an outline of pain measurement tools. Due to the nature of rheumatological conditions, the psychosocial aspects of pain are particularly relevant and these will be discussed in depth.

PAIN MECHANISMS

Although man has formed many ideas through the ages about how pain is generated and perceived, the major progress in pain theory has occurred over the last 300 years with advances in anatomy and physiology. Only a brief overview of recent pain theory can be given here; for further information, an excellent summary is given in Melzack & Wall (1991).

By the beginning of the 20th century, three major theories of pain were proposed: specificity, pattern and affect. Elements of all of these have been incorporated in the pain gate theory.

SPECIFICITY THEORY

This theory stated that pain impulses travelled along a dedicated pathway from receptors in the periphery to a specialised 'pain centre' in the brain. A specific role was proposed for each type of nerve ending, free nerve endings being identified as 'pain receptors'. This theory can be supported to the extent that there is some specialisation of receptors but that others are not specialised; for instance, the free nerve endings in the cornea which can detect all modalities of sensation. The theory also does not explain the variable nature of pain, or why surgical lesion of the pathway often fails to abolish pain. In addition, no pain centre has been identified; current research indicates that several different parts of the brain are involved in pain perception, and the precise mechanism is not clear (Johnson, 1997).

PATTERN THEORY

According to pattern theory, the quality of sensation was dependent not on the type of receptor giving rise to the sensation but on the pattern of stimuli reaching the brain. The brain then decoded this pattern into the various sensations. Pain could be modified by the intensity of receptor stimulation and 'summation', the cumulative effect of rapid repeated volleys of impulses. Receptors were considered to be identical. This theory ignores the specialisation of some receptors, for instance Pacinian corpuscles which only give rise to a sensation of pressure no matter how much they are stimulated.

AFFECT THEORY

This theory progressed from the Aristotelian idea of pain as an emotion. Pain was thought to be an emotive quality that modulated sensation, and was an integral part of pain perception. It was the unpleasant quality to the sensation.

THE PAIN GATE THEORY

This theory (Melzack & Wall, 1965) is now widely accepted as the best explanation for the mechanism by which pain is perceived (Figure 4.1). This theory proposes that afferent nerve impulses (stimuli from nociceptors travelling along the peripheral fibres in the direction of the spinal cord and then to the brain) are modified or blocked by a 'gate' within the dorsal horn of the spinal cord. The gate is affected by the pattern of afferent impulses reaching the gate, and by descending (efferent) mechanisms such as the release of endorphins and other physiological changes that occur in nervous tissue. These changes may either enhance or impede nerve impulse transmission.

At its simplest, the pain gate can be thought of as the balance between activity in the large diameter Aβ fibres which inhibit transmission through the relay and 'close the gate', and the small diameter Aδ fibres/C fibres which excite the relay and 'open the gate'. In addition descending control from various structures in the brain can also inhibit the relay and close the gate. Once the electrical impulses reach the brain, they are further modified and integrated with other sensory input. It is at the level of the brain that the electrical impulses are perceived as pain.

It is important to understand that afferent fibres do not have a fixed response, but are subject to modification even before they reach the pain gate and after they have reached the brain. Jones & Derbyshire (1996) found that rheumatoid arthritis (RA) patients showed less cortical and subcortical activity in response to thermal pain than normal pain-free controls and a generally damped response, indicating a cortical adaptation to pain.

PERIPHERAL PAIN MECHANISMS

INTRA-ARTICULAR MECHANISMS

Table 4.1 summarises innervation of joints. Under normal conditions, large numbers of articular nerve fibres are nonresponsive to noxious stimuli and only react following inflammation. Inflammatory mediators such as prostaglandins and bradykinins alter the sensitivity of afferent fibres; some sensitise the receptors, while some act directly on them. Sensitivity of activated joint mechanoreceptors gives rise to pain on normal movement or light pressure.

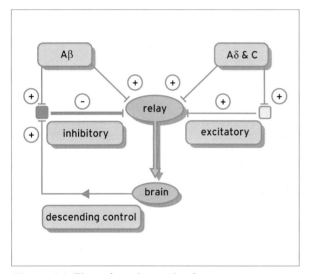

Figure 4.1 **The pain gate mechanism.**

Table 4.1 **Innervation of joints.**

Innervation of joints		
Fibre	Number(%)	Properties
Aβ	<10	Mainly low threshold innocuous stimuli e.g. proprioception
Aδ	>10	Mainly noxious, sensitive to movement; after inflammation may give rise to pain at rest. A small number are mechano-insensitive. After inflammation these become active and sensitive to mechanical stimuli
C	40	As Aδ. Unmyelinated. About a third are mechano-insensitive but activated by inflammation
Sympathetic	40	Unmyelinated postganglionic efferent fibres. Other afferent fibres are not normally responsive to sympathetic stimulation, but become responsive after local trauma or inflammation

Endogenous opioids were thought only to affect central mechanisms such as the pain gate, but are now believed to act on peripheral nerves as well. Intra-articular injections of morphine before arthroscopy have been shown to decrease the need for post operative analgesia (Kidd *et al.*, 1996). In addition, conditions inside the inflamed joint are hypoxic and acidotic. Inflammatory exudates are also acidic, and may contribute to inflammatory pain.

SPINAL MECHANISMS

The responsiveness of spinal neurones may also be increased or decreased. Repetitive or prolonged C fibre firing leads to progressively greater activity in dorsal horn neurones, known as 'wind up'. This results in central sensitisation—dorsal horn neurones have a lowered threshold and exaggerated responses to normal stimuli. This may lead to allodynia, where normal stimuli are perceived as pain. Spinal neurones are also affected by prostaglandins, neurokinin, nitrous oxide, opioids and adrenergic agonists, although the exact mechanism of receptor interactions in spinal neurones is not fully understood.

Spinal mechanisms may also be responsible for referred pain, and pain and tenderness (hyperalgesia) of normal tissues around inflamed or damaged joints. It is important to note that pain may not follow dermatomes; for instance, patients with hip pathology will often complain of pain in the knee region.

Neurogenic Inflammation

Neurogenic inflammation is a local inflammatory response as a result of unmyelinated nerve stimulation. It is sometimes referred to as the axon reflex, and causes the familiar weal and flare response in skin. It is thought that peptides such as substance P, neurokinin A and somatostatin are synthesised in the dorsal root ganglion and transported to the peripheral tissues via unmyelinated nerves. Experimentally induced arthritis has been found to increase levels of these peptides. Substance P causes vasodilatation and plasma extravasation, and possibly also activates the immune system. Also during inflammation nerve growth factor concentration rises and may be responsible for development of long-term changes in the spinal cord.

CLINICAL RELEVANCE

Pain in rheumatological conditions tends to be variable and unpredictable. Symptoms may occur independently of the underlying condition, sometimes in the absence of demonstrable clinical pathology. Conversely, obviously damaged joints may be pain-free (Kidd *et al.*, 1996). The patient's description of his or her pain may be useful in differential diagnosis; for instance, RA pain is usually steady and aching. If the patient describes it as agonising, terrifying or excruciating, it may be due to sepsis, nerve entrapment or non-organic causes. This however needs to be viewed in the light of the patient's ethnic background or desire to be believed out of frustration (Russell & Piercy, 1993).

Pain in osteoarthritis (OA) may arise from subchondral bone, synovium, capsule, ligaments, entheses, marginal bone and periosteum, most probably due to mechanical stimuli. Periarticular tender spots may be bursitis or enthesopathy due to an unstable joint (McCarthy *et al.*, 1994). Nocturnal pain may be neurogenic, vascular, infectious, crystalline or from severe structural damage, tendinitis or bursitis. Synovitis without structural damage rarely wakes the patient (Liang & Sturrock, 1994).

Sensitisation of mechanoreceptors may explain use-related 'incident' pain which occurs on movement and is absent at rest. This type of pain can be difficult to treat, and the dose of analgesic needed to control the level of pain experienced on movement may have unacceptable levels of toxicity for pain free periods (Kidd, 1996, Kidd *et al.*, 1996).

The flare response is increased in chronic pain syndromes with tender muscle points. It is also increased over inflamed rheumatoid wrists compared with control points on the rest of the arm, and decreased in patients with spinal degenerative pain compared to patients with non-organic pain. This may indicate central sensitisation.

PSYCHOSOCIAL FACTORS

The body's perception of stimuli is part of an on-going learning process, and pain is no exception. Pain is perceived against a background of experience, positive or negative role models, knowledge, beliefs and culture (Gifford, 1998). The physiology of pain is inextricably linked with psychological and socio-economic issues that affect pain perception and coping mechanisms. Pain will affect people in different ways depending on such factors as the influence of family and peers, social and employment situations, education and the likelihood of the pathology being chronic or short-term.

CONTROL

Most of us enjoy control over various aspects of our life; the concept of Locus of Control and self-efficacy is well researched and may be affected by the chronicity of many rheumatological conditions. This may alter the perception of pain and its relief. Control over pain through patient controlled analgesia (PCA) is increasing for various conditions, and many therapeutic interventions also offer patient control through buttons to stop equipment or by the therapist offering to stop a procedure if it is too uncomfortable. PCA abuse and the continuous use of panic buttons are negligible with good patient–therapist relationships; it is interesting to note that perceived control is frequently as effective as actual control. Roche & Klestov (1995) suggest that the most positive therapeutic interventions in RA include increasing the patient's perception of self control.

SOCIAL SUPPORT

Social support is seen as one of the coping mechanism for pain control. It can be positive or negative; pain behaviour may be unwittingly reinforced by the patient's carer, through their own actions and behaviour. It can be lacking in the disabled and elderly, where although pain complaint may be reduced, it is thought they maybe suffer more—the mechanism of this may be related to physiology and/or psychology (Gibson *et al.*, 1994). This is worth bearing in mind as many rheumatology conditions are related to the older population, and this may influence both assessment and treatment. Social relationships may change; patients may become isolated and unable to talk about their pain as others are tired of listening. Coping with the pain experience becomes an added demand to daily life, sometimes resulting in depression and anger. These trends can be reversed when the pain is relieved, but repeated failed attempts to decrease the pain compound the problems (Large, 1996).

COGNITIVE AND AFFECTIVE ASPECTS

Cognition of pain is important as a survival method in relation to the searching for a memory of pain, to know whether or not it is life threatening, how to deal with it etc. It is also important in terms of communication. Young children often lack the language to describe their pain and may have no frame of reference for it in terms of its severity or type. However, adults frequently describe pain in a way in which they are unlikely to have experienced it—for instance, 'it is like red hot needles burrowing'.

Painful sensations may indicate further damage or pathology, and this in itself can lead to anxiety. A consequence of this is that the patient avoids movement fearing it may aggravate the pain. If this continues it leads to deconditioning which in itself may become a cause of pain, loss of confidence and increase in disability. Roche & Klestov (1995) maintain that activity should be encouraged during the non-inflammatory phase of disease to demonstrate that pain does not equate with damage. These authors also identify that pain is often inconsistent with disease severity and that there may be some difficulty in introducing a psychologically based programme while reassuring the patient of the real physical factors contributing to pain.

The relationship between the cognitive component, emotional component and physical aspects of pain cannot be easily divided: patients who are highly anxious may complain of more intense pain which is not easily alleviated. Cognitive behavioural approaches may be particularly applicable to patients with chronic pain and therapists may be involved in group or individual programmes that aim to help patients re-evaluate their pain and what it means to them.

PATIENT EDUCATION

Patient education is a cornerstone of therapy intervention and enables patients to be an active participant in their management. Part of this approach is through the knowledge given to the patient. This knowledge should not be jargonised and should be delivered at the appropriate time. Knowledge works within the cognitive dimension of pain and may well influence the downward moderation of pain through the peri-aqueductal grey area. While knowledge

itself can be a coping mechanism, other coping mechanisms are often needed such as breathing exercises or simply knowing that pain relief will be offered to them regularly after a procedure. Education needs to include explanation of the purpose of drugs; patients may be on drug regimes that include anti-depressants used for their pain relieving properties and not their psychotropic effects. It should not be assumed that they are depressed.

DISEASE-RELATED ISSUES

The psychological effects of pain may vary with the patient's condition and whether it is perceived as long-term or of short duration and how it will impinge on the various aspects of the individual life. Ahern *et al.* (1995) found that patients with RA are more preoccupied with their illness and its effects, and more worried about their general health, than patients with OA. They admit more readily to other problems in their lives, and perceive psychological factors to play a more important role than OA patients. However, they are not more depressed, do not feel more vulnerable, have no more angry feelings and interpersonal frictions, and have no more difficulty expressing personal feelings than OA patients. One of the important roles for the clinician is to enhance coping mechanisms, and their efficacy, utilised by a patient group (Keefe *et al.*, 1997).

DISABILITY-RELATED ISSUES

Disability related to pain is a complex entity to assess, influenced not just by the severity, location, frequency etc. of that pain but by the same variables that were mentioned at the beginning of this section, such as finance, experience, education, personal value systems and ethnocultural background. The level of disability however does not always equate with severity of the pain experienced, but rather with the persistence of pain (Bennett, 1996). It has also been suggested that the medical profession may unwittingly contribute to disability by 'medicalising' pain syndromes such as fibromyalgia (Bennett, 1996). Predicting impairment and disability for patients with chronic pathologies such as RA and low back pain has enormous economic implications (Brena *et al.*, 1979) and research is often commissioned to this end. However, the relationship between physical and psychosocial variables needs careful exploration (Flor & Turk, 1988).

ORGANIC FACTORS

Psychophysiological processes may have a role in the cause of pain; muscle tension is a widely cited example, and contributes to the development of trigger points, but the theory that prolonged postural tension leads to ischaemic pain has not been conclusively established (Large, 1996). Pain in muscle tension may be due to excessive bracing and agonist/antagonist activity. The emotional responses of fear and stress, which many patients experience as well as pain, may also contribute to the psychophysiological relationship between pain and its perception and expression.

MacFarlane *et al.* (1996) identified several risk factors for persistent pain. They found that pain was more prevalent in females with low educational achievement; there was also a strong association with sleep disturbance, fatigue and problems with micturition, abdominal pain or headaches. These patients also tended towards a high score on the General Health Questionnaire and a high fatigue score on the Health and Fatigue questionnaire. Care must be taken when looking at pain in relation to gender as some of the pain responses may be due to social conditioning and may disappear with education.

THE PLACEBO RESPONSE

Just as the definition of pain is complex and varied, so this is the case for the terms placebo and placebo effect. Shapiro & Morris (1978) define it as 'any therapy or component of therapy that is used for its non specific psychological or psychophysiological effect, or for its presumed specific effect, but is without specific activity for the condition being treated'. This definition, although commonly cited, is frequently challenged by others. However, it is a powerful concept that is frequently underestimated and underutilised by clinicians. Placebos are often given in medical drug trials, but it is not necessary to give a placebo in order to elicit a placebo effect. This can be seen in the many interactions therapists have with patients—the interaction itself may exert a strong placebo effect. Turner *et al.* (1994) reviewed the literature relating to pain and placebo and concluded that placebo effects and the natural history of the pathology contribute to good management outcomes, and care must be taken not to attribute everything to specific treatment effects. Placebo has been shown to produce positive results in pathologies ranging from asthma to diabetes, ulcers, low back pain and the common cold, and the chronicity of signs and symptoms does not necessarily influence the response. The response rate is frequently reported to be around 35% but can be as high as 70%. The possibility that specific personality types are placebo responders is unsupported; patients who have a clinical need may be high responders, but what seems more relevant is patient expectation, including the use of expensive equipment or experiencing a degree of discomfort to relieve pain. Other important factors are related to the therapist's characteristics (Richardson, 1994) such as empathy, friendliness and positiveness about the intervention, and for some patients the status of the therapist is pertinent. Patients who have had a previous positive health interaction are also likely to be more positive. Therefore effective therapeutic intervention is more than just being technically proficient and therapists, whether acting as individuals or as part of a multidisciplinary team (MDT), have the potential to enhance the placebo effect.

The placebo effect should therefore be seen as a beneficial adjunct to intervention. It cannot and must not be used to differentiate between organic and inorganic pain.

Understanding psychological and physical factors in pain is important and will influence the choice of interventions that are available to therapists. Figure 4.2 summarises some of the interventions and where they may be acting in the modulation of pain. Above all, the therapist

needs to acknowledge and believe the patient's report of pain and be aware of its impact on both the patient's and carer's lives (Large, 1996). Many patients do not expect the pain to be cured and often the knowledge that their pain is accepted as real can have a powerful placebo effect on the individual. Health professionals have been known to focus on the physical aspects of rheumatic conditions and underestimate depression and anxiety in their patients. This is not fulfilling patients' needs (Ahern *et al.*, 1995).

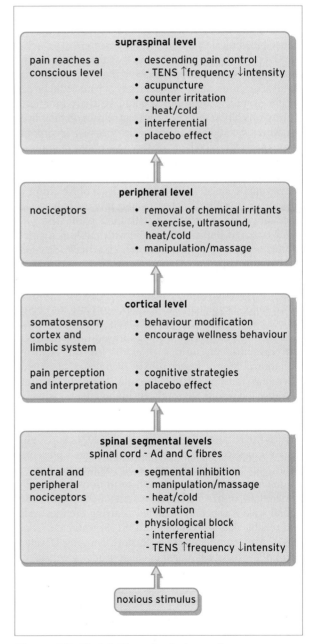

Figure 4.2 Modulation of pain by various interventions.

MEASUREMENT

The complexity of pain as defined at the beginning of this chapter means that its measurement is far from straightforward. Various components such as intensity can be measured in isolation, or a more composite measure may be utilised such as the McGill Pain Questionnaire (Melzack, 1975), which records data on some of the qualitative aspects of pain. Measurement tools can vary from a simple numerical rating scale (NRS), which has the ability to be generic in its application, to specific measures such as the foot function index (Saag *et al.*, 1996), or disease specific measures such as the body chart in ankylosing spondylitis (Dziedzic *et al.*, 1995). Table 4.2 summarises some of the better known pain measures that may be utilised in clinical situations, and in research.

Overall, what is important is that the aspect of pain measured is the most appropriate to monitor the patient's needs. For some patients the intensity of pain could be part of the overall picture, but it could be their functional activity which best reflects the impact of pain on their lives; for others it could be a psychosocial measure incorporating aspects of mood or anxiety. Assessment tools or methods that quantify pain and the result of therapeutic intervention are primarily utilised by therapists, but qualitative data collection methods, such as observation or interviews, may reveal richer insights into the pain experience and how patients cope with their pain. One such study is that by Borkan *et al.* (1995) which utilises a variety of methods to explore issues in low back pain. Studies such as this may help therapists understand the relationship between disability and pain. Measures that take account of physical, emotional and cognitive components may be much more useful than isolated measures and may better reflect the therapeutic approach taken. It is worth noting that pain measures may also be utilised in conjunction with disability measures such as the Juvenile Arthritis Functional Status Index (JASI) (Wright *et al.*, 1996). Therapists must be aware of the value of the tool in order to utilise the results appropriately in therapeutic activity.

Measures should be as reliable and valid as possible but they must also be easy to use as well as having some meaning for the patient (Sim & Waterfield, 1997). Apparently minor issues, such as the way in which a scale is presented to the patient, may be of considerable importance. A visual analogue scale, for example, can be presented vertically, horizontally, or in a curvilinear manner; however, the horizontal scale is generally regarded as giving the most valid and reliable data (Dixon & Bird, 1981, Sriwatanakul *et al.*, 1983). A thermometer scale (Burford Nursing Development, 1984) may be favoured by children and older patients, as it is presented in terms of an object familiar to most people and has verbal descriptors. Pain measurements may be linked in with patients' self assessment of their disease activity (Hanley *et al.*, 1996), giving the advantage of patients taking some control over their disease management; however, this type of self assessment raises other issues for consideration before adopting it.

Measures frequently used for pain research might not be feasible in a busy physiotherapy department or in the community. While measures useful for acute pain may have little value used with a chronic pain patient, physical manipulation of a self administered pain measurement tool is also important to consider in rheumatological patients (Waterfield & Sim, 1996).

Many other aspects of the patient's background, such as culture and the words used to describe pain, must also be considered when deciding on a measurement tool. Age may be a factor in the choice of measure, as already illustrated, and the assessment of pain in paediatric rheumatological conditions will call upon an understanding of both the pathology and the developmental stage of the patient. As already discussed, anxious patients may well express higher scores on pain measurement tools and their memory of previous pain episodes may be distorted (Roche & Gijsbers, 1986). In a study by Keefe & Williams (1989) patients with RA were poorer at recalling long periods of disease related pain compared to a single episode of experimental pain.

The timing of pain measurements may be particularly pertinent as pain may be related to either a diurnal or a nocturnal pattern depending on the pathology. In addition, if one is looking for the amount of relief a patient gains from an intervention such as a drug regime it is useful to know the parameters of the drug's life and the timing of the dose. Many patients with rheumatological conditions are assessed over a period of time and there is some debate as regards whether they should have access to their previous pain scores (Scott & Huskisson, 1979).

CONCLUSION

Pain is a complex problem for patients and therapists alike. Pain is induced and enhanced by inflammation as well as being moderated by various other physiological and psychosocial processes. It is necessary to address all these to improve patients' well-being. Pain management in the rheumatological patient is an extensive and complex topic, and impossible to cover in a chapter of this length. For information on the management of pain, please see texts such as Ellis (1994), Oosterveld (1994), Low & Reed (1994), Lehmann & Lateur (1994) or Walsh (1997). It is vital to remember that the patient is an integral part of his or her own pain management, and wherever possible it is the patient who should be in control.

ACKNOWLEDGEMENT

With thanks to Mrs C Fenelon for her contribution to the initial drafts for this chapter.

Summary of pain measurement instruments		
Instrument	**Description**	**Strengths and weaknesses**
Verbal rating scale	A hierarchical adjectival scale (usually four- or five-point) of pain intensity or pain affect	Easy to administer, complete and score, but with low responsiveness; poor content validity owing to its unidimensionality; data are ordinal
Visual analogue scale	A 10 cm continuous line anchored at each end with statements representing the extremes of the dimension being measured (most often pain intensity)	A high degree of reliability with certain client groups, but may pose challenges to others; poor content validity owing to its unidimensionality (though use of two or more visual analogue scales may counter this shortcoming); potentially highly responsive, and may produce interval/ratio level data
Box scale	An 11-point discrete scale of pain intensity, with extreme values labelled as for a visual analogue scale	Less responsive than the visual analogue scale, but easier for some patients to complete; data are ordinal
Numerical rating scale	A discrete visual analogue scale that is usually divided into 11 numbered scale points; labelled as for a visual analogue scale	Less responsive than the visual analogue scale, but easier for some patients to complete; data are ordinal
Behavioural rating scale	Pain intensity is expressed in terms of its self-reported impact on everyday function	Scores do not necessarily represent the impact of pain intensity alone, or indeed any component of the pain experience; scores are highly relevant to assessments of disability
McGill Pain Questionnaire (long form)	A composite measure which taps the sensory, affective, evaluative and other dimensions of pain, in both qualitative and quantitative terms; pain location is also recorded	A fair degree of reliability, if completion is supervised, and good content validity, but rather time-consuming to complete and complex to score; suitable for both chronic and acute pain, of various origins; can be administered either orally or in written form, and is available in a number of languages
McGill Pain Questionnaire (short form)	A shortened variant of the original McGill Questionnaire which covers the same areas, except for pain location	Easier and quicker to administer than the long form McGill, but the choice of descriptors is more restricted; suitable for both chronic and acute pain, of various origins; available in a number of languages
Pain diary	A self-completion instrument which can tap a number of dimensions of pain over time	A high degree of content validity, but may present problems in terms of reliability and compliance; careful instruction is required
Pain perception profile	A sophisticated form of pain diary which gathers quantitative ratings of the intensity, unpleasantness and nature of pain, by means of a total of 37 verbal descriptors	A sophisticated and somewhat complex instrument, not suitable for self-completion and requiring a degree of training in its use; probably too complex for routine clinical use
Descriptor differential scale	Consists of twelve 10-point bipolar scales representing pain intensity or pain affect	A high degree of internal consistency reliability; rather complex to administer, and thus most suited to specialist situations
Pain drawing	This usually takes the form of a body chart, on which the location of pain can be marked	Possesses a high degree of validity and reliability; allows the distribution of pain to be quantified where appropriate

Table 4.2 **Summary of pain measurement instruments.**

REFERENCES

Ahern MJ, McFarlane AC, Leslie A *et al*. Illness behaviour in patients with arthritis. *Ann Rheum Dis* 1995, **54**:245-250.

Bennett R. Fibromyalgia and the disability dilemma. A new era in understanding a complex multidimensional pain syndrome. *Arthritis Rheum* 1996, **39**:1627-1634.

Borkan J, Reis S, Hermoni D *et al*. Talking about the pain: A patient-centred study of low back pain in primary care. *Soc Sci Med* 1995, **40**:977-988.

Brena SF, Chapman SL, Stegall PG *et al*. Chronic Pain States: their relationship to impairment and disability. *Arch Phys Med Rehabil* 1979, **60**:387-389.

Burford Nursing Development: Nurses and pain. *Nurs Times* 1984, **18**:94.

Dixon JS, Bird HA. Reproducibility along a 10cm vertical visual analogue scale. *Ann Rheum Dis* 1981, **40**:87-89.

Dziedzic K, Hay EM, Jackson SE *et al*. *An assessment of the body chart in ankylosing spondylitis*. Proceedings of the 12th International Congress of the World Confederation for Physical Therapy. Washington DC, USA; 1995.

Flor H, Turk D. Chronic back pain and rheumatoid arthritis: Predicting Pain and Disability from cognitive variables. *J Behav Med* 1988, **11**:251-265.

Gibson SJ, Katz B, Corran TM, Farrell MJ. Chronic and acute pain syndromes in pateints with multiple sclerosis. *Acta Neurol* 1994, **16**:97-102.

Gifford L. Pain, the tissues and the nervous system: a conceptual model. *Physiotherapy* 1998, **84**:27-36.

Hanley JG, Mosher D, Sutton E *et al*. Self Assessment of disease activity by patients with rheumatoid arthritis. *J Rheumatol* 1996, **23**:1531-1538.

International Association for the Study of Pain: Pain terms: A list with definitions and notes on usage. *Pain* 1979, **6**: 249.

Johnson MI. The physiology of the sensory dimensions of chronic pain. *Physiotherapy* 1997, **83(10)**:526-535.

Jones AKP, Derbyshire SWG. Cerebral mechanisms operating in the presence and absence of inflammatory pain. *Ann Rheum Dis* 1996, **55**:411-420.

Keefe FJ, Affleck G, Lefebvre JC *et al*. Pain Coping strategies and daily coping efficacy in rheumatoid arthritis: a daily analysis. *Pain* 1997, **69(1-2):**35-42.

Keefe FJ, Williams DA. New directions in pain assessment and treatment. *Clin Psychol Rev* 1989, **9**:549-568.

Kidd BL, Morris VH, Urban L. Pathophysiology of joint pain. *Ann Rheum Dis* 1996, **55**:276-283.

Kidd BL. Problems with pain - is the messenger to blame? *Ann Rheum Dis* 1996, **55**: 275.

Large RG. Psychological aspects of pain. *Ann Rheum Dis* 1996, **55**:340-345.

Liang M, Sturrock RD. Evaluation of musculoskeletal symptoms. In: Klippel JH, Dieppe P, eds. *Rheumatology*. London: Mosby Year Book Europe; 1994, 2:1.

MacFarlane GJ, Thomas E, Papageorgiou AC *et al*. The natural history of pain in the community: a better prognosis than in the clinic? *J Rheumatol* 1996, **23**:1617-1620.

McCarthy C, Cushnaghan J, Dieppe P. Osteoarthritis. In: Wall PD, Melzack R, eds. *Textbook of Pain, 3rd edition*. Edinburgh: Churchill Livingstone; 1994:387-396.

Melzack R. The McGill Pain Questionnaire: Major properties and scoring methods. *Pain* 1975, **1**:277-299.

Melzack R, Wall P. *The Challenge of Pain, 3rd edition*. London: Penguin; 1991.

Melzack R, Wall PD. Pain mechanisms - a new theory. *Science* 1965, **150**:971.

Richardson PH. Placebo effects in pain management. *Pain Rev* 1994, **1**:15-32.

Roche PA, Gijsbers K. A comparison of memory for induced ischaemic pain and chronic rheumatoid pain. *Pain* 1986, **25**:337-343.

Roche PA, Klestov AC. Anxiety, depression and the sense of helplessness: their relationship to pain from rheumatoid arthritis. In: Shacklock MO, ed. *Moving in on pain*. Australia: Butterworth-Heinemann; 1995, 90-96.

Russell AS, Piercy JS. Assessment and management of the adult patient. In: Maddison PJ, Isenberg DA, Woo P, Glass DN, eds. *Oxford Textbook of rheumatology*. Oxford: Oxford Medical Publications; 1993: 3-8.

Saag KG, Saltzman CL, Brown CK *et al*. The foot function index for measuring rheumatoid arthritis pain: evaluating side to side reliability. *Foot Ankle Int* 1996, **17**:506-510.

Scott J, Huskisson EC. Accuracy of subjective measurements made with or without previous scores: an important source of error in serial measurement of subjective states. *Ann Rheum Dis* 1979, **38**:558-559.

Shapiro AK, Morris LA. The placebo effect in medical and psychological therapies In: Bergin AE, Garfield S, eds. *Handbook of psychotherapy and behavioural change, 2nd edition*. Chichester: John Wiley; 1978:369-410.

Sim J, Waterfield J. Validity, reliability and responsiveness in the assessment of pain. *Physiother Theory Pract* 1997, **13**: 23-37.

Sriwatanakul K, Kelvie W, Lasagna L *et al*. Studies with different types of visual analog scales for measurement of pain. *Clin Pharmacol Ther* 1983, **34**:234-239.

Turner JA, Deyo RA, Loeser JD *et al*. The importance of placebo effects in pain treatment and research. *JAMA* 1994, **271**:1609-1614.

Walsh D. Nociceptive pathways - relevance to the physiotherapist. *Physiotherapy* 1991, **77**:317-321.

Waterfield J, Sim J. Clinical assessment of pain by the visual analogue scale. *Br J Ther Rehabil* 1996, **3**:94-97.

Wright FV, Kimber JL, Law M. The Juvenile Arthritis Functional Status Index (JASI) A validation study. *J Rheumatol* 1996, **23**:1066-1079.

GENERAL READING

Adams N. *The psychophysiology of low back pain*. Edinburgh: Churchill Livingstone; 1997.

Ellis N. *Acupuncture in clinical practice: a guide for health professionals*. London: Chapman & Hall; 1994.

Gerber LH. Non pharmacological modalities in the treatment of rheumatic diseases. In: Klippel JH, Dieppe P, eds. *Rheumatology*. London: Mosby Year Book Europe; 1994: 8:4.

Lehmann JF, Lateur JF. Ultrasound, shortwave, microwave, laser, superficial heat and cold in the treatment of pain. In: Wall PD, Melzack R, eds. *Textbook of pain, 3rd edition*. Edinburgh: Churchill Livingstone; 1994:1237-1249.

Low J, Reed A. *Electrotherapy explained - principles and practice*. Oxford: Butterworth-Heinemann; 1994.

Oosterveld FGJ. *Heat and cold treatment in rheumatic diseases*. Cip-Gegevens Koninklijke Bibliotheek, Den Haag; 1994.

Walsh D. *TENS: clinical applications and related theory*. Edinburgh: Churchill Livingstone; 1997.

5

D Pratt

BIOMECHANICS AND GAIT IN RHEUMATOLOGY

CHAPTER OUTLINE

- Methods of studying gait
- Gait changes due to chronic arthritis
- Biomechanical examination
- The use of walking aids
- Orthotic gait

INTRODUCTION

This section deals with a description of ideal gait motions and the effects of some rheumatological conditions, their treatment, and walking aids. A knowledge of the ideal motions is valuable when considering the effects of treatments or the likely effects of a specific intervention. This is because gait is amongst the most highly automated movements in the body and displays considerable synergy between central and peripheral nervous system processes. The specific motions taking place within the gait cycle are determined by the body's need to absorb shock loading (Pratt, 1989), adapt to surface irregularities and move the body forward. Saunders *et al.* (1953) refer to locomotion as 'the translation of the centre of mass through space along a path requiring the least expenditure of energy'.

In describing gait it is usual to examine one of the repetitive gait cycles and consider this to be representative of the act of walking (Figure 5.1); one cycle is defined as the period between successive ipsilateral heel strikes (HS). This cycle is formed from two phases, stance taking about 60% of the total time and swing taking the remaining 40%. Within these phases there are events which are used to identify sections of the cycle. These have been defined as HS, foot flat (FFL), midstance (MSt), heel lift (HL), toe off (TO) and midswing (MSw). However, if the gait pattern is not ideal then these specific events may not occur and many now prefer less specific terms, such as initial contact, loading response, midstance, terminal stance, pre-swing, initial swing, midswing and terminal swing (Perry, 1985). From these basic events it is possible to identify timings of, for example, double support intervals (when both feet are in contact with the ground) or swing times. In addition it enables distance factors such as stride length (the distance between successive ipsilateral heel strikes) and step length (the distance between successive contralateral heel strikes) to be calculated.

Motions of the joints and the body are also characteristic of a person's walking, and well defined patterns are evident (McHugh, 1993). The accuracy with which these data can be recorded has increased with the advent of modern technology and this will be outlined later on. In addition, the body exerts a varying force between the foot and the ground. Clearly, if a person is not to fall through the floor it will have to apply a force exactly equal in magnitude and in the opposite direction to that between the foot and the ground, this being called the ground reaction force.

Muscles are used to control the limbs during walking and as such the study of electromyographic (EMG) patterns is also used to assess gait. However, as muscles contract and the body moves, energy is both consumed and generated. Techniques to measure these aspects of gait have been developed and these will be outlined later in the chapter.

METHODS OF STUDYING GAIT

The topic of gait analysis is huge and only a brief overview can be presented here. For more in-depth information on the topics of gait and gait analysis the interested reader is directed to Smidt (1990), Oberg *et al.* (1994) and Whittle (1996).

OBSERVATION

This is the simplest form of gait analysis, and often the only form readily available. It has drawbacks as it relies on our imperfect memory for historical comparisons and assessment, and it is not possible to carry out any meaningful measurements. Simple observation can be significantly enhanced by the use of a video camera and recording facility. Despite this assistance even the most experienced observer will still have difficulties in differentiating the numerous details of a person's gait, and quantitative data are still not available. In addition, no details of forces, pressures or EMG activity are available. With these major disadvantages in mind, many techniques have been developed to provide objective quantitative data on gait. It is best to deal briefly with each of these in relation to the main components of gait as mentioned above.

TIME AND DISTANCE MEASUREMENTS

Foot switches are a common way to record these parameters, these switches being either inserted into the shoe or attached to the outside and usually connected to a belt-worn recording device. They are typically used to record when the heel and the toe part of the shoe are in contact with the ground. Timing circuitry may also be included in the system so that not only the sequence of contact can be recorded but also the timing. Portability is a great advantage here as subjects can walk, run, climb stairs etc. and have their performance recorded. Poor mechanical reliability of the switches has prevented this simple technique from becoming more popular—however, newer foot switch designs are available which are more reliable, more complicated and more expensive. Instrumented walkways or mats have also been developed to record these parameters. These systems are usually fixed flush to the ground which may limit the activities studied but are very quick and reliable. They are, however, able to record not only timings but distance parameters, which in-shoe systems are unable to do. The accuracy of the distance measurements is usually low as this is limited by the spacing of the transducers in the mats. If the spacing is large the measurements are less accurate but the system will be quicker and cheaper—a balance has to be found.

KINEMATIC MEASUREMENTS

These relate to the quantification of the motion of the body and its limbs and this study is often termed motion analysis. Historically this was carried out by photography, either using cine film or by stroboscopic exposures on a single plate. However, the time taken to collect manually

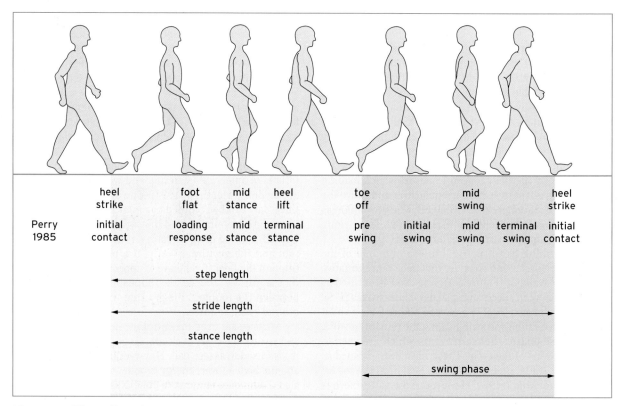

Figure 5.1 **The gait cycle.**

all the data from the pictures was very long and this limited the techniques from regular use. The advent of high quality video cameras meant that data collection and analysis was easier but most of these systems can still only be relied upon to give qualitative information as they are too inaccurate for reliable quantitative use. This is because they produce only a two-dimensional image of a three-dimensional activity, and rotations out of the plane of the camera give false angular values. They do, however, have a valuable role in providing temporal aspects of gait (Wall & Crosbie, 1997) and a quick method of recording motion and offering historical comparisons to aid in assessment of the progress of a treatment or intervention.

Many systems have been developed to record accurate three-dimensional positions of markers attached to people walking. They use a variety of techniques such as reflection of light from the markers (infra-red and visible), emission of light by the markers (infra-red and visible), changes in polarisation of light due to marker motion, ultrasound emitted by markers and motion of accelerometers and magnetometers attached to the body (Granat *et al.*, 1995, Carrera *et al.*, 1996, Dickstein *et al.*, 1996). These systems tend to be used for selected assessment of patients as they all take considerable time to set-up the markers or sensors and collect representative data. Once collected, they have to be interpreted and conclusions drawn which also takes time. This is why many of the initial systems were reserved for research.

All of these systems have their advantages and disadvantages and now the most reliable and accurate clinical systems employ three-dimensional arrays of high quality video cameras and computers with sophisticated software. This means that vast amounts of data can be collected and analysed more quickly. However, they are still very time consuming processes and not usually amenable for regular use in the clinic but reserved for specific patients with, perhaps, a complicated problem needing a higher level of assessment to determine viable treatment.

Examples of current sophisticated motion analysis systems which represent the best of the current techniques are the Elite™ system (BTS srl, Milan, Italy) and the Vicon™ system (Oxford Metrics, Oxford, England). Here, body mounted retro-reflective markers are used to record limb positions by reflecting strobed infra-red light back to special television cameras (Figure 5.2). The strobing is at between 50 and 200 Hz and has the effect of 'freezing' the image of the moving marker. The computer can identify the markers in real time and work out from several camera views the actual position of the marker within the required three-dimensional space to a high level of accuracy (the absolute accuracy is limited by skin movement causing markers to move, although newer software and marker arrays can eliminate some of these) (Ehara *et al.*, 1995). These marker positions are used, together with patient-specific anthropometric data, to calculate joint centres. The results from these newer systems are better than the photographic techniques.

The use of electro-goniometers attached to the person being studied has been used in the past. For a full three-dimensional assessment these are bulky items which can affect the very motion being studied and the alignment of the transducers with anatomical joint axes is difficult (Pratt, 1991). Cheaper systems using just one or two axes of measurement are of value and may, in selected joints with primarily single plane motion (such as the knee), be sufficient for some useful interpretation of the effects of therapy or surgery (Ball & Johnson, 1993). However, they still need careful alignment with the joint and are not always as reliable and repeatable as would be liked.

KINETIC MEASUREMENTS

These studies are concerned with the causes of motion such as ground reaction forces, joint and muscle forces and kinetic and potential energies of the body and its segments and also include the study of under-foot pressure patterns.

Ideal walking produces a characteristic pattern of forces between the foot and the floor, acting about three axes which are at 90^0 to each other. Devices called force plates, which are sunk flush with the floor, record these forces, measured in percentages of body weight for comparison between individuals. These force plates are very accurate but have the disadvantage that they can produce gait deviations when the person attempts to hit the plate as requested. That is why several manufacturers and

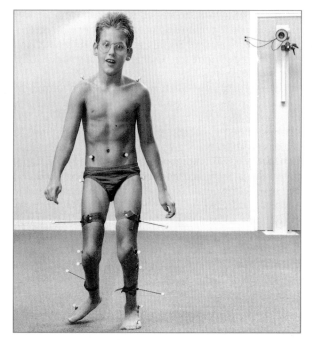

Figure 5.2 Markers used in kinematic measurement of gait. Photograph of a typical array of markers used in the kinematic assessment of gait. This system uses 20 markers located on the legs and trunk to provide three-dimensional marker positions which are then used to calculate actual joint positions with the aid of specific anthropometric patient data.

researchers have developed in-shoe devices which currently record only vertical forces (Lord & Hosein, 1994), but newer multicomponent devices are being developed (Warren-Forward *et al.*, 1992). They have the advantage that they are part of the patient's footwear but generally their accuracy and reliability is less than the fixed plates.

A useful addition to gait analysis is the video vector generator. This device enables the ground reaction force vector to be superimposed on the positional information of the body and is used to help in assessing the benefits of orthotic intervention or results of therapy (Butler *et al.*, 1992). It does this by showing the external moments on the joints caused by the distance between the force vector and the joint; as this increases, the flexion or extension effect of the force also increases. In normal gait the external moments acting on the leg pass very close to joint centres thus minimising the internal moments that muscles have to exert to counterbalance the effects of the external moments. A qualitative assessment of the effects of orthoses, therapy or surgery can be visualised and corrective measures taken. Even a first-order quantification of the effects of the external moments can be made by measuring the perpendicular distance from the joint centre to the line of the force vector and multiplying it by the value of the force (moment = force × perpendicular distance between the line of action of the force and the centre of rotation). However, this value must be treated with caution as it will not take account of the out-of-plane angle of the force vector (Figure 5.3).

As walking is carried out with minimum energy expenditure this requires an energy conservation mechanism to be operative. By this process both kinetic and potential energies are interchanged between various segments of the body.

Energy consumption can be measured either by monitoring oxygen consumption (Waters & Yakura, 1990) or by using the force plate (Kodadadeh, 1993). There are clear patterns of energy consumption which show an increase with increasing walking speed and age. In addition, pathological conditions also affect energy consumption and total body mechanical energy is a good indication of the efficiency of walking. A parameter known as the Physiological Cost Index (PCI) is also used to monitor energy consumption (MacGregor, 1978). The disadvantage of this system is that it is less sensitive to the differences between individuals than the other techniques. It is calculated as:

PCI = [heart rate (walking) – heart rate (resting)] / speed

Heart rate is measured in beats per minute (or second) and speed in metres per minute (or second) and has found favour as an indicator of physical handicap (Butler *et al.*, 1984).

EMG patterns produced during gait are also repeatable and may be used to diagnose problems. Generally, surface mounted electrodes are used which is quicker and less painful for the patient but produces less specific outputs than needle electrodes. The work by Inman *et al.* (1981) provides a good description of the general muscle functions with differentiation between concentric and eccentric actions. There are many ways to process the raw data such as on/off patterns or by analysing the data mathematically and producing outlines or patterns reflecting the muscle activity (Shiavi & Green, 1983). Most often the on/off patterns are used simply to indicate whether a muscle is acting or not. It is perhaps not surprising that population variability is high with distal muscles being the most consistent and two-joint muscles exhibiting the greatest variability. Walking speed and conditions also affect the signals and because of this specifics of EMG patterns are not included here.

The specific study of pressure distribution between the foot and the floor has been used to quantify gait and assess the effects of treatments, particularly in the diabetic foot (Duckworth *et al.*, 1985). Systems to study this are either worn inside the shoe, like the EMED F system (Hughes *et al.*, 1991, Cavanagh *et al.*, 1992) or are based on a mat with sensing elements in a matrix which is placed on the floor, such as the Musgrave Footprint (Preston Communications, Llangollen, Wales) (Bennett & Duplock, 1993). The sensors used vary but they all

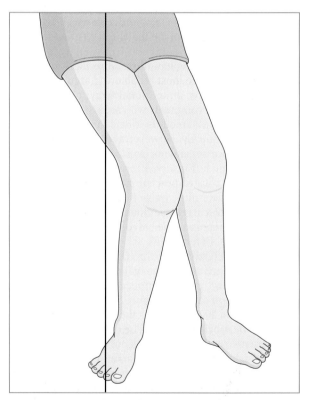

Figure 5.3 Force vector in valgus knee. A force vector superimposed on an image of someone walking with a valgus knee deformity. This clearly shows the position of the force lateral to the joint which produces an external valgus moment tending to reinforce the deformity.

produce a pressure distribution map of the foot. The devices worn in the shoe tend to be less accurate, more prone to distortion artifacts but better represent the actual conditions imposed on a foot. The mat-based systems are more accurate, less prone to artifacts but require patients to walk barefooted across the mat. As they usually walk in shoes, this technique may not actually provide the clinician with the most appropriate information.

As always in the field of medicine, a choice has to be made as to what the clinician requires and what accuracy is relevant before selecting an investigative procedure, and gait analysis is no exception.

GAIT CHANGES DUE TO CHRONIC ARTHRITIS

As a large percentage of the people with rheumatoid disease are elderly, many of the gait changes seen may be those associated with increasing age as well as those due to the condition itself. Older, healthy people tend to walk slower with a decreased stride length and increased cadence (Cunningham *et al.*, 1982). There is also reduced joint motion in the sagittal plane in hips, knees and ankles during walking in the elderly together with less vertical displacement of the head and reduced transverse rotation of the pelvis.

Differences in the kinetics of gait are less noticeable. Larish *et al.* (1988) found that the differences in the vertical ground reaction force were in the range 1.0 to 3.0% of body weight and a difference of between 0.1 and 0.4% of body weight in the fore-aft ground reaction force. They also found that there were no significant differences between the young and elderly in relation to energy consumption when normalised for body weight and distance walked.

THE HIP

There has been more research into the arthritic hip than any other joint in the body, notably the work of Bombelli (1983). His analyses show that the osteoarthritic hip is most likely to have a dislocating shear force producing extra stresses on the superolateral aspect of the joint capsule, due to the alignment of the femur and pelvis. This work also shows how the shift of the centre of gravity of the person can lead to reductions in these shearing forces and thus reduce pain. This is true whether the osteoarthritis (OA) is produced by mechanical, metabolic or combined processes.

An antalgic gait, often seen in chronic arthritis, is characterised by excessive lateral displacement of the head and upper trunk towards the involved weightbearing side. It is a self-protective gait used to minimise the discomfort in the hip, knee, ankle or foot. The stance phase on the affected side is shorter than that on the unaffected side as the patient attempts to remove weight from the affected side as quickly as possible. In addition, the painful region is often supported by one hand, if it is within reach, whereas the other arm is outstretched as a counterbalance. The shift of the body over the painful hip results in a decrease in the activity of the abductors and a consequent

reduction in joint loading. This action is thought to reduce the load on the femoral head from twice body weight to approximately body weight as the load is now more vertical over the joint. A limping individual such as this has a greater transfer of kinetic and potential energy on the involved limb and thus has to work harder to walk.

The gait deviations from ideal can be summarised as follows. Patients of any age with OA and rheumatoid arthritis (RA) of the hip tend to walk slower and tend to spend a disproportionate amount of time in single limb stance. Angular hip motion is reduced particularly in the sagittal plane (Figure 5.4), and the ground reaction forces in all three orthogonal directions are reduced on the affected side. James *et al.* (1994), in a study of monoarticular hip arthritis, found that asymmetries in loading and unloading rate were the most sensitive indicators of gait dysfunctions. They also noted a plateau in the vertical ground reaction force thought to indicate that the patients were attempting to reduce hip joint force and thus reduce pain.

Murray *et al.* (1971) summarised the gait abnormalities as irregularity and asymmetry, comparing sound and affected limb, in duration of the weight bearing periods, step length, vertical and forward motion of the head, lateral displacement of the head, trunk, upper limbs or some combination of the three and sagittal plane motion of the

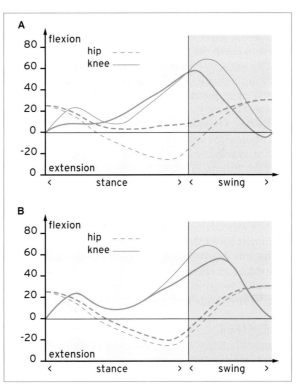

Figure 5.4 Hip and knee joint motions in both limbs in men with unilateral hip pain normalised for the differences between the swing and stance times. The light lines indicate the normal traces and the dark lines indicate the study data. Adapted from *Murray et al.*, 1971.

shoulders and elbows. In addition, the following parameters were significantly reduced compared to ideal:
- Walking speed.
- Step length.
- Cadence.
- Maximum extension of both hips and ankles during late stance.
- Maximum flexion of both knees during swing.
- Shoulder flexion during the forward part of arm swing.
- Elbow extension during the backward part of arm swing.

An increase in some parameters was noted:
- Lateral motion of the head.
- Anterior pelvic tilting.
- Transverse rotation of the pelvis.

Whilst some of the above deviations from the ideal can be attributed to pain, the alleviation of pain does not restore ideal walking patterns. Joint deformity, neural control deficits and multiple joint involvement can still cause some of the gait deviations to persist. The replacement of the affected hip(s) can however lead to significant improvements in gait. Nearly all of the measurable gait parameters improve either in symmetry or magnitude following hip arthroplasty but the resulting gait is still considerably short of ideal. Patients with RA tend to be more severely involved and so often improve proportionately more than those with OA. Despite this they do not usually reach the level of gait performance of the patients with OA.

The major gait improvements following hip replacement are increased angular hip motion, mainly in the sagittal plane, increased ground reaction forces, decreased displacement of the head and centre of gravity and less energy being required (Iida & Yamamuro, 1987). Walking endurance also increases.

For an ankylosed hip, the most 'normal' gait is obtained with the hip in 15^0 flexion, $3–5^0$ adduction and $5–10^0$ external rotation (Hauge, 1965). Studies claim that walking speed improves following this procedure to 80% of ideal with concomitant improvements in walking distance.

Non steroidal anti-inflammatory drugs (NSAIDs) are commonly used to improve comfort in rheumatoid disease. In the only study located, 16 patients were administered aspirin and its effects on pain and gait measured. As well as improved comfort their walking speed increased from 85 to 93 cm/s with lower heart rates (Steven et al., 1983).

THE KNEE
In general, patients with RA or OA of their knees walk slower, with increased asymmetry, less motion of the affected joint, with less forward and lateral smoothness during progression and the rates of limb loading and unloading are decreased. Andriacchi et al. (1977) found that there was typically a shorter step length, higher cadence, decreased swing and stance times and the medially directed ground reaction force was higher. In addition, Chao et al. (1980) found decreased joint motion

in three planes during stance and three aspects of the ground reaction force were changed (magnitude of the first peak, and locations of the trough and second peak). Murray et al. (1985) studied men with unilateral knee disability compared to normal and found that walking speed was lower, cadence had decreased, stride length had decreased and stride width had increased.

As with the hip, joint replacement is the likely treatment for chronic arthritis of the knee and there are eventual improvements seen in walking performance following surgical intervention. However, as with the hip, patients with RA do not usually reach the same level of gait performance as those with OA.

The functional benefits of total knee replacement (TKR) seem to depend upon whether one or both knees are involved. In a study by Berman et al. (1987) three groups were identified:
- Unilateral TKR with no evidence of rheumatoid disease in the contralateral knee.
- Unilateral TKR with asymptomatic rheumatism in the contralateral knee.
- Bilateral TKR.

The gait of all three groups improved, with group 2 improving significantly less than the others. It was concluded that asymptomatic arthritis can impair gait. As arthritis of the knees usually results in a varus deformity in OA and a valgus deformity in RA, tibial plateau loads are significantly affected. Prodromos et al. (1985) showed that a high tibial osteotomy can improve the weight bearing pattern of the plateaux, but soft tissue effects have been found to be very significant in determining the long-term durability of TKRs (Wilton et al., 1994). These effects are associated with the tightness of tissues around the knee on the side which is under compression, i.e. the lateral side with a valgus knee. When the knee is placed in a corrected position during surgery these tissues should be released to restore the normal tensions and balance of forces in the knee. This is thought to improve durability not only from the improvements in the mechanics of the joint but also on the restoration of joint proprioception.

THE ANKLE (THE TALOCRURAL JOINT)
The usual surgical treatment for OA or RA of the ankle is arthrodesis. This is found to produce less compensation for lost motion and less stress on the knee if the foot is held at 90^0 to the tibia with between $0–5^0$ of rearfoot valgus and between $5–10^0$ of external rotation (Buck et al., 1987). In a long-term follow-up of 12 patients with ankle arthrodeses some small differences in stance phase times were noted (Mazur et al., 1979). They found that these small differences disappeared once the patients walked in shoes, which also increased their walking speed.

The results of total ankle joint replacement are disappointing (Demottaz et al., 1979) when compared with other lower limb joints. Very little is published about the effects on gait except to indicate that abnormal gait patterns are produced principally as a consequence of weak plantarflexors.

Ankle joint replacement did not seem to offer pain relief as 81% of their study group still had pain. The EMG patterns showed excessive muscle action, particularly in the triceps surae (of both legs), medial hamstrings and glutei. The patients had a wider base of gait than usual which was thought to be the cause of the force vector passing medially to the tibia, compared to along and parallel to it. They concluded that this operation was not successful and ankle fusion was the preferred option.

BIOMECHANICAL EXAMINATION

Examination of the lower limb requires a full assessment of the relationship between the various segments of the limb and the supporting surface. This section will deal with supine, prone, standing and dynamic evaluations. Examination should start with the establishment of any fixed deformities and other joint dysfunctions. The foot is particularly important as it responds to stresses caused by proximal functional problems, and conversely deficits of foot structure give rise to proximal effects. Assessment should follow the procedures laid down by Root *et al.* (1971), which are outlined below.

SUPINE EXAMINATION

In supine, the following can be assessed:

- Hallux range of motion, together with the range of first ray motion and the position of the first metatarsal head relative to the other metatarsal heads.
- Ankle dorsiflexion, both with the knee flexed and extended. Ensure that the subtalar joint is prevented from pronating.
- Forefoot motion about the longitudinal midtarsal joint axis whilst holding the rearfoot in neutral to determine what range of forefoot compensation is available.
- Tibial torsion and the range of internal and external femoral rotation. Note any findings such as the increased range of femoral rotation due to excess subtalar pronation, when the knee is flexed between 0 and 30° (Coplan, 1989).
- Muscle strength.

Ranges of motion at the knees and hips can now be assessed in the usual way and any leg length discrepancy noted. Note any pain during motion which may limit function and any other factors which might affect the person's ability to walk, such as previous surgery or trauma.

PRONE EXAMINATION

In prone, the forefoot to rearfoot relationship can be assessed. This is fundamental to the function of the foot and the whole leg. For the best results the calcaneus is bisected and a line drawn on the skin together with a bisector of the lower third of the calf. Using these marks the alignment of the rearfoot to the leg and the forefoot to the rearfoot can be assessed by measuring the angle between the two lines for the former and between the rearfoot bisector and the forefoot plane for the latter (Pratt, 1995). From such measurements it can be determined if the foot is functioning within normal limits or not (Root *et al.*, 1971).

STANDING EVALUATION

With the patient standing it is easy to see if the foot presents as 'normal' or not, i.e. to see if the longitudinal arch collapses or the calcaneus adopts a more valgus or varus position (Figure 5.5). The foot position can be compared in its relaxed or usual position (relaxed calcaneal stance) with the position it adopts with subtalar joint in neutral (neutral calcaneal stance). With experience, this observation will indicate how the foot is adapting to compensate for either its own mechanical abnormalities or for those imposed by proximal deficits, for example valgus or varus angulation at the knee. The many causes of foot compensation are detailed in Anthony (1991), Michaud (1993) and Pratt *et al.* (1993).

At this stage the effects of any leg length discrepancies found earlier can be checked. Not all differences in leg length will produce symptoms, but sometimes a small, apparently insignificant, difference in conjunction with other factors may produce symptoms. These are easily remedied by adding an appropriate shoe raise.

An additional test to carry out whilst standing is the equinus compensation test if limited ankle motion has been detected at an earlier stage. The patient is asked to stand with the subtalar joint in neutral and with the knees fully extended. The examiner places his or her fingers beneath the midtarsal joint and asks the patient to flex the knees: a true equinus secondary to a bony restriction or a soleus contracture will produce compensatory midtarsal motion as the knees flex. If the contracture is in the gastrocnemius then compensatory midtarsal motion will occur if the body is moved forward over the straightened leg.

DYNAMIC EVALUATION

After these assessments the next stage is to watch the patient walking and to add the examination findings to the walking observations. This will give a complete picture of any abnormal motions and their cause. It must be remembered that dynamic evaluation needs to take into account all three planes of motion to get the full picture. As assessment of gait in the clinic is difficult (for reasons already mentioned, and due to the speed with which some actions take place), a video camera is a very useful tool. This will

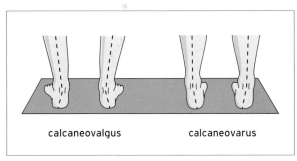

Figure 5.5 Biomechanical examination: standing evaluation.

enable the examiner not only to keep a record for future comparisons but to examine the walking patterns at leisure without requiring the patient to walk for a long time, something which may be painful and tiring.

To help with the assessment of step and stride lengths, simple grid markings on the floor will be useful. For the assessment of the kinematics of gait it is helpful to have a system or checklist so that a particular sequence is gone through each time and nothing is left out.

THE USE OF WALKING AIDS

Sticks are commonly used by the patient to reduce hip pain by reducing the load on the head of the femur. When a patient with one diseased hip walks he or she is told to use one stick on the opposite side. The effect on hip joint loading in such a situation can be described thus. The muscles around the hip which are controlling joint motion under the effects of body loading produce a force at the hip joint. If this load is too high the easiest way to reduce the joint loading in this situation is to provide external stabilisation via a cane or stick. If this cane is used on the opposite side to the affected hip it can provide support for the trunk which would usually come from the hip abductors. Thus, high stabilising hip abduction muscle forces are not required and the joint is loaded less. It is clear that the use of the stick on the diseased side would be less beneficial as it would provide a smaller lever arm over which to off-load the hip.

The patient may use two walking aids to off-load the hip totally by raising the leg off the ground. This is very difficult as it requires significant effort from the upper limbs and trunk but extra load can be taken by the second stick at a level lower than this maximum and still reduce the hip joint loading and give further pain relief.

One strange effect of the interdependence of muscle and joint forces is that somebody with unilateral OA of the hip may experience a reduction in joint pain when they carry a load on the diseased side! Mathematically, however, this is quite logical and is easy to explain. If the load is carried so as to produce a moment which acts in the same way as the hip abductors, this extra external force can reduce the requirements of the hip abductors to aid stabilisation of the joint. This would mean that the load would have to be carried on the affected side on the lateral side of the body at a distance greater than that between the hip joint and the hip abductors. The load would have to be small, as too large a load would itself overload the hip joint thus negating the reduction in muscle force.

ORTHOTIC GAIT

In many cases of RA in the ankle and subtalar joints, orthoses are used to reduce pain and allow a greater walking speed and distance and produce a more normal single limb support time. Orthoses for the foot and ankle specifically for RA are often rigid, inducing compensation for

	Orthotic causes of observeable gait deviations	
---	---	
Deviation	**Probable orthotic cause**
Lateral trunk bending	Excessive height of medial upright of knee ankle foot orthosis (KAFO); Excessive abduction of hip joint; Insufficient shoe raise (in leg length discrepancy)
Hip hiking/circumduction	Pes equinus uncompensated by contralateral shoe raise; Inadequate plantarflexion stop or dorsiflexion-assist spring; Hip or knee lock uncompensated for with contralateral shoe raise
Abnormal hip rotation	Transverse plane malalignment
Wide base of gait	Excessive height of medial upright of KAFO; Excessive abduction of the hip joint; Knee lock uncompensated with a contralateral shoe raise
Abnormal side foot contact	Transverse plane malalignment
Anterior trunk bending	Inadequate knee lock
Posterior trunk bending	Inadequate support from the brim of a weight-relieving KAFO
Hyperextended knee	Incorrect angle of the orthotic foot section relative to the leg; Pes equinus uncompensated for by a shoe raise
Knee instability	Inadequate knee lock; Inadequate dorsiflexion stop
Inadequate dorsiflexion control	Inadequate dorsiflexion-assist spring or plantar-flexion stop
Vaulting	Hip or knee lock uncompensated for with contralateral shoe raise; Inadequate plantarflexion stop or dorsiflexion-assist spring

Table 5.1 **Likely orthotic causes of some observable gait deviations.** Note that these deviations may also be observed in the absence of orthoses as compensation for muscle function deficit or pain. Adapted from Edelstein, 1988.

this elsewhere in the legs and trunk. One orthosis, the Cherwell splint, has resolved this by using a single, usually medially placed, ankle hinge (Merritt, 1987). Since this orthosis was developed many hinged orthoses are now available (Pratt, 1994). Orthoses affect gait even in an individual without a functional deficit, but this has to be balanced with the advantages such devices provide. Often the goal of orthotic management is not ideal gait but optimal performance within the user's limitations. The interested reader is directed to Bowker *et al.* (1993) for in-depth information on the biomechanics of orthoses and their effect on the function of the body. Table 5.1 is a brief overview of some probable orthotic causes of gait deviations when using orthoses, taken from the work of Edelstein (1988).

CONCLUSION

Biomechanics has shown, both in this instance and elsewhere, that it can provide valuable assistance in determining what forces or motions take place under normal and pathological conditions. These parameters are then used by clinicians and paramedical staff to help evaluate treatments, develop new approaches and assess the outcomes of interventions. However, the reader must be cautioned not to think that gait analysis can provide all the answers relating to walking problems. There are still many assumptions made for such analyses, such as the assumption of principal muscle actions. It is well known that muscles do not provide one simple action but work with others and often provide varying motions or work under differing control strategies. But the level of analysis available currently *has* to assume that simplified actions introduce errors into the final results. This cannot be avoided but should be recognised. This is only one example of many possible sources of error.

REFERENCES

Andriacchi TP, Ogle JA, Galante JO. Walking speed as a basis for normal and abnormal gait measurements. *J Biomech* 1977, **10**:261-268.

Anthony RJ. *The manufacture and use of the functional foot orthosis*. Basel: Karger; 1991.

Ball P, Johnson GR. Reliability of hindfoot goniometry when using a flexible electrogoniometer. *Clin Biomech* 1993, **8**:13-19.

Bennett PJ, Duplock LR. Pressure distribution beneath the human foot. *J Am Podiatr Med Ass* 1993, **83**:674-678.

Berman AT, Zarro VJ, Bosacco SJ, Israelite C. Quantitative gait analysis after total knee arthroplasty for monoarticular degenerative arthritis. *J Bone Jt Surg* 1987, **69A**:1340-1345.

Bombelli R. *Osteoarthritis of the hip*. Berlin: Springer-Verlag; 1983.

Bowker P, Condie DN, Bader DL, Pratt DJ, eds. *Biomechanical basis of orthotic management*. Oxford: Butterworth Heinemann; 1993.

Buck P, Morrey BF, Chao EYS. The optimum position of arthrodesis of the ankle: a gait study of the knee and ankle. *J Bone Jt Surg* 1987, **69A**:1052-1062.

Butler PB, Englebrecht M, Major RE *et al*. Physiological cost index of walking for normal children and its use as an indicator of physical handicap. *Dev Med Child Neurol* 1984, **26**:607-612.

Butler PB, Thompson N, Major RE. Improvement in walking performance of children with cerebral palsy: preliminary results. *Dev Med Child Neurol* 1992, **34**:567-576.

Carrera DJ, Sharpe MH, Pearcy MJ, Frick RA. The reliability of postural sway measures using the 3SPACE Tracker. *Clin Biomech* 1996, **11**:361-363.

Cavanagh PR, Hewitt FG, Perry JE. In-shoe plantar pressure measurement: a review. *The Foot* 1992, **2**:185-194.

Chao EY, Laughman RK, Stauffer RN. Biomechanical gait evaluation of pre- and postoperative total knee replacement patients. *Arch Orthop Traum Surg* 1980, **97**:309-317.

Coplan JA. Rotational motion of the knee: a comparison of normal and pronating subjects. *J Orthop Sports Phys Ther* 1989, **10**:366-369.

Cunningham DA, Rechnitzer PA, Pearce ME, Donner AP. Determinants of self-selected walking pace across ages 19 to 66. *J Gerontol* 1982, **37**:560-564.

Demottaz JD, Mazur JM, Thomas WH, Sledge CB, Simon SR. Clinical study of total ankle replacement with gait analysis: a preliminary report. *J Bone Jt Surg* 1979, **61A**:976-988.

Dickstein R, Abulaffio N, Geleernter I, Pillar T. An ultrasonic-operated kinematic measurement system for assessment of stance balance in the clinic. *Clin Biomech* 1996, **11**:173-175.

Duckworth T, Boulton A, Betts R *et al.* Plantar pressure measurement and the prevention of ulceration in the diabetic foot. *J Bone Jt Surg 1985,* **76B**:79-85.

Edelstein JE. Orthotic assessment and management. In: O'Sullivan SB, Schmitz TJ, eds. *Physical rehabilitation: assessment and treatment procedures, 2nd edition.* Philadelphia: F.A. Davis; 1988.

Ehara Y, Tanaka S, Fujimoto H, Miyazaki S, Yamamoto S. Comparison of the performance of 3D camera systems II. *Gait Posture* 1995, **3**:166-169.

Granat MH, Maxwell DJ, Bosch CJ, Ferguson ACB, Lees KR, Barbenel JC. A body-worn gait analysis system for evaluating hemiplegic gait. *Med Eng Phys* 1995, **17**:390-394.

Hauge MF. The gait with an ankylosed hip. *Acta Orthop Scand* 1965, **36**:348-356.

Hughes J, Pratt L, Linge K, Clark P, Klenerman L. Reliability of pressure measurements: the EMED F system. *Clin Biomech* 1991, **6**:14-18.

Iida H, Yamamuro T. Kinetic analysis of the centre of gravity of the human body in normal and pathological gaits. *J Biomech* 1987, **20**:987-995.

Inman VT, Ralston H, Todd F. *Human walking.* Baltimore: Williams and Wilkins; 1981.

James PJ, Nicol AC, Hamblen DL. A comparison of gait symmetry and hip movements in the assessment of patients with monarticular hip arthritis. *Clin Biomech* 1994, **9**:162-166.

Kodadadeh S. Energy methods for the clinical monitoring of pathological gait. *Gait Posture* 1993, **1**:23-25.

Larish DD, Martin PE, Mungiole M. Characteristic patterns of gait in the healthy old. *Ann NY Acad Sci* 1988, **515**:18-32.

Lord M, Hosein R. Pressure redistribution by moulded inserts in diabetic footwear: a pilot study. *J Rehab Res Dev* 1994, **31**:214-221.

MacGregor J. The objective measurement of physical performance with long- term ambulatory physiological surveillance equipment (LAPSE). In: Stoot FD, Rafferty EB, Goulding L, eds. *Proceedings of the 3rd International Symposium on Ambulatory Monitoring.* London: Academic; 1978:29-39.

Mazur JM, Schwartz E, Simon SR. Ankle arthrodesis. *J Bone Jt Surg* 1979, **61A**:964-975.

McHugh B. A description of gait. In: Bowker P, Condie DN, Bader DL, Pratt DJ, eds. *Biomechanical basis of orthotic management.* Oxford: Butterworth-Heinemann; 1993:38-57.

Merritt JL. Advances in orthotics for the patient with rheumatoid arthritis. *J Rheumatol* 1987, **14**:62-67.

Michaud TC. *Foot Orthoses and other forms of conservative foot care.* Baltimore: Williams and Wilkins; 1993:27-56.

Murray MP, Gore DR, Clarkson BH. Walking patterns of patients with unilateral hip pain due to osteoarthritis and avascular necrosis. *J Bone Jt Surg* 1971, **53A**:259-264.

Murray MP, Gore DC, Sepic SB, Mollinger LA. Antalgic maneuvers during walking in men with unilateral knee disability. *Clin Orthop* 1985, **199**:192-200.

Oberg T, Karsznia A, Oberg K. Joint angle parameters in gait: Reference data for normal subjects. *J Rehabil Res Dev* 1994, **31**:199-213.

Perry J. *Atlas of orthotics, 2nd edition.* St Louis: C.V. Mosby; 1985.

Pratt DJ. Mechanisms of shock attenuation via the lower limb. *Clin Biomech* 1989, **4**:23-34.

Pratt DJ. Three dimensional electrogoniometric study of selected knee orthoses. *Clin Biomech* 1991, **6**:67-72.

Pratt DJ. Some aspects of modern orthotics. *Physiol Meas* 1994, **15**:1-27.

Pratt DJ. Functional foot orthoses. *The Foot* 1995, **5**:101-110.

Pratt DJ, Tollafield DR, Peacock JC, Johnson GR. Foot Orthoses. In: Bowker P, Condie DN, Bader DL, Pratt DJ, eds. *Biomechanical basis of orthotic management.* Oxford: Butterworth-Heinemann; 1993:124-145.

Prodromos CC, Andriacchi TP, Galante JO. A relationship between gait and clinical changes following high tibial osteotomy. *J Bone Jt Surg* 1985, **67A**:1188-1194.

Root MC, Orien WP, Weed JH. *Biomechanical examination of the foot, volume 1.* Los Angeles: Clinical Biomechanics Corp; 1971.

Saunders JB, Inman VT, Eberhart HT. The major determinants in normal and pathological gait. *J Bone Jt Surg* 1953, **35A**:543-558.

Shiavi R, Green N. Ensemble averaging of locomotor electromyographic patterns using interpolation. *Med Biol Eng Comput* 1983, **21**:573-578.

Smidt GL. Rudiments of gait. In: Smidt GL, ed. *Gait in rehabilitation.* New York: Churchill Livingstone; 1990:1-20.

Steven MM, Capell HA, Sturrock RD, MacGregor J. The physiological cost of gait (PCG): a new technique for evaluating non steroidal anti-inflammatory drugs in rheumatoid arthritis. *Br J Rheumatol* 1983, **22**:141-145.

Wall JC, Crosbie J. Temporal gait analysis using slow motion video and a personal computer. *Physiotherapy* 1997, **83**:109-115.

Warren-Forward MJ, Goodall RM, Pratt DJ. Three dimensional displacement and force transducer. *IEE Proc A* 1992, **139**:21-29.

Waters R, Yakura J. Energy expenditure of normal and abnormal ambulation. In: Smidt GL, ed. *Gait in rehabilitation.* New York: Churchill Livingstone; 1990:65-96.

Whittle MW. *Gait analysis – an introduction.* Oxford: Butterworth-Heinemann; 1996.

Wilton TJ, Sambatakakis A, Attfield SF. Soft tissue balance at the time of knee replacement; rationale and method. *Knee* 1994, **1**:111-116.

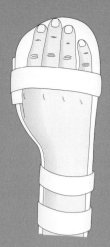

6

M Wade &
S Rimmer

JOINT PROTECTION ADVICE AND SPLINTING

CHAPTER OUTLINE

- Joint protection
- Joint protection principles
- Energy conservation
- Common functional problems and solutions

- Splinting
- Common splints for rheumatoid arthritis

INTRODUCTION

Joint protection advice is given with the aim of maintaining independence and reducing the impact of rheumatological disease on the patient's function. The intention is to reduce stress and pain on joints, reduce inflammation and help preserve the correct structure of the joints. Energy conservation techniques attempt to help the patient conserve physical resources and improve functional endurance. Splinting can also play an important role in the management of rheumatological conditions.

JOINT PROTECTION

The concept of joint protection was originally proposed by Cordery in 1965, based on a theoretical understanding of anatomy, biomechanics, pathology of rheumatoid disease and the consequences of inflammation.

At the time it was hoped that diligent application of this knowledge could prevent deformity, but the difficulty of achieving long-term compliance has limited the ability to demonstrate this. Barry *et al.* (1994) showed that patients' knowledge of joint protection techniques increased following a single education session with an occupational therapist and that this improvement was sustained over 6

months. Behavioural change proved more difficult to assess. Hammond (1994) demonstrated that joint protection education can lead to a change in attitudes, but that behavioural changes would require greater input than is normally devoted to this process. Research studies (Furst *et al.*, 1987, Lorig, 1992, Hammond, 1996) have concluded that the use of cognitive behavioural strategies is the most effective way of ensuring greater compliance. This involves regular repetition of verbal and written information, repeat demonstration and practice of techniques with weekly review and goal setting. This can be carried out on an individual basis or within a group. Small group programmes enable members to support and encourage each other which leads to increased compliance. Weekly sessions of 1–2 hours for 4–6 weeks in groups of 4–8 people have proved most effective (Hammond, 1996).

Joint protection techniques are not only a means of maintaining function but also enable the patient to achieve a sense of control over the disease and a positive, proactive approach. Rheumatoid disease can lead to feelings of fear, helplessness, anxiety, stress and depression. Blalock & De Vellis (1992) suggest that information seeking, problem solving, self management and social support are all linked with better psychological adjustment and physical function.

JOINT PROTECTION PRINCIPLES

RESPECT FOR PAIN

Patients with rheumatoid arthritis (RA) experience both acute and chronic pain. It is essential therefore to be able to understand and distinguish between the two and respond accordingly. Many patients experience background pain all the time, and therefore if this was seen as a need to rest then there would be a decrease in functional activities, a reduction in range of movement and deformities would develop. However, when patients are experiencing a flare-up, and joints are acutely inflamed, rest is needed in order to reduce inflammation. Such acute pain should be respected. When performing an activity and pain becomes acute, patients should stop the activity as soon as possible. If they carry on until the pain becomes such that they have to stop, this will increase inflammation and put undue pressure on the joints. There is some evidence that pain can be relieved in the short-term by using a joint protection technique to do a task (Agnew, 1987).

BALANCE BETWEEN ACTIVITY AND REST

The patient needs to learn the importance of activity and rest and how to achieve a balance between them in daily life. (See Energy Conservation below.)

AVOID POSITIONS OF DEFORMITY

It is recommended that certain positions should be avoided as they could lead to deformities. For example, if there is a tendency towards ulnar deviation in the hand then alternative grips or techniques such as using the palm of the hand or gadgets to open jars should be employed to avoid this. In the lower limb the deformity to be avoided is flexion of the knees. Therefore patients must not put pillows under the knees when sleeping.

USE THE LARGEST JOINT POSSIBLE

When carrying out an activity the weight and stress should be distributed to the largest joint as it is protected by stronger muscles. For example, a shopping bag should be carried over the forearm rather than the fingers, a plate or tray should be carried underneath with the palms taking the weight rather than the finger tips, doors should be opened with the hips rather than the hands.

DISTRIBUTE THE STRAIN OVER SEVERAL JOINTS

When holding an item, even a cup, the patient should use both hands in order to distribute the load over several joints.

AVOID SUSTAINED POSITIONS OR REPETITIVE ACTIVITIES

Staying in one position for a length of time can cause pain and stiffness on movement, therefore patients need to regularly change their position. Carrying out an activity which requires a sustained position or is repetitive, e.g. holding a pen when writing, holding a book to read or standing to iron, can cause muscle fatigue leading to extra force and pressure on the joints. Therefore patients need to rest frequently or adapt their technique, e.g. using a pen holder, book stand or sitting to iron.

AVOID CARRYING HEAVY OBJECTS

Patients should try to avoid carrying heavy objects as this can place extra stress on the joints. They should be encouraged to slide heavy objects across work surfaces and buy lightweight versions of equipment. The use of a trolley can be advantageous.

CHANGE ACTIVITY FROM ONE GROUP OF JOINTS TO ANOTHER

Patients need to be aware of which joints they use to carry out activities. This awareness highlights the need to change activities regularly to avoid undue stress on a particular group of joints.

CONSERVE ENERGY

Patients should be encouraged to use the energy they have available in the most effective way. (See Energy Conservation below.)

MAINTENANCE OF RANGE OF MOVEMENT AND MUSCLE STRENGTH

Each patient should be given a specific exercise programme designed to put each joint through a full range of movement to maintain mobility, muscle strength and length and to prevent contractures occurring. Brighton *et al.* (1993) carried out a study which demonstrated the effects of a long-term exercise programme on the rheumatoid hand. This was a randomised controlled trial which showed an increase in grip strength and a smaller reduction in range of movement in the test group which had carried out the exercises. Unsworth (1997) outlines a comprehensive exercise programme in pictorial form and stresses the importance of balancing exercise and rest.

USE OF ASSISTIVE EQUIPMENT AND SPLINTS

By using assistive equipment patients may avoid unnecessary strain in their joints. (See Assistive Equipment below.) Splinting is used to maintain a position of function by active reinforcement of weakened muscles and to protect joints. (See Splinting below.)

ENERGY CONSERVATION

Patients with RA recognise the articular features of the condition but often do not associate systemic symptoms with the disease. They need to understand that their feelings of tiredness, fatigue and lack of energy may be due to an increase in disease activity. Other contributory factors to fatigue are lack of sleep due to pain and stiffness, and the extra effort required to use weakened muscles. Energy conservation techniques encourage patients to maximise the use of limited energy resources; such techniques include work simplification, pacing and the use of assistive equipment.

WORK SIMPLIFICATION

This is analysis of an activity within an environment to ensure that it is carried out in the most efficient way. It can be achieved by asking questions such as:

• How well is the environment organised?
• Are items/equipment used regularly easily accessible?
• Is equipment light and easy to use?
• Are the surfaces at the correct height?
• Would it be better to sit down to do the task?
• Can the job be eliminated (e.g. ironing sheets)?
• Can the job be made more simple (e.g. to cook and serve from same dish)?
• Can the number of journeys be reduced (e.g. across a room or up and down stairs)?
• Can labour saving devices be used (e.g. washing machine, tumble dryer, food processor)?
• Can someone else help with the task?

PACING

This is the achievement of a balance between rest, exercise and activity. The patient needs to learn the importance of each of these and how to incorporate them into their daily routine. Rest can mean:

• Resting one joint that is inflamed, which is usually done by splinting. The efficacy of splinting is discussed under Splinting below.
• Resting the whole body, for limited periods, if there is exacerbation of the disease.
• Resting the mind and body through relaxation.

Furst *et al.* (1987) showed that an improvement in pacing could be achieved through an occupational therapy education programme. As a result of resting during physical activity and achieving a balance between rest and physical activity, the overall time spent physically active increased.

The value of self relaxation was demonstrated by O'Leary *et al.* (1988) as part of a cognitive behavioural strategy in the treatment of people with RA. It reduced pain and joint inflammation and improved the psychosocial functioning of those in the treatment group. This approach is based on the biopsychosocial model of pain.

The need to rest is often seen by the patients as failure on their part, and the therapist needs to explain its benefits. The main benefit is that it enables more to be achieved by the end of the day without excess tiredness. Resting for short, frequent periods can actually increase overall functional activity. Patients are often forced to rest when they have carried out an activity to the degree which has resulted in pain. They should be encouraged to recognise this and to rest before the pain becomes so unbearable they have to stop.

Patients need to recognise the difference between specific exercise programmes and general activities. Exercise programmes are usually provided by physiotherapists to maintain muscle strength, length and range of movement.

Activity relates to anything that a patient does at home, work or during leisure time. Patients should be encouraged to look at these activities and try to alternate a demanding task with a less demanding one.

The concept of pacing is obviously easier to apply when patients are in control of their day. It can be difficult to achieve in an employment situation particularly if employers or colleagues are inflexible. The therapist needs to support patients and help them adjust and establish a routine that specifically suits their situation.

ASSISTIVE EQUIPMENT

Assistive equipment is used when a patient is experiencing a particular functional difficulty which cannot be solved using a different technique. Figures 6.1–6.4 show examples of different pieces of equipment. This equipment may be needed long-term or for a short time while experiencing a flare-up or following surgery. There are conflicting views on whether it should be used as a preventative measure or a last resort (Melvin, 1989). Rogers

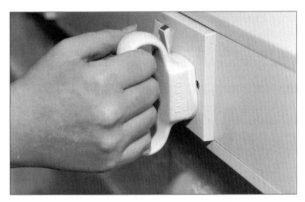

Figure 6.1 Handiplug.

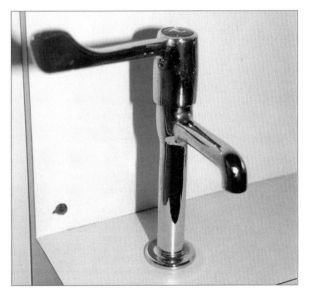

Figure 6.2 Lever tap.

& Holm (1992) carried out a literature review on the use of assistive technology devices in patients with rheumatic disease, highlighting the lack of scientific study on the prescription, provision and use of assistive devices. Physical, psychological, financial and environmental issues all need to be considered.

The mechanism for the provision of such equipment varies from area to area, therefore the therapist needs to be clear on the procedures. It may be possible to loan equipment from hospitals and social services. Some patients may wish to purchase their own and there are a number of ways of doing this; information on suppliers is included at the end of the chapter.

It is very important that each patient and his or her situation is assessed individually. It is vital for the therapist to find out the patient's needs and priorities and not assume that the patient wants to achieve independence in all aspects of daily life. For example, a patient may prefer to have help getting dressed in the morning so as to conserve energy for another task which is perceived as more rewarding. Carers also need to be involved or they may feel that they cannot provide what the patient expects, but not want to relinquish their carer role. Communication is therefore central to the whole process.

The therapist must understand the psychological effects equipment may have on a patient, some of whom may see its use as reflecting a deterioration in function and a progression of the disease and therefore try to manage without for as long as possible. Some may see it as giving in and others may find the presence of the equipment in their home as highlighting their disability to visitors. It is therefore important for the therapist to explain the rationale behind each piece of equipment to the patient and carer so that its use can be seen positively. For example, some equipment reduces the strain on joints, so lessening the pain and inflammation and potentially preventing further deterioration.

When the functional needs have been established, the therapist can then identify equipment which can be of benefit. The therapist should demonstrate the equipment and the patient given an opportunity to try it out. It is also worthwhile for the therapist to re-evaluate the equipment after a period of use to check that it is being used correctly and solving the difficulty. If not, then an alternative could be tried if available. This ensures all equipment is utilised well, which is particularly important with restricted budgets.

COMMON FUNCTIONAL PROBLEMS AND SOLUTIONS

Table 6.1 suggests some ideas to solve problems commonly encountered by people with rheumatoid disease. It is by no means exhaustive. The principles of joint protection can be applied to any problem highlighted by the patient. This can be a creative problem solving exercise for the therapist and the patient. Some gadgets have already been shown to make tasks easier and less painful for people with RA, for example, electric can openers and vegetable peelers (Bradshaw, 1982, 1986) and lever taps (Sweeney et al., 1994). However, much more research is required on the efficacy of assistive devices.

SPLINTING

Splinting can be a valuable part of the management of RA. It is essential that the therapist has a thorough knowledge of anatomy and that a full assessment is carried out on each patient for each splint.

RATIONALE FOR SPLINTING

The main functions and indications for splinting in RA are outlined in Table 6.2. These examples are representative of the type of splint included in each rationale. However,

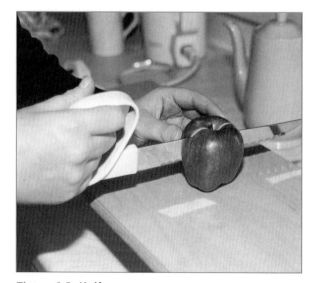

Figure 6.3 **Knife.**

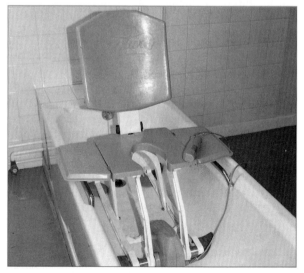

Figure 6.4 **Bath lift.**

research on the efficacy of splinting in the management of RA has been limited and conflicting.

Gault & Spyker (1969) showed that inflammation was reduced while wearing resting splints but not afterwards. Falconer (1991) reviewed the literature on hand splinting in RA and cites studies providing evidence for the reduction in disease activity while wearing splints with only a transient loss of range of movement and strength. She also points out the dangers of prolonged use of splints in reducing bone mass and strength and the development of contractures. This illustrates the importance of clear instructions of when to wear splints and when to exercise.

Nocturnal resting splints have been shown to significantly reduce pain (Johnsson *et al.*, 1992), while wrist supports have been shown to reduce pain during activity but there is conflicting evidence regarding their effect on hand function and grip (Anderson & Maas, 1987, Backman & Dietz, 1988). Mercer & Davis (1995) carried out a survey on satisfaction with prefabricated wrist and thumb supports and found that those fitted according to a standard protocol were used regularly and were reported to reduce pain and increase function.

A small study by Palchik *et al.* in 1990 demonstrated that splinting was able to resolve boutonniere deformities. Noaker *et al.* (1988) conducted a follow-up study of silver ring splints for swan-neck deformity and results indicated improvement in hand function. There is no empirical evidence, as yet, though, for the prevention of deformity by using splints. As for the correction of deformity, Williams (1990) proposed that prolonged passive stretch on a contracted joint may elongate tight soft tissues.

MATERIALS

There are a wide range of materials available for splint making. Some examples of thermoplastic materials and their properties are given in Table 6.3. These materials are

Common functional problems and solutions	
Activities of daily living	**Solution**
Preparing and draining vegetables	Large handled, swivel blade peeler; spike board to hold vegetable still; place vegetables inside a cooking basket in the pan and then drain by lifting basket out and deal with water when cold
Opening bottles and jars	Many different types of bottle/jar openers on the market, non-slip mat to keep bottle/jar still
Lifting kettle	Fill with lightweight jug; kettle tipper – for jug or conventional electric kettles (nothing available at present for cordless kettles)
Turning taps	Lever-action tap turners can be fitted to existing taps or lever taps can be used as replacements
Standing	High seat stool or perching stool
Carrying items	A trolley can reduce strain on joints and reduce number of trips between rooms
Cooker knobs	Special turners are available; gas and electricity boards offer a range of alternative controls
Holding cutlery	Adapted cutlery is available, for example, larger, lightweight and/or angled handles
Holding cup or mug	Lightweight, large handled and insulated mugs
Dressing	Loose fitting, front fastening clothes are much easier and lightweight ones are more comfortable
Socks/stockings/tights	Sock/stocking/tights gutter
Shoes	Long handled shoe horn and elastic laces
Pants/trousers/skirts	Helping hand/easy reach
Cardigans/shirts	Dressing stick
Buttons	Button hook or Velcro replacement
Bathing	Non-slip mats, bath board and seat; mechanical bath equipment is available – some enable the patient to be independent and others assist the carer; shower - either over the bath, used in combination with a bath board, or a separate 'walk-in' type with a seat

Table 6.1 **Common functional problems and solutions.**

	Common functional problems and solutions (continued)
Activities of daily living	**Solution**
Tooth care	Increase grip of toothbrush by enlarging handle with dense foam tubing; wall mounted toothpaste dispensers
Shaving	Increase grip of razor by enlarging handle with dense foam tubing; Use an electric razor
Reading	Use of a book rest
Hairbrushing/combing	Long-handled brush/comb
Toileting	Raised toilet seats, rails, frame that combines seat and arms; commode – may be necessary if mobility is reduced and so unable to get to toilet (particularly useful at night); long-handled bottom wipers; 'Clos-O-Mat' toilet enables a person with severe limitations to operate a switch which sprays warm water to cleanse and then warm air to dry handles may need to be adapted in order for clients to be able to grip and flush the toilet
Seating	Raise existing chair to a suitable height or obtain a high seat chair; ejector cushion or chair (spring loaded or motorised); mechanised riser and/or recliner chairs; suitable chair required for work to ensure good posture
Bed	Raise bed to suitable height; leg lifters available – manual or mechanised; duvets are lighter than sheets and blankets, which reduces pressure on joints and it is easier to make the bed; bed cradle to get the weight of the bed clothes off feet; pressure relieving mattresses to reduce the risk of pressure sores if turning is difficult; firm mattress is easier to turn over on and stand up from
Opening doors	Key turner gives a better grip; Yale knob turner can assist in opening the door from the inside
Writing	Increase grip of pen by enlarging handle with dense foam tubing or use of a pen holder
Driving	Automatic transmission; power assisted steering; steering wheel grip can be enlarged using dense foam tubing or a steering knob can be used; extra mirrors can compensate for limited neck movement; patients should be aware that they should inform the Driving and Vehicle Licensing Agency of any disability

Table 6.1 (continued) **Common functional problems and solutions.**

available in a variety of thicknesses and some have a memory and are therefore remouldable. The choice of material depends on the type of splint being made, the area to be splinted and the condition of the patient's skin. Dry heating can be done in an oven or with a heat gun, while water baths are used for wet heating. Representatives from the companies that supply these materials and equipment are usually more than happy to demonstrate existing and new products.

COMMON SPLINTS FOR RA

PADDLE SPLINT

The paddle splint is designed to extend from approximately two-thirds of the length of the forearm to the tips of the fingers (Figure 6.5). It is designed to rest joints, relieve pain and to prevent/correct deformity. In an attempt to achieve the latter it is essential that all joints are positioned carefully. The positions to aim for are approximately $20–30^0$ extension at the wrist and avoiding radial deviation; metacarpophalangeal (MCP) joints in maximum flexion and avoiding ulnar deviation; the interphalangeal joints in maximum extension and the thumb in abduction and extension. It is important to have an ulnar ridge on the splint to maintain correct alignment of the MCP joints.

The splint should be worn at night when the patient has inflammation of the hand or while trying to correct a deformity. It can be worn during day time rest periods but it is vital that it is removed regularly for gentle exercises to prevent loss of movement, strength and function.

WRIST SUPPORT

This splint is used to rest the wrist, provide support, alleviate pain, improve function and prevent deformity. Patients often find it beneficial when carrying out activities of daily living as it immobilises the wrist but leaves the fingers and thumb free to work. It is very important that the patient realises that the splint should not be worn all the time as it can result in a reduction in movement and muscle strength.

The wrist support is available commercially from many different companies and can be made out of strong elastic material or neoprene rubber. It is essential that these splints are fitted correctly. The metal bar should be bent to ensure the wrist is in approximately 30^0 extension and should not extend beyond the proximal palmar crease as this can impair hand function.

If the ready-made standard splint does not fit or a more rigid type is required, the therapist can make one from a thermoplastic material (Figure 6.6).

Indications for splinting		
Indication	**Splint function**	**Applicable splints**
To rest a joint	splint prevents movement of the affected joint and so alleviates pain and inflammation	paddle, wrist support
To provide support	support and stabilisation of some joints can facilitate movement in others	metacarpophalangeal ulnar deviation (MUD) splint, thumb post, wrist support
To protect and immobilise joint	may be necessary after surgery	paddle, extension outrigger after meta-carpophalangeal joint replacement, collar after cervical spine surgery
To prevent deformity	maintaining a position of function during active disease	paddle, wrist support
To alleviate pain	by resting and supporting joint	paddle, wrist support, MUD splint, swan-neck deformity splint, thumb post
To improve function	provides a fulcrum from which distal joints can function more effectively	wrist support, thumb post, MUD splint, swan-neck deformity
To correct deformities	regaining joint alignment by functional positioning of joints. Serial splinting to correct fixed, flexed or deviated joints	wrist support, thumb post, swan-neck deformity splint, paddle splint, elbow resting splint, serial plasters for fixed flexion at the knee

Table 6.2 **Indications for splinting.**

Properties of splinting materials							
Material	**Description**	**Medium to heat all at 72°C/160°F**	**Working time (minutes)**	**Rigidity**	**Stretch**	**Conform-ability**	**Supplier**
San-splint (Eeziform)	Suitable for large/ resting splints	water	3–5	high	low	low	Smith and Nephew
San-splint XR	Suitable for small hand splints	water	3–5	medium	medium	high	Smith and Nephew
Aquaplast	Suitable for small hand splints	water or dry heat	1–10 (depends on thickness)	medium	high	high	Smith and Nephew
Orthoplast	Suitable for large/ resting splints	in water or dry heat	8–10	medium	low	low	Johnson & Johnson
Orthoplast II	Suitable for small hand splints	water or dry heat	3–4	high	high	high	Johnson & Johnson
X-lite	Thermoplastic impregnated on a cotton mesh which allows for aeration Suitable for resting splints	water or dry heat	3–4	high	medium	medium	Orthopaedic Systems

Table 6.3 **Properties of splinting materials.**

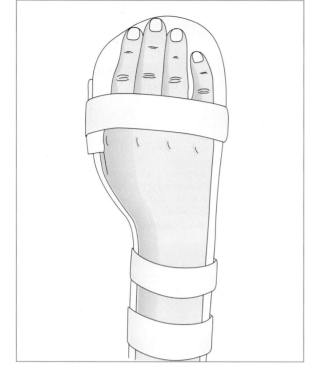

Figure 6.5 Paddle splint.

IMPORTANT POINTS IN SPLINTING

There are some essential points that a therapist must consider to ensure correct and effective splinting techniques:

- Therapists need to know why they are making the splint and ensure patients know why they need it.
- The patient should be able to put the splint on and take it off independently.
- The splint should be as light, comfortable and aesthetically pleasing as possible. It should not have any corners or sharp edges.
- Therapists should provide instruction, both verbal and written, on when to wear the splint and how to care for it. Patients should also know how to contact the therapist if the splint needs altering, is broken or uncomfortable.
- Follow-up appointments to check the splint and evaluate its efficacy are vital.

All these points are considered essential for achieving compliance in splint wearing. Research shows that education on the benefits of splints and comfort are key issues in improving compliance (Agnew & Maas, 1995). The use of standardised protocols for splint prescription and education are advocated in studies by Spoorenberg *et al.* (1994) and Mercer & Davis (1995). Splinting is most effective when used as part of the total programme for the holistic management of RA (Falconer, 1991).

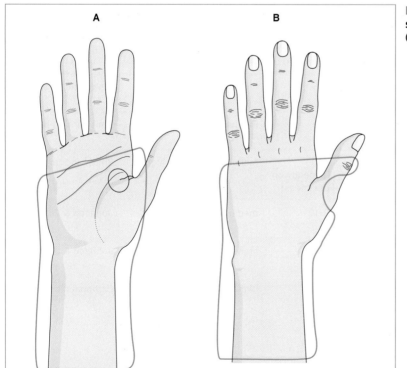

Figure 6.6 Patterns for wrist supports. (A) Wrist gauntlet. (B) Wrist extension split.

CONCLUSION

This chapter has summarised the key principles of joint protection and splinting. The application of these principles to the daily life of people with rheumatological conditions makes an important contribution to successful multidisciplinary management.

COMPANIES SELLING SPLINTING MATERIALS AND EQUIPMENT

- Camp Product Supplies, 30–32 Sovereign Road, Kings Norton Business Centre, Birmingham, B30 3HN. Tel: 0121 433 4411 (ready-made splints only).

- Johnson & Johnson Professional, The Braccans, London Road, Bracknell, Berkshire, RG12 2AT. Tel: 01344 864050.
- Kettering Surgical Appliances, 73 Overstone Road, Northampton, NN1 3J. Tel: 01604 22886 (ready-made splints and Velcro only).
- Nottingham Rehab*, 17 Ludlow Hill Road, West Bridgford, Nottingham, NG2 6HD. Tel: 0115 9452345.
- Orthopaedic Systems, 22–23 Oldgate, St Michaels Ind Est, Widnes, Cheshire WA8 8TL. Tel: 0151 420 3250.
- Promedics Limited, Clarendon Road, Blackburn, Lancashire BB1 9TA. Tel: 01254 57700.
- Smith & Nephew Homecraft *, Low Moor Estate, Kirkby-in-Ashfield, Nottingham, NG17 7J2. Tel: 01623 754047.
    * Also supply assistive devices.

REFERENCES

Agnew PJ. Joint protection in arthritis: fact or fiction? *Br J Occup Ther* 1987, **50**:227-230.

Agnew PJ, Maas F. Compliance in wearing wrist working splints in rheumatoid arthritis. *Occup Ther J Res* 1995, **15**:165-180.

Anderson K, Maas F. Immediate effect of working splints on grip strength of arthritis patients. *Aust J Occup Ther* 1987, **34**:26-31.

Backman CL, Dietz JC. Static wrist splint: its effect on hand function in three women with rheumatoid arthritis. *Arthritis Care Res* 1988, **3**:151-169.

Barry MA, Purser J, Hazelman R, McLean A, Hazelman BL. Effect of energy conservation and joint protection education in rheumatoid arthritis. *Br J Rheumatol* 1994, **33**:1171-1174.

Blalock SJ, De Vellis RF. Rheumatoid arthritis and depression: an overview. *Bull Rheum Dis* 1992, **41**:6-8.

Bradshaw ESR. *Food preparation aids for rheumatoid arthritis patients. Screw top jar and bottle openers, can openers, vegetable peelers, stabilizers*. London: DHSS Aids Assessment Programme; 1982.

Bradshaw ESR. *Assessment of cooking utensils for rheumatoid arthritis patients. Saucepans, cooking baskets and steamers*. London: DHSS Disability Equipment Assessment Programme; 1986.

Brighton SW, Lubbe JE, Van der Merwe CA. The effect of a long-term exercise programme on the rheumatoid hand. *Br J Rheumatol* 1993, **32**:392-395.

Cordery JC. Joint protection: a responsibility of the occupational therapist. *Am J Occup Ther* 1965, **19**:285-294.

Falconer J. Hand splinting in rheumatoid arthritis: a perspective on current knowledge and directions for research. *Arthritis Care Res* 1991, **4**:81-86.

Furst GP, Gerber CC, Fisher S, Shulman B. A program for improving energy conservation behaviors in adults with rheumatoid arthritis. *Am J Occup Ther* 1987, **41**:102-111.

Gault S, Spyker J. Beneficial effects of immobilisation of joints in rheumatoid and related arthritides: a splint study using sequential analysis. *Arthritis Rheum* 1969, **12**:34-44.

Hammond A. Joint protection behavior in patients with rheumatoid arthritis following an education program: a pilot study. *Arthritis Care Res* 1994, **7**:5-9.

Hammond A. Rheumatoid arthritis. In: Turner A, Foster M, Johnson S, eds. *Occupational therapy and physical dysfunction: principles, skills and practice, 4th edition*. London: Churchill Livingstone; 1996:747-765.

Johnsson PM, Sandkvist G, Eberhardt K, Liang B, Herrlin K. The usefulness of nocturnal resting splints in the treatment of ulnar deviation of the rheumatoid hand. *Clin Rheumatol* 1992, **11**:72-75.

Lorig K. *Patient education: a practical approach*. St Louis: CV Mosby; 1992.

Melvin JL. *Rheumatic disease in the adult and child: occupational therapy and rehabilitation, 3rd edition*. Philadelphia: FA Davis Company; 1989.

Mercer C, Davis M. A survey of the uses and benefits of prefabricated wrist and thumb supports. *Br J Ther Rehab* 1995, **2**:599-603.

Noaker J, Garty MK, Kwoh CK. A follow-up evaluation of silver ring splints. *Arthritis Rheum* 1988, **31**:S160.

O'Leary A, Shoor S, Lorig K, Holman HR. A cognitive-behavioral treatment for rheumatoid arthritis. *Health Psychol* 1988, **7**:527-544.

Palchik NS et al. Non-surgical management of boutonniere deformity. *Arthritis Care Res* 1990, **3**:227-232.

Rogers JC, Holm MB. Assistive technology device use in patients with rheumatic disease: a literature review. *Am J Occup Ther* 1992, **46**:120-127.

Spoorenberg A, Boers M, van der Linden S. Wrist splints in rheumatoid arthritis: what do we know about efficacy and compliance? *Arthritis Care Res* 1994, **7**:55-57.

Sweeney GM, Catchpool N, Clarke AK. Choosing lever taps for people with arthritis. *Br J Occup Ther* 1994, **57**:263-265.

Unsworth H. *Coping with rheumatoid arthritis*. Nottingham: Nottingham Rehabilitation; 1997.

Williams P. The use of intermittent stretch in the prevention of serial sarcomere loss in immobilised muscle. *Ann Rheum Dis* 1990, **49**:316.

GENERAL READING

Barr NR, Swan D. *The hand: principles and techniques of splintmaking, 2nd edition*. London: Butterworths; 1988.

Brattstrom M. *Joint protection and rehabilitation in chronic rheumatic disorders*. London: Wolfe Medical Publications Ltd; 1987.

Cannon NM, Foltz RW, Koepfer JM, Lauck MF, Simpson DM, Bromley RS. *Manual of hand splinting*. New York: Churchill Livingstone; 1985.

Copard BM, Lohman H. *Introduction to splinting*. London: Mosby; 1996.

Fess EE, Gettle KS, Strickland JW. *Hand splinting: principles and methods*. St Louis: The CV Mosby Company; 1987.

Malick MH. *Manual on static hand splinting, 4th edition*. Pittsburgh: Harmaville Rehabilitation Centre; 1980.

Palmer P, Simons J. Joint protection: a critical review. *Br J Occup Ther* 1991, **54**:453-458.

Sandles L. *Occupational therapy in rheumatology: an holistic approach*. London: Chapman and Hall; 1990.

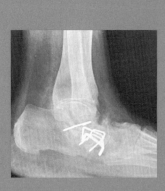

7 K West & E Hall

SURGERY FOR RHEUMATIC PROBLEMS

CHAPTER OUTLINE

- Surgical procedures
- Indications for surgery
- Pre-operative planning
- Pre-operative physiotherapy

- Post-operative rehabilitation
- Psychological aspects
- Surgery in children

INTRODUCTION

This chapter will identify some of the more common procedures and factors involved in the surgical management of rheumatic problems. A more detailed account of specific surgical procedures can be found in orthopaedic textbooks.

Surgical management of rheumatic disease has become a well established speciality within orthopaedics. However, surgical intervention should not be viewed as a medical failure or as an isolated event in the disease process but rather as a continuum of treatment (Figgie, 1994). The result of this intervention has enabled patients to become as independent as possible by reducing or eliminating pain and improving function. Inflammatory polyarthritis, though, presents the surgeons with a multitude of problems due to the ongoing and destructive nature of the disease.

Sub-specialisation within orthopaedics is growing and care is needed to ensure that the patient with an inflammatory condition is assessed and treated holistically. Failure to follow this advice can lead to expensive but useless surgery, for example delicate hand surgery with excellent isolated outcomes is a waste of time if the patient's shoulder and elbow joints are so severely damaged that the arm has limited function.

Early evaluation and good communication between the rheumatology and orthopaedic teams is paramount to ensure that the results of surgical intervention produce the optimum outcomes in terms of pain relief and restoration of function. Early intervention by using more minor surgical procedures may delay or even prevent more major procedures.

SURGICAL PROCEDURES

The main surgical procedures used in the treatment of inflammatory arthritis are:
- Arthroscopy.
- Synovectomy.
- Arthrodesis.
- Arthroplasty.

ARTHROSCOPY

This simple procedure can be used as a diagnostic tool as well as a treatment modality. An arthroscopy is an internal visual examination of a joint using a fibreoptic arthroscope. Probes, forceps and cutting tools can be passed down the arthroscope to the tissues in view for further procedures to take place. Persistently inflamed joints (i.e. the knee) may benefit from an arthroscopic washout, with saline, and removal of loose bodies. An injection of cortisone may also be administered. The arthroscope additionally enables the surgeons to assess the amount of joint damage by direct inspection of the joint surfaces. The reduction in inflammation results in less pain, increased mobility and enhanced quality of life. This procedure can delay the need for more aggressive surgery and gives an opportunity to plan any future surgical management for the patient.

SYNOVECTOMY

There are two types: surgical, and radiation (Yttrium). Synovectomy is the removal of the synovial membrane of joints and tendon sheaths. This can be performed either arthroscopically or by an open procedure.

Surgical Synovectomy

The most common sites are the knee and the wrist. Joint synovectomy is usually performed on patients with minimal or no erosions radiologically, and two-thirds of the synovium is removed. The synovium regenerates within 3 months but results indicate that there is long-lasting pain

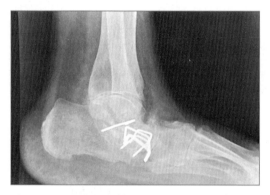

Figure 7.1 Triple arthrodesis of the hindfoot to restore a plantigrade weightbearing base.

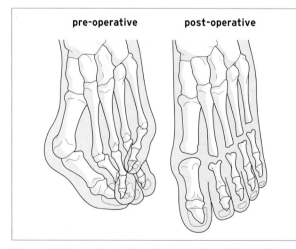

pre-operative   post-operative

Figure 7.2 A schematic diagram of metatarsal head excision (Fowler's procedure).

relief and restoration of function (Adolfsson & Nylander, 1993, Fiocco et al., 1996). However, Ochi and colleagues (1991) found no evidence of any delay in bony destruction due to the ongoing disease process. Jensen et al. (1991) concluded that synovectomy in the knee joint is a valuable palliative procedure and may in some cases postpone joint replacement.

Tenosynovectomy (removal of the tendon sheath) can prevent the tendons from rupturing, improve function and reduce pain.

Radiation Synovectomy

This alternative to surgery has been found to be efficacious for the treatment of rheumatoid arthritis (RA). However, the procedure is not widely used due to the fears of radiation leakage and oncogenesis (Deutsch et al., 1993).

ARTHRODESIS

This operation is designed to produce a bony ankylosis or fusion of a diseased joint or joints (i.e. triple arthrodesis of the hindfoot, see Figure 7.1). This procedure is carried out when the joints are severely damaged and are causing pain and functional difficulties. It may also be the only option for failed joint replacements. It is imperative that the joint is fused in a position of optimum function. Surgical advances have now made it possible to convert some hip and knee arthrodeses to satisfactory arthroplasty in later life.

ARTHROPLASTY

This procedure involves the refashioning of a joint and is performed primarily for pain, loss of joint range and subsequent loss of function. The main types of arthroplasty are:
• Excision.
• Replacement.

Excision Arthroplasty

This is where one or both aspects of the joint are excised. Some common examples in rheumatology are the removal of the metatarsal heads for severe pain and deformity (Fowler's procedure, see Figure 7.2) and the removal of the ulnar styloid for pain and where the extensor tendons are being compromised (Darrach procedure). For failed hip replacements the Girdlestone arthroplasty is the main alternative. The 'joint space' fills with fibrous tissue and a pseudarthrosis develops.

Replacement Arthroplasty

This is where the joint surfaces are excised or refashioned and then replaced or covered with artificial material to create a new joint. Examples of the procedure include a total replacement of the hip (Figure 7.3), knee (Figure 7.4), elbow (Figure 7.5) and shoulder (Figure 7.6). In the patient with inflammatory arthritis and multiple joint involvement there may need to be an ongoing programme of joint replacements. McDonagh et al. (1994) found that though this group of patients remained very disabled they were still ambulant and living in the community therefore indicating that a programme of multiple joint replacements is a worthwhile policy.

INDICATIONS FOR SURGERY

Surgical intervention will be considered for the reduction of pain, the preservation of joints and tendons and the restoration or improvement of function. The decisions about the timing, the sites and the order of surgery are complex ones and there needs to be discussion between the orthopaedic surgeon, the rheumatologist, the therapists and the patient.

Depending on the procedure used the surgery can be described as:
- Preventative (i.e. synovectomy and arthroscopic debridement).
- Preservative (i.e. excision arthroplasty and synovectomy).
- Corrective (i.e. replacement arthroplasty).
- Salvage (i.e. arthrodesis).

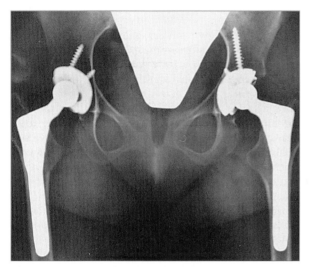

Figure 7.3 **Total hip replacement.**

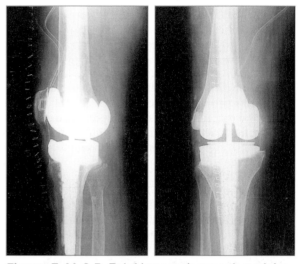

Figures 7.4A & B **Total knee replacement: modular constrained implants with metal augmentation trays to build up the lateral tibial condyle.**

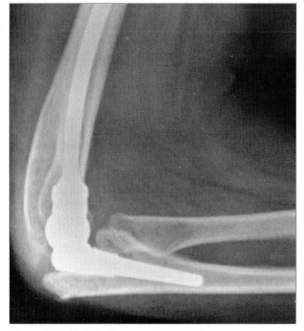

Figure 7.5 **Total elbow replacement.**

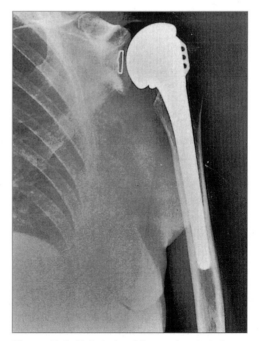

Figure 7.6 **Total shoulder replacement.**

In the early stages of the disease, preventative and preservative measures may be the treatments of choice. Judicious use of such measures may increase the efficacy of medication and rehabilitation treatments as well as prolonging periods of good function therefore delaying the need for replacement surgery (Gerber & Hicks, 1995). In the later stages when there has been significant joint destruction and loss of function, corrective and salvage procedures may be more appropriate interventions.

PRE-OPERATIVE CONSIDERATIONS

The systemic nature of rheumatic disease and the multiplicity of problems that may be encountered can delay or even prevent much needed surgical procedures. Factors to be considered are given below.

Anaemia

Low haemoglobin (Hb) levels, common in inflammatory disease, can delay surgery because the amount of blood lost during orthopaedic surgery is relatively high and can therefore put the patient in a high risk category. Anaemia also leads to increased fatigue which can hinder post-operative rehabilitation.

Vasculitic Lesions

These lesions indicate the possibility of widespread systemic inflammation and can delay or prevent surgery. Vasculitis may delay wound healing because of poor tissue viability and if the lesions become infected there is an increased risk of the joint replacement being compromised.

Generalised Flare Up

This will delay surgical intervention as the patients are generally unwell and not fit enough for surgery or the post-operative regime.

Medication

Many patients with an inflammatory arthropathy are prescribed immunosuppressant drugs to control the disease process. This compromises the immune system, lowers the white cell count and reduces the body's resistance to infection. Some drugs may need to be discontinued prior to surgery. The long-term use of steroids results in patients having thin, papery and easily damaged skin which is difficult to heal. Care needs to be taken before, during and after surgery to minimise the trauma to the skin. These two factors may not delay or prevent surgery but may have a bearing on the overall outcome.

Bone Quality

Patients with long-standing disease and/or long-term steroid users usually develop poor bone quality. This may make joint replacement surgery unfeasible as the bone is not strong enough to withstand the fitting of the joint prosthesis (i.e. the femur may fracture during a total hip replacement procedure). Consulting the orthopaedic surgeon at an early stage should ensure that it is not too late to perform the required surgery and that a constructive and not just a salvage procedure can be offered.

Cervical Spine

Involvement of the cervical spine in RA is well documented. Instability and subluxation, especially at the atlanto-axial joint, is a common feature of rheumatoid disease. This may occur in the later stages or early in very aggressive disease and can delay or prevent surgery. The anaesthetists may have difficulty intubating the patients due to loss of neck extension or cord damage may be caused due to the instability. It is therefore paramount that all rheumatoid patients undergoing a surgical procedure with a general anaesthetic have an X-ray of their cervical spine (postero-anterior (PA) and lateral planes) to assess the spinal state (see Chapter 8). All patients should wear a soft collar to theatre as a reminder of the potential for cervical spine instability.

EFFICACY OF SURGICAL PROCEDURES

Rheumatoid patients with severe multiple joint destruction may require a series of joint replacements to improve their quality if life. It is necessary to prioritise the operations to obtain the best functional outcomes. The priority of the procedures is:
• Cervical spine.
• Lower limb.
• Upper limb.

If the stability of the cervical spine is compromised, a fusion to stabilise the neck has to be undertaken prior to any peripheral joint replacement.

The lower limbs are operated on before the upper ones to maintain mobility; some surgeons also prefer their patients not to use mobility aids immediately post elbow or shoulder replacement. An exception to this may be if the patient is unable to use mobility aids as a result of severe upper limb dysfunction. The order of surgery in the lower limb is:
• Foot.
• Hip.
• Knee.
• Ankle.

For effective rehabilitation and restoration of mobility following hip and/or knee surgery it is necessary to have a stable plantigrade foot with minimal pain. This can be achieved with surgery, orthotics or a combination of both. The overall aim of lower limb surgery is to restore mobility by providing pain relief and improving the mechanical axis of the leg by correcting the malalignments which commonly occur in RA. Deviations from this axis lead to gait abnormalities and early failure of the prosthesis due to loosening (Figgie et al., 1989).

In the upper limb the order of surgery is:
• Shoulder.
• Elbow.
• Wrist.
• Hand.

A painfree stable wrist with good functional alignment is important for effective rehabilitation of the hand. Subluxation and radial deviation of the wrist causes increased stress on the metacarpophalangeal joints and encourages further ulnar deviation. This may compromise the surgical outcomes of joint replacement. (A more detailed account of hand and wrist surgery can be found in Chapter 17.)

The relief of pain and an increased range of movement (ROM) in the elbow joint can enable a patient to attain reasonable upper limb function despite poor shoulder movement. Shoulder replacements require the rotator cuff to be intact to achieve a functional ROM. In many rheumatoid patients requiring total shoulder replacement the rotator cuff is damaged; therefore this surgery is usually performed for pain relief only as there is little likelihood of restoring ROM. Other surgical procedures for the shoulder complex include acromionectomy and decompression.

It is therefore of extreme importance to evaluate the biomechanics of all the limbs when considering a surgical option and then plan the surgical procedures accordingly.

PRE-OPERATIVE PLANNING

Prior to any surgical intervention, especially multiple joint replacements, there needs to be a thorough assessment of the patient's medical, physical and psychological state. To obtain the optimum outcome from surgery, the patient has to be as medically fit and psychologically prepared as possible for the surgery and the post-operative rehabilitation. Newman (1990) states that results from even the most sophisticated surgery can be improved by an intensive rehabilitation programme, appropriate use of appliances and an optimisation of medical therapy.

Once the decision to operate has been taken, involvement of the multidisciplinary team (MDT) can ensure that the appropriate advice support and practical help is available. This can include pre-operative maintenance therapy including hydrotherapy, exercises, provision of walking aids and pain relieving electrical modalities from the physiotherapists. The provision of extra gadgets, as appropriate, both pre- and post-operatively and discussions on alternative ways of performing every day tasks requires the involvement of the occupational therapist. It is also important to involve the family and/or carers so that all people concerned have a clear picture of what the surgery and post-operative recovery and rehabilitation period entails. The patient and family must be encouraged to discuss and plan these matters to ensure that the recovery period is as smooth as possible and that the eventual outcomes are maximised.

PRE-OPERATIVE PHYSIOTHERAPY

Physiotherapists have an important role pre-operatively. Ideally, the therapist will spend time with the patient discussing the impending surgery and its implications. An explanation of what is involved at the different stages (pre-operative, immediately post-operative and rehabilitation). This should be accompanied by suitable information leaflets to reinforce the verbal information. Advising the patient of expected and realistic outcomes needs to be discussed, with emphasis on the fact that these can be achieved with effective post-operative rehabilitation.

Baseline data on the patient's functional abilities prior to surgery are recorded and an appropriate pre-operative regime is implemented. This ensures that the overall musculoskeletal system is conditioned to assist with the post-operative rehabilitation. It is important to assess all limbs and not just the one for surgery. For example, strengthening of the upper limbs will help mobility following total hip replacement due to the more effective use of a frame or crutches.

Prior to surgery any patients with pre-existing chest conditions and those at risk (i.e. smokers and obese patients) should be assessed and shown breathing exercises to decrease the risk of chest complications post-operatively. General maintenance exercises for all upper and lower limb joints should be taught to encourage the maintenance of muscle tone and reduce joint stiffness while the patients are immobile.

POST-OPERATIVE REHABILITATION

The physiotherapist's role in the rehabilitation of these patients following surgery is an important one. The aims of therapeutic intervention are to:
- Reduce pain.
- Reduce swelling.
- Increase ROM.
- Increase muscle strength.
- Restore function.

The therapist may also provide suitable mobility aids, i.e. crutches, frames, sticks etc. Assessment of the patient for appropriate splints and braces may be required.

Prior to the commencement of any post-operative regime the orthopaedic surgeon's instructions must be established. The therapist must ascertain whether the patient is to be fully weightbearing or not, what movements need to be avoided and for how long and if there were any operative complications. Once all these factors are known, then a progressive rehabilitation regime can be planned and implemented. The regime should include strengthening and ROM exercises, gait re-education, stairs and functional activities in conjunction with the occupational therapist. The use of ice therapy and electrical modalities may be needed for the reduction of pain and swelling.

In several studies, the use of continuous passive motion (CPM) in patients following total knee arthroplasty was found to be beneficial. It achieved more rapid and successful outcomes in terms of improving ROM, decreasing swelling and earlier discharge from hospital (Johnson & Eastwood, 1992, McInnes et al., 1992). Gotlin et al. (1994) indicated that the addition of electrical stimulation to the quadriceps muscle during CPM treatment significantly reduced the extensor lag, consequently decreasing the length of stay in hospital and rehabilitation time.

The rehabilitation of patients following surgery, who have multiple joint pathology, can be a complicated task. The therapist must have an appreciation of the potential pain, weakness and loss of function in the non-operated joints. For example, mobilising a patient with upper limb involvement following lower limb surgery can be difficult. Transfers may be difficult if not impossible and the patient may require the use of a forearm support (gutter) frame for walking. Overall these patients will require a greater input from other members of the MDT to enable them to be safe at home.

An interdisciplinary approach to inpatient rehabilitation following hip or knee replacement surgery enables patients to reach functional outcomes sooner and decreased their length of stay in hospital (Erickson & Perkins, 1994).

PSYCHOLOGICAL ASPECTS

Rheumatology patients undergoing surgical procedures have numerous issues to contend with which can cause stress and disruption to family life and routine.

Pre-operatively, the patients have problems of increasing disability due to pain and deteriorating joint function. They also have to organise themselves and other family members so that all concerned can adjust to and cope with the forthcoming surgery and rehabilitation period. The patients may also need an opportunity to express their own fears and worries about the surgery; this may involve a member of the MDT, as some patients may not talk openly to their spouses or children.

Unrealistic expectations can cause psychological distress. Patients' frustration can become more evident as the rehabilitation programme progresses because they are not attaining the goals they had set for themselves. It is therefore important that the patients discuss expectations and possible outcomes prior to the surgical procedure, especially joint replacement surgery, to ensure that these expectations and goals are realistic.

In the longer term the psychological aspects will be more positive due to decreased pain and increased function. Adjustments within the whole family have to be made as the roles people adopted pre-operatively will change. Carers may not have to care so much or may care in a different way; they may feel their role or job is no longer needed, perhaps leading to feelings of redundancy which can create their own psychological emotions and stresses.

Despite the short-term stresses and upheavals, the effect of joint replacement surgery for patients with RA and osteoarthritis (OA) is good. Surgery for OA leads to significant improvement for pain, mobility and quality of life. The impact of surgery in RA is not so marked (Borslap *et al.*, 1994).

Improvements in pain, disability and psychological state have been reported in patients undergoing surgery for both OA and RA. This is despite the polyarticular nature of RA where overall improvements tend to be less noticeable (Kirwan *et al.*, 1994, Petre *et al.*, 1994).

SURGERY IN CHILDREN

Surgery for children with a rheumatic disease is not undertaken lightly. If possible, any prosthetic surgery is delayed until the child is older or a young adult. This is when growth has stopped, the child has reached skeletal maturity and attained full stature. An exception to this is when the child's physical capacity, especially mobility, is severely limited. The joints usually replaced are hips and/or knees, with pain often the major deciding factor. Another consideration that may lead to early joint replacement would be if the damaged joint was causing a more rapid deterioration in other joints.

Those children who require early prosthetic surgery are usually seropositive and have polyarticular involvement. They may have a stunted skeleton and require custom made implants which are made using precise radiographic measurements. Despite the high incidence of radiographic evidence of loosening and complications, the quality of life for these patients is improved dramatically (Cage *et al.*, 1992).

Children with juvenile chronic arthritis commonly have persistent flexion contractures of hips and knees. These result in gait abnormalities and altered joint biomechanics leading to poor mobility and potentially faster joint destruction. Soft tissue release of hip flexoadductors with possible capsulotomy and knee flexors has been shown to improve, if not correct, the deformity, alleviate pain and improve function. It should be remembered that these children will require a comprehensive rehabilitation programme following this procedure to gain the best results (Moreno Alvarez *et al.*, 1992). Potential poor compliance to any postoperative rehabilitation programme may preclude the child from undergoing such a procedure as the outcome will not be effective or satisfactory.

Some other procedures in children include lower jaw extension for micrognathia. This is performed for functional as well as cosmetic reasons. A persistent monarthritis of the knee may result in overgrowth of one side of the epiphyseal plate. It may be necessary to staple this side to prevent continued overgrowth and the resultant valgus or varus deformity.

CONCLUSION

Patients with a rheumatic disease may require joint surgery at some stage during their disease course and often involving more than one procedure. As therapists, it is necessary to be aware of the pain and dysfunction in all joints and tailor the planned rehabilitation programmes accordingly.

Despite the many potential problems and complications, the overall outcomes are favourable, even in those patients with severe multiple joint pathology as a result of RA. Comprehensive rehabilitation is important for all rheumatological patients and a long-term study found that there was greater improvement in functional ability in those patients who had undergone joint replacement surgery compared with those undergoing rehabilitation alone (McCarthy et al., 1989).

REFERENCES

Adolfsson L, Nylander G. Arthroscopic synovectomy of the rheumatoid wrist. *J Hand Surg* 1993, **18**:92-96.

Borslap M, Zant JL, Van Soesbergen M, Van der Korst JK. Effects of total hip replacement on quality of life in patients with osteoarthritis and in patients with rheumatoid arthritis. *Clin Rheumatol* 1994, **13**:45-50.

Cage DJ, Granberry WM, Tullos HS. Long-term results of total hip arthroplasty in adolescents with debilitating polyarthropathy. *Clin Orthopaed Rel Res* 1992, **283**:156-162.

Deutsch E, Brodack JW, Deutsch KF. Radiation synovectomy revisited (review). *Eur J Nucl Med* 1993, **20**:1113-1127.

Erickson B, Perkins M. Interdisciplinary team approach in the rehabilitation of hip and knee arthroplasties. *Am J Occup Ther* 1994, **48**:439-441.

Figgie MP, Inglis AE, Sobel M, Goldberg VM, Figgie HE 111. Correction of angular deformities in primary total knee arthroplasty. *Orthop Trans* 1989, **12**:589.

Figgie MP. Introduction to the surgical treatment of rheumatic diseases. In: Klippel JH, Dieppe PA, eds. *Rheumatology*. London: Mosby; 1994:8:20.1-8:20.6.

Fiocco U, Cozzi L, Rigon C et al. Arthroscopic synovectomy in rheumatoid and psoriatic knee joint synovitis. *Br J Rheumatol* 1996; **35**:463-470.

Gerber LH, Hicks JE. Surgical and rehabilitation options in the treatment of the rheumatoid arthritis patient resistant to pharmacologic agents. *Rheum Dis Clin North Am* 1995, **21**:19-39.

Gotlin RS, Hershkowitz S, Juris PM et al. Electrical stimulation effect on extensor lag and length of hospital stay after total knee arthroplasty. *Arch Phys Med Rehab* 1994, **75**:957-959.

Jensen CM, Poulsen S, Ostergren M, Hansen KH. Early and late synovectomy of the knee in rheumatoid arthritis. *Scand J Rheumatol* 1991, **20**:127-131.

Johnson DP, Eastwood DM. Beneficial effects of continuous passive motion after total condylar knee arthroplasty. *Ann R Coll Surg Engl* 1992, **74**:412-416.

Kirwan JR, Currey HL, Freeman MA, Snow S, Young PJ. Overall long-term impact of total hip and knee joint replacement surgery on patients with osteoarthritis and rheumatoid arthritis. *Br J Rheumatol* 1994, **33**:356-360.

McCarthy G, Egan S, Fitzgerald O, Bresnihan B. Severe disability in rheumatoid arthritis: assessment following comprehensive rehabilitation. *Irish J Med Sci* 1989, **158**:225-227.

McDonagh JE, Ledingham J, Deighton CM et al. Six-year follow-up of multiple joint replacement surgery to the lower limbs. *Br J Rheumatol* 1994, **33**:85-89.

McInnes J, Larson MG, Daltroy LH et al. A controlled evaluation of continuous passive motion in patients undergoing total knee arthroplasty. *JAMA* 1992, **268**:1423-1428.

Moreno Alvarez MJ, Espada G, Maldonado-Cocco JA, Gagliardi SA. Long-term follow up of hip and knee soft tissue release in juvenile chronic arthritis. *J Rheumatol* 1992, **19**:1608-1610.

Newman RJ. Major joint replacement surgery for rheumatoid arthritis. *J R Soc Health* 1990, **110**:194-198.

Ochi T, Iwase R, Kimura T et al. Effect of early synovectomy on the course of rheumatoid arthritis. *J Rheumatol* 1991, **18**:1794-1798.

Petrie K, Chamberlain K, Azariah R. The psychological impact of hip arthroplasty. *Austral New Zeal J Surg* 1994, **64**:115-117.

SECTION 2

COMMON CONDITIONS

Rheumatology (roo mat ol o je). Branch
of medicine which is concerned with the
diagnosis and treatment of rheumatic
disorders.

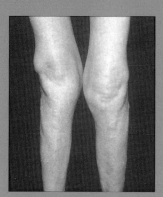

8

J Lloyd

RHEUMATOID ARTHRITIS

CHAPTER OUTLINE

- **Incidence**
- **Aetiology**
- **Clinical Features**

- **Diagnosis**
- **Management**
- **Case history**

Rheumatoid arthritis (RA) will be introduced as a model of the inflammatory process. The incidence, aetiology and pathology of this fascinating condition will be presented. In addition, assessment procedures, management and some outcome tools will be discussed as relevant to the physiotherapist.

INTRODUCTION

RA has been described as the 'commonest potentially treatable cause of disability in the western world' (Emery & Salmon, 1995). It is an inflammatory polyarthritis with systemic manifestations, reflected in its alternative name of rheumatoid disease. The name was first used by Sir Alfred Garrod in 1850 in a book 'On gout and rheumatic gout'. Historical evidence of the existence of the classic rheumatoid deformities is provided by paintings, particularly those of Peter Paul Rubens, one of which hangs in the entrance of the National Hospital for Rheumatic Diseases in Bath. The condition is enormously varied both in its manifestations and in its severity and progression, hence functional deficits are difficult to predict with any accuracy. It is a condition characterised by exacerbations and remissions, some of which may be prolonged.

As well as discussing the disease in terms of pathology and management, consideration must be given to the disability and loss of working days that ensue following onset. Rheumatoid suffering has been described as 'pain, stiffness, swelling, deformity, related diseases, frustration, anxiety, depression and iatrogenic'.

The remarkably varied pattern of the disease produces differing pictures of disability according to the population studied. Around 50% of patients will have little or no residual deformity, 40% will have some disability and 10% will have severe disability (Hickling & Golding, 1984). Males tend to have a better prognosis than females unless they have the severe systemic manifestations of the disease. Life expectancy may be reduced by up to 4 years in men and by up to 10 years in women (Akil & Amos, 1995).

INCIDENCE

Females are affected more than males (3:1) with 1% of the population affected in all, although estimates vary according to the diagnostic criteria used and whether figures relate to only definite RA or whether probable RA is also included, e.g. 2–4% (Golding, 1988, Carson-Dick, 1972). These figures increase to 6% in males over the age of 75 years and 16% in females over 65 years (Barnes, 1980).

The annual incidence of new cases is approximately 0.02%, although this varies according to the diagnostic criteria used. Age at onset tends to follow a normal distribution with a peak in the 5th decade.

Since this is a predominantly female condition one could attempt to link the condition with the role of the female hormones, particularly as it is reported that cases declined in the years following widespread use of the oral contraceptive pill and 75% of rheumatoid patients improve during pregnancy (Dieppe *et al.*, 1985). This issue is still in debate and conflicting studies have been reported but it seems that oral contraceptives may mitigate or postpone the onset of RA slightly, although they are not likely to alleviate the symptoms of the condition (Spector *et al.*, 1991). In addition breast feeding in the post partum period has been linked with an increased risk for developing RA, possibly due to increased prolactin production (Brennan & Silman, 1996).

There appears to be familial aggregation of patients with rheumatological conditions and many show association with human leukocyte antigen (HLA)–DR4 (Walker, 1995). Such individuals may develop RA if they possess the correct HLA typing and are exposed to certain environmental factors, although research is inconclusive.

Worldwide distribution is said to be fairly uniform, although some claim prevalence for temperate climates (Hickling & Golding, 1984), others that erosions are as common in Jamaica as they are in wetter climes (Carson-Dick, 1972). It may be true, however, that symptoms are increased in areas of less attractive climates and patients are increasingly induced to complain of their problems!

AETIOLOGY

The cause of RA is unknown, but genetic factors clearly play a part since up to 10% of patients with the condition report a first degree relative with the condition. There is no evidence to suggest that diet, trauma, stress or climate are at all involved although it is possible that they could act as a trigger along with other environmental factors in genetically susceptible individuals who are exposed to other circumstances concurrently. Other initiating theories include the possibility of infection from a virus such as Epstein–Barr virus, or gut related toxins or viruses, or a micro-organism yet to be identified.

In addition, the pathology seems to have an autoimmune focus. There appears to be an association between RA and the tissue-typing marker HLA–DR4, which was identified in 60–80% of RA patients compared with 20% controls. The D locus genes influence immunological processes. The presence of DR4 in Caucasian patients seems to indicate the likelihood of severe disease or susceptibility to disease, whilst DR2 may suggest a milder disease and an increased chance of response to second line drug therapy (Panayi, 1986). The fact that severity is possibly predictable assists the rheumatologist and health professionals in organisation of a suitable management programme.

PATHOLOGY

The initial changes of inflammation occur in the synovial membrane, possibly following invasion of the synovium by an antigen (e.g. viral or toxin from the bowel) which triggers an antibody–antigen reaction and activates complement. The synovial blood vessels proliferate, dilate and become congested, possibly provoked by an increase in glycosaminoglycan production which causes a mucoid change in the outer synovial tissue with vasculitis and perivasculitis.

The hypertrophic and hyperplastic synovial membrane is infiltrated with chronic inflammatory cells such as macrophages, T- and B-lymphocytes and plasma cells, thus increasing its thickness and possibly its surface area. Lymphocytes, interleukins, lymphokines and other inflammatory mediators encouraged by T4 and T8 (the helper, inducer phenotype) provoke differentiation into plasma cells. 70% of the plasma cells produce immunoglobulin (Ig)G and IgM rheumatoid factors; IgG presents as phagocytosed extracellular and intracellular immune complexes. The synovial cells increase in height and in number, and increase the production of synovial fluid.

However, other workers have indicated that hypertrophy and hyperplasia of B cell areas occur releasing activated macrophages, which in turn release interleukin 1 onto the synovial membrane producing the local and systemic effects (Gardner, 1986). Persistent disease is the result of antigen or inadequate T-lymphocyte suppression causing chronic self-perpetuating inflammation.

Chronic inflammatory responses after a time are exudation, destruction, proliferation and repair. There is multiplication by mitotic division of synovial cells, which are normally a single cell layer and become five or seven cells in thickness. As inflammation persists and synovium swells, villi of synovial tissue are formed and tend to project into the joint surface at the articular margins and over the bone ends. These finger like projections of inflamed synovium and granulation tissue are called pannus. This pannus gradually eats into the adjacent cartilage and bone forming erosions and contributing to joint destruction. Further information on inflammation is to be found in Chapter 2.

ONSET

The condition is typically described as a symmetrical polyarthritis, classically starting peripherally and spreading proximally. However, in rare cases the condition can present with a generalised systemic illness or with one of the extra-articular manifestations.

Onset can be acute where the patient will wake one morning with swelling and stiffness of many joints; or onset could be insidious with a general feeling of stiffness and weariness, with maybe the odd joint swelling which may then develop over a period of weeks or months. Those with insidious onset are said to have a worse outcome and this onset is also identified as the most usual form, affecting 60– 70% of patients (Akil & Amos, 1995).

Alternatively the disease can develop from palindromic rheumatoid where the patient will present with acute arthritis of one or two joints which resolves completely in 2 to 3 days, but may occur again after a variable period. This presentation may evolve into typical RA in 25–35% of patients.

Other forms of presentation also exist, particularly in the elderly where shoulder joints may present the first signs and the onset may be heralded by polymyalgia rheumatica (see Chapter 14).

CLINICAL FEATURES

Since the early stage of the condition is one of inflammation the presenting features are those associated with the cardinal signs of inflammation: pain, swelling, heat, loss of function and possibly erythema. These features are related to the joints involved.

The joints of the hand often show the earliest signs of the disease, especially in proximal interphalangeal joints (PIPs) and metacarpophalangeal joints (MCPs). The distal interphalangeal joints (DIPs) are rarely involved in true RA. The carpus, radiocarpal and ulnarcarpal joints are also affected early. Similar joints in the feet are attacked and evidence of the first erosions is often seen in the metatarsophalangeal joints (MTPs). About 10–20% of patients have foot involvement first (Brower, 1995).

Pain

This is the symptom that affects patients most and it is the one towards which many of the interventions selected by the physiotherapist will be directed. Patients will experience pain at rest which may intensify with activity, but which may also lessen after a period of activity. It is often found difficult to separate the pain and the stiffness of RA.

Nature of Pain (Shipley, 1995)
- Localised or diffuse.
- Unilateral or bilateral.
- Aching or sharp.
- Present only with use.
- Present constantly.
- Worse at night or at rest.
- Associated with sensory symptoms.

Much research is currently under way into mechanisms provoking and perpetuating pain. During inflammation, the nervous system undergoes changes that modify the processing of painful stimuli. Exaggerated nervous responses may result from normally non-noxious stimulation such as movement or pressure (Schaible, 1996, Kidd et al., 1996). This sensitisation of pain fibres is a major component of inflammatory joint pain and is induced by inflammatory mediators such as prostaglandins and bradykinins (Schaible & Grubb, 1993). Sensory nerve endings may be irritated by chemical mediators (Kidd, 1996) and by raised pressure within the joint—a mechanism which also occurs in osteoarthritis (OA) (Marks, 1992). Furthermore, it seems that sensory nerves may play an active part in the inflammatory process (Kidd et al., 1996). Anxiety and frustration may also have their effect on the pain perpetuation cycle.

Tenderness

In addition to the presence of pain, tenderness may also be elicited on palpation. This may be due to abnormal intra-articular pressure and sensitisation of nerves leading to secondary hyperalgesia. The presence of tenderness around an affected joint is one of the diagnostic criteria of RA and there are standardised scales available for its measurement, e.g. the Ritchie articular index (Ritchie et al., 1968).

Swelling

Swelling is a characteristic sign of the inflammation of rheumatoid disease. It occurs around the joints and synovial membranes affected and is closely related to the anatomy of the synovial membrane like the disease itself. It is usually symmetrical and peripheral initially involving the MCPs, PIPs, wrists and MTPs. It is caused by synovitis, which results in hypertrophy of the synovial membrane and increased production of synovial fluid.

The synovial swelling of chronic inflammation is typically 'boggy' and may be warm and tender on palpation. The extent of the swelling, its relation to the synovium and the soft boggy feel help to distinguish the swelling of RA from that of other causes, e.g. trauma. Characteristic profiles of many joints and bursae are caused by the synovial swelling, e.g. spindle fingers where PIP joints are affected.

Heat

Joints in an acute inflammatory phase and affected by RA may feel warm to the touch. However, this is not always obvious; patients may report that their joints feel warm, but on objective examination this is undetectable.

Erythema

Erythema is occasionally visible over superficial joints in a stage of acute inflammation and is due to an increase in blood flow in the affected area and chemotaxis.

Loss of Function

Patients with RA will be unable to function at the same level as was possible before the onset of the condition, leading to frustration or despair. The loss of functional ability can be linked directly with pain, deformities, joint instability, muscle weakness, active synovitis, tendon rupture, fatigue and neurological complications, along with early morning stiffness (EMS) for morning functional loss. Physiotherapists and occupational therapists are directly involved with assessing and intervening to amend this affect of rheumatoid disease. This will be discussed further below.

Stiffness

A feature of inflammatory joint disease is EMS, and its duration is used as a measure of the activity of the inflammatory process; the longer the EMS, the more active the disease. In RA, EMS tends to be prolonged (greater than 30 minutes) as compared to the EMS of degenerative conditions which is relatively short-lived (5–10 minutes).

It is also highly incapacitating for patients, rendering them fairly incapable in the morning. The cause of EMS is not fully understood but is thought to be caused by accumulation of oedema containing cells and chemicals in inflamed joints during a relatively still period. These are dispersed with movement during the morning and the patient will start to feel a little easier. The stiffness may return again during the evening. Patients who have poor sleep patterns report that their EMS is lessened following an unsettled night.

Deformity

This occurs in a characteristic pattern according to the joint involved and is due to joint damage altering the joint biomechanics. For example, altered muscle pull may result from an effusion inhibiting the muscles acting on that joint and joint mechanics may be changed due to erosions and subluxation. Tendons and ligaments may be stretched from their anatomical position due to synovial swelling.

Additionally, protective muscle spasm may hold a joint in a position of relative ease, and due to shortening of extra-articular soft tissues such as the capsule or ligaments a fixed deformity may occur. For example, a fixed flexion deformity of the knee joint can easily result from this pattern of events (particularly if the uneducated or non-compliant patient chooses to rest the painful joint in a position of relative ease with a pillow under the knee).

Deformity also can result from an uneven pattern of erosion, for instance in the lateral compartment of the knee, causing a valgus deformity. Frequently a combination of factors is involved. Table 8.1 summarises the common deformitites in RA.

Muscle Wasting

Atrophy of muscles around the affected joints is a feature of RA and also has the effect of enhancing and highlighting deformities and swelling. It is known that muscles are inhibited by the presence of an effusion (Hurley & Newham, 1993) and also that pain prevents full action of muscle. In addition, as joints may not move through their full range of movement it is possible that a part of the muscle is not acting at the full potential and thus preventing the maintenance of power.

Patients may be fearful of moving their joints due to the pain experienced and possibly also for a fear of causing further damage. This may cause muscle wasting through lack of use. Additionally patients occasionally have tender muscles and a low-grade myositis.

Decreased Range of Movement

Loss of joint mobility occurs in RA both directly due to the disease process and to the sequelae of the disease. It occurs in the affected joints as soon as inflammation starts. Inflammation causes pain, thus inhibiting movement.

Hypertrophy and swelling of the synovial membrane may physically prevent a full range of motion being achieved. When inflammation is fully established, end-range movement will be prevented by oedema in the tissues, the growth of the pannus over the bone ends and intra-articular fibrosis. Protective spasm in surrounding muscles further reduces movement.

In addition to these factors, joint motion may be further impeded by involvement of the surrounding soft tissues in the inflammatory process, e.g. tenosynovitis of the extensor tendons passing over the carpus. Muscles weakened by disuse and inhibition may no longer possess the strength to move a painful and stiff joint through a range of motion. Movement may be prohibited

Table 8.1 **Common deformities in rheumatoid arthritis.**

Common deformities in rheumatoid arthritis	
Shoulder girdle	Protracted
Shoulder	Flexion, adduction, medial rotation
Elbow	Flexion, increased carrying angle
Forearm	Pronation
Wrist	Volar subluxation, flexion, radial deviation
Metacarpophalangeal	Volar subluxation, flexion, ulnar deviation
Proximal interphalangeal and distal interphalangeal	Boutonniere (flexed proximal interphalangeal joints, hyperextended distal interphalangeal joints) Swan-neck (hyperextended proximal interphalangeal joints, flexed distal interphalangeal joints)
Hips	Flexion, adduction, lateral rotation
Knees	Flexion, valgus
Ankles	Valgus
Metatarsophalangeal	Plantar subluxation, hyperextension
Proximal interphalangeal and distal interphalangeal	Flexion

mechanically by subluxation of the joint and by the nature of the instability caused by erosions and ligamentous laxity. Patients may also be afraid of movement due to pain or lack of knowledge of the disease.

EXTRA-ARTICULAR MANIFESTATIONS OF RA

RA is a systemic disorder and the disease can manifest itself in a number of different organs. Whilst these areas are not specifically the province of the physiotherapist, it must be recognised that in order to adopt a holistic approach to management of the patient with RA these features should be considered and may affect intervention.

Extra-articular manifestations of the disease tend to occur in those patients with long-standing and severe disease and in those who are sero-positive to rheumatoid factor (RF), particularly those possessing high titres of RF (see Chapter 2). Occasionally systemic manifestations of RA may be the presenting feature and could present something of a diagnostic dilemma.

Fatigue

Patients with RA may complain of profound fatigue or unexplained tiredness. Some patients may not recognise this feature as part of the disease and dismiss their fatigue as one of the problems of trying to function with constant pain. This feeling of weariness can contribute to other features of the disease such as general malaise, which is an unexplained and perhaps unusual feeling of generally being unwell, possibly also with anorexia and weight loss, although this could be multifactorial. It may also contribute to mild depression.

Anaemia

Around 50% of patients with RA will have measurable anaemia that tends to reflect disease activity. The haemoglobin (Hb) content of the red cell may run as low as 6 g/dl and frequently the rheumatoid patient will have a Hb which will not rise above 9 g/dl, where the healthy adult Hb is 12–14 g/dl in males and 10–12 g/dl in females. The severity of the anaemia generally varies inversely with the erythrocyte sedimentation rate (ESR) (Turnbull, 1995). It is usually normochromic and normocytic, meaning that the red blood cells are the normal size and colour.

Causes of Anaemia in Rheumatoid Arthritis

The mechanism of anaemia of chronic disease is complex but indicates that the red cells are unable to incorporate and utilise any iron, so attempting to treat with iron supplements would be futile.

- Iron deficiency – frequently related to drug therapy (particularly non steroidal anti-inflammatory drugs (NSAIDs)) causing gastro-intestinal bleeding, but may also be caused by poor diet or poor absorption.
- Folic acid deficiency is less common and mainly as a result of pregnancy in RA or reduced intake through diet.
- Vitamin B deficiency in RA is generally the combination of RA with pernicious anaemia.

- Autoimmune haemolytic anaemia is occasionally seen in patients with Feltys syndrome (see below).
- Bone marrow hypoplasia is a rare but serious complication of Felty's syndrome or of drug treatment (Turnbull, 1995).

The anaemia may improve with disease control and rectification of deficiencies, e.g. vitamin B12. Folic acid can also help to elevate the Hb but iron supplements are not helpful. Blood transfusions may be required in some severely anaemic patients prior to surgery.

Felty's Syndrome

This condition, named after the physician who first described it in 1924, occurs in around 1% of the rheumatoid population (Campion & Maddison, 1986). It is typically a combination of RA, leucopenia and splenomegaly; it is postulated that the condition does not occur by chance but represents the patient with many extra-articular manifestations and particularly severe disease. Patients are prone to infections and may have hyper pigmentation of the skin or liver abnormalities. These patients are more likely to develop vasculitis (Matteson *et al.*, 1995). Management is aimed at the rheumatoid disease but can involve splenectomy. Morbidity and mortality are high with infection being the main cause of death (Campion & Maddison, 1986).

Nodules

Subcutaneous nodules may affect around 20% of patients with RA (Figure 8.1). They occur mainly in the sero-positive person and tend to mirror the disease, often disappearing when the condition is inactive. They are not tender and can occur anywhere although the commonest sites are pressure areas of fibrous connective tissue and include the extensor surfaces of the forearm, the posterior aspect of the Achilles tendon, the spines of the scapulae, the ischial tuberosities and the sacrum. The histology is typical and diagnostic, consisting of a central area of fibrinoid necrosis with a rim of pallisade cells (mainly histocytes) surrounded with chronic inflammatory cells; occasionally the central portion may become fluid and suppurate discharging pus. Similar nodules may occur in the heart and lung.

The Eye

Patients with evidence of vasculitis may be susceptible to episcleritis, which usually resolves. Scleritis however is much more serious and can lead to visual impairment and blindness. It is an inflammation of the sclera, causing an initial redness and often has an insidious onset although pain, sometimes severe, is a later feature. Eventually the choroid layer takes on a bluish tinge and is visible through the sclera. Rheumatoid nodules can form in the sclera and sloughing of a nodule in this position can cause a hole through which the contents of the eye can herniate. This is an unpleasant condition called scleromalacia perforans (Buchanan & Keen, 1986).

Keratoconjunctivitis sicca can occur in around 10% of rheumatoid patients. It is a condition caused by a failure of the lachrymal gland to secrete, causing a dry eye that feels

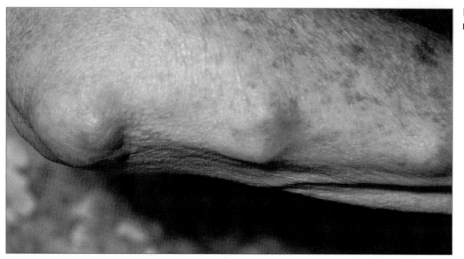

Figure 8.1 **Rheumatoid nodule.**

sore and gritty; untreated, this can lead to conjunctivitis or erosions of the cornea (see Sjögrens syndrome, Chapter 16).

The Skin

Thinning of the skin is common in RA and reflects the duration of the disease and the age of the patient, although it may also be due to steroid therapy. Atrophy and bruising of the skin of the forearms and the shins may be apparent and spontaneous ulceration of the lower leg can occur. Palmar erythema is an unexplained feature of RA. Vasculitis also manifests itself with skin lesions (see below).

The Heart

Involvement of the heart is rarely diagnosed in life, although 40% patients may show evidence of chronic pericarditis at post-mortem (Sokoloff, 1953). Pericarditis has been found in sero-positive patients with nodules (Hara *et al.*, 1990). Valves can be involved with nodules on the cusps interfering with opening; deposits in the myocardium can cause conduction defects (Carpenter *et al.*, 1967).

The Lung

Pleurisy is a common finding at post-mortem (Butler, 1990) and patients often have a higher incidence of chest infections than the general population. Pleural effusions have been observed in 10% of patients with rheumatoid pneumoconiosis (Caplan, 1953), especially in sero-positive males; sometimes these were extensive, causing pleural thickening. Fibrosing alveolitis can also occur, causing progressive dyspnoea and cough. Rheumatoid nodules in the lung are diagnosed by excluding other causes, e.g. tuberculosis and carcinoma; again males are affected more often than females and they also often exhibit other nodules elsewhere (Matteson *et al.*, 1995).

Bone

Peri-articular osteoporosis is an early diagnostic feature of RA on X-ray. Generalised osteoporosis is also common in RA and there are many ways of explaining its aetiology. This issue is explored further in Chapter 15.

Vasculitis

Inflammation of blood vessels occurs mainly in those patients who are sero-positive for rheumatoid factor, who have been previously treated with several disease modifying anti-rheumatic drugs (DMARDs), are middle aged, and smokers (Breedveld, 1997). It causes necrosis of the vessel walls and can present as splinter haemorrhages or small nailfold lesions, about 0.5–1 mm in diameter, indicating an area of tissue necrosis distal to the inflamed artery. These lesions, showing digital endarteritis, are found in around 8% of patients with RA. They usually present on the side of the fingernail and in themselves are harmless and insignificant, although they may be painful. They are however an indication of possible serious systemic involvement and should always be taken seriously. The physiotherapist should warn the medical staff of the presence of nail fold lesions since drug therapy may require alteration. Those with minor manifestations of vasculitis will probably be monitored regularly. The patients with medium/large vessel vasculitis are treated with prednisolone and either azathioprine or cyclophosphamide (Breedveld, 1997).

Additionally vasculitis may present as skin necrosis, leg ulcers, areas of peripheral gangrene or as mononeuritis multiplex. The latter is caused by interruption of the blood supply to the nerve, and can present as a sensory neuropathy in a 'stocking and glove' distribution or as wrist drop and foot drop.

Clinical manifestations may thus range from benign nailfold infarcts to mononeuritis multiplex, gangrene and internal organ infarction. Around 10% of patients with RA develop peripheral neuritis due to vasculitis (Chakravarty, 1997). The presentations of systemic vasculitis are many and clearly vary with the vessels involved and their distribution (see Chapter 14).

Raynaud's Phenomenon

Raynaud's is a vasospasm of the vaso vasorum of the digital vessels. It is usually provoked by a change in temperature, emotional disturbance, trauma and certain chemicals (particularly those in cigarette smoke), and may precede the RA by many years. Classically Raynaud's is a tricyclic phenomenon where the skin exhibits three different colours, i.e. pallor, cyanosis and rubor (Belch, 1987), associated with pain. The physiotherapist should be alert to these changes since their presence may affect the choice of intervention. The management of Raynaud's is described in Chapter 13.

Amyloidosis

Amyloid is a protein crystal that can be deposited in organs such as the kidney, heart or gut, hampering the function of that organ. It used to be associated with tuberculosis, bronchiectasis and osteomyelitis although RA is now the most common cause, particularly severe long-standing illness. The occurrence of amyloidosis is rare and the outcome is usually poor due to organ dysfunction.

DIAGNOSIS

Diagnosis is usually based on history, clinical findings, X-ray examination and blood tests. For the purposes of research and in order to standardise the diagnostic criteria various standards have been drawn up; the American Rheumatism Association (Arnett et al., 1988) and the New York Criteria (Bennett & Burch, 1967) are two sets of criteria commonly used although they often yield different results.

NEW YORK CRITERIA FOR RA (EPIDEMIOLOGICAL) 1968

- A history of an episode of joint pain involving three or more joints (PIPs, MCPs, MTPs of one side count as a single joint).
- Swelling, limitation of motion or subluxation of at least three limb joints, observed by the physician, two of which are symmetrical. One of the involved joints must be in the hand or foot.
- X-ray evidence of erosive arthritis in the hands or feet of grade 2–4 severity.
- A positive serological reaction for rheumatoid factor determined by a method which is controlled by periodic testing of reference sera.

The revised American Rheumatism Association (ARA) criteria of 1987 are listed in Table 8.2.

Radiological Examination

Radiological examination can be very revealing both in terms of the diagnosis of the condition and in its subsequent management. X-rays will show any bony damage along with soft tissue swelling and deformity, and will hence highlight disease progression with possible consequences for management. X-rays remain the radiological examination of choice for diagnosis and monitoring of the rheumatoid patient despite the development of more technologically sophisticated techniques.

The hands and the feet are normally examined along with other symptomatic areas. Evidence of RA is usually initially apparent in the peripheries; in addition, when X-rays of the hands and feet are taken many more synovial joints are shown than in an examination of the knee for example. X-rays of hands and feet are sometimes performed for exclusion purposes. The X-ray changes in RA are:

- Juxta-articular osteoporosis.
- Soft tissue swelling.
- Deformity.
- Erosions at joint margins.
- Decreased joint space.

X-ray examination is a requirement for patients with potential cervical spine disease who are about to undergo anaesthesia (Soar & Handel, 1995). As a base line marker for these patients, any subsequent progression of subluxation

Table 8.2 **The revised American Rheumatism Association criteria of 1987.**

The revised American Rheumatism Association criteria of 1987	
Morning stiffness	Duration: at least 1 hour, lasting 6 weeks
Arthritis of at least 3 areas	Soft tissue swelling or exudation >6 weeks
Arthritis of hand joints	Wrist, metacarpophalangeal or proximal interphalangeal lasting >6 weeks
Symmetrical arthritis	At least one area, lasting >6 weeks
Rheumatoid nodules	As observed by physician
Serum rheumatoid factor	As assessed by a method positive in less than 5% of control subjects

can be detected. It is important that atlanto-axial instability is measured and monitored. The distance of the arch of the atlas from the odontoid process is measured in flexion and extension on a lateral view of the cervical spine. The stability of the cervical spine is of particular importance to the physiotherapist since flexion and extension should be avoided in those patients with potential and actual instability. Protection may also be required in the hydrotherapy pool during floating procedures.

Other methods of imaging are also available to evaluate difficult problems, e.g. magnetic resonance imaging (MRI, see Figure 8.2), computerised tomography, ultrasound, scintigraphy etc.

Examination of Blood Parameters

Blood tests will reveal evidence of inflammation which is indicative of RA although not specific to the disease, e.g. high ESR, low Hb. Other markers in the serum indicate the presence of RA with a higher degree of accuracy, e.g. C-reactive protein (CRP), plasma viscosity and Ig estimation including RF; these tests are described in Chapter 2.

MANAGEMENT

Management of the patient with RA is a multidisciplinary process and as such is an excellent example of patient centred teamwork. Features of the multidisciplinary team (MDT) in RA have been discussed in Chapter 1. Early referral to experts and early intervention is currently seen as the key to success in prevention of major functional incapacity in the patient with RA (Emery & Salmon, 1995). Delay in therapy is likely to result in some loss of functional status

(Emery, 1994). Emery also indicates that 'inflammation is both treatable and reversible, the degree to which functional status can be improved is dependent on both its duration and its extent'.

The rheumatologist will be keen to select the optimal drug management for the patient based on results of biochemical and immunological data. Therapy aims to slow down or halt the rheumatological processes and help to preserve joint integrity and function. Adequate pain relief will enable the patient to comply with the physiotherapy programme and to maintain some part of a normal life. The rheumatologist will manage the patient's condition and refer on to other agencies such as the therapy professions. The team will review the patient at regular intervals to assess the efficacy of drug therapy and monitor the progress of the disease. This assessment is variously conducted in the outpatient clinic, in the community clinic, the patient's home or the physiotherapy clinic. In addition the patient may also be referred to the clinical nurse specialist who runs a nurse led clinic alongside the physician and monitors the patient for side effects of any drug therapy as well as offering general advice about the condition and considering referral to other professionals if necessary.

Some discussion concerning the distribution of tasks within the team may have occurred. It could also be the duty of the rheumatologist or the nurse to administer certain health assessment questionnaires and disease profiling tools, which will be briefly mentioned below. Patient global assessment, pain score and articular index can be completed at each attendance (Symmons, 1994). Simple measures of disease activity that may affect delivery of physiotherapy modalities include EMS, ESR and Hb.

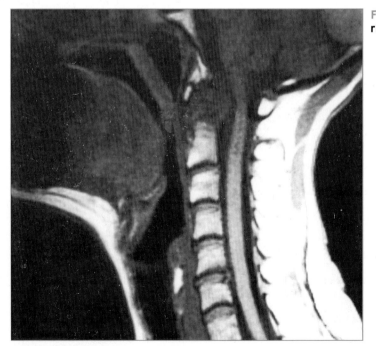

Figure 8.2 Magnetic resonance image of rheumatoid cervical spine.

PHYSIOTHERAPY

Ideally, the physiotherapist needs to meet the patient as soon as possible after diagnosis, often being present in clinic with the rheumatologist when the diagnosis and possible management of the condition is revealed to the patient.

The involvement of the MDT at the earliest possible time is advantageous to both the patient and the professional since coping strategies and good joint protection habits can be introduced. In some units, it is the duty of the physiotherapist to co-ordinate referrals to other professionals, or the consultant may assume this responsibility. In other units, it is the duty of the rheumatology nurse to plan the patient's care (Maycock, 1991). Health professionals then have the opportunity of early assessment and intervention to instruct the patient in joint care and protection before poor patterns of joint use have been allowed to develop. In addition, education shortly after onset has been shown to be beneficial in prevention of anxiety and assists in compliance (Tucker & Kirwan, 1991). Early intervention is currently seen as the key to success in prevention of functional loss and enabling patients to manage their disease themselves (Emery, 1994).

ASSESSMENT

Accurate assessment is clearly an essential requirement prior to any intervention. In most patients this should be geared towards function since some restriction in joint range is often inevitable and acceptable to both patient and practitioner. Self report questionnaires, e.g. the Health Assessment Questionnaire (HAQ) or Arthritis Impact Measurement Scale (AIMS), can aid assessment and are less demanding of time than demonstration. The patient may, in addition, be required to demonstrate skills and methods of working to the occupational therapist at some stage during the initial fact-gathering period.

Subjective Assessment

This can be a very time consuming procedure and it may be necessary to conduct the interview over several sessions, enabling the physiotherapist and the patient to develop a rapport which may facilitate the disclosure of further important facts.

As well as the usual details such as general medical history and history of the present complaint, it is vital that the therapist ascertains a picture of the patient's ability to cope within his or her own boundaries since rectification of these problems will be the goal of the therapeutic intervention. An accurate account of the nature, severity and diurnal variations of the individual's pain must be obtained, as advice and therapeutic options to alleviate and assist in managing pain are available. Patient's perceptions of their worst problems will assist the setting of priorities and, along with their functional aspirations, may help dictate some goals. Quality of life issues must also be considered. Some indication of change over time may corroborate this information. Duration of EMS may indicate disease activity, although it is highly subjective and variable. It may however give the physiotherapist some idea of functional problems.

Some indication from the patient of the previous therapy along with previous medication and the efficacy of the total package is a useful gauge for future therapy. It also serves as a very crude assessment of the patient's attitude to the disease—for example, how well does the patient recollect details of drugs previously administered? Does the patient leave everything to the doctor or can he or she recall all drugs taken and any side effects? What information is forthcoming regarding previous physiotherapy—have any exercises or advice been continued?

A succinct social history is of great importance in the rheumatoid patient, as family members may ultimately become carers who also will require support from the MDT. Additionally rheumatoid patients should be spared an over protective family and ideally strive to maintain their independence.

Measurement Tools

These are reliable valid scales to assess various aspects of the life of rheumatoid patients in addition to their attitude to the disease. The oldest disability measurement tool is the Steinbrocker functional index (Steinbrocker, 1949), revised by Hochberg and colleagues in 1992. This index categorises patients into four functional classes; it lacks sensitivity to change and has thus been superseded by instruments that are more sensitive.

The modified Stanford HAQ (Kirwan & Reeback, 1986) is a reliable measure of functional ability listing 20 everyday tasks and asking the patient to grade the difficulty in performing these jobs, from 'without any difficulty' to 'unable to do so'. Standardised methods of scoring are used. The modified HAQ is widely used in the UK. It is easily understood by the patient and requires only a few minutes to complete.

Other methods of measuring the effect of joint disease include the AIMS (Meenan et al., 1992) and monitor general well-being as well as function and disease activity. The AIMS when used in drug trials is able to detect clinically meaningful differences between groups (Bell et al., 1990). Bell also indicates that the best measure has yet to be developed, one which is sensitive, reliable and valid and assesses function, health status and utility for the individual patient (Bell et al., 1990).

Psychological measurements are utilised quite widely to assess the effect of the disease on patients and their coping strategies. The Hospital Anxiety and Depression scale (HAD) (Zigmond & Snaith, 1983) measures emotional status and attitude to illness. This is a major consideration in patients with chronic illness. Assistance with coming to terms with disability and in developing coping strategies may be necessary. The Beck depression inventory is also used, although mainly for research purposes with specific patient groups (Beck et al., 1988).

Other scales provide a comprehensive range of facts. The SF36 (Ware & Sherbourne, 1992) and the Nottingham Health Profile (McEwen, 1993) are generic measures and may not be considered specific enough for people with RA in certain circumstances (Bowling, 1995).

Recently Quality of Life assessment procedures have received growing interest. A measurement tool has been developed to identify specific aspects of RA not previously considered (Whalley *et al.*, 1997). The RA Quality of Life (RAQoL) instrument measures pain and fatigue along with other disease specific issues. It was developed using a qualitative approach to produce a quantitative tool from the results of interviews with patients with RA. It has been found to have good face and content validity and is well accepted by patients, taking about 6 minutes to complete (De Jong *et al.*, 1997)

Examples of Items in the RAQoL

- I have to go to bed earlier than I would like to.
- I'm afraid of people touching me.
- It's difficult to find comfortable shoes that I like.
- I avoid crowds because of my condition.
- I have difficulty dressing.
- I find it difficult to walk to the shops.
- Jobs about the house take me a long time.
- I sometimes have problems using the toilet.
- I often get frustrated.
- I have to keep stopping what I am doing to rest.
- I have difficulty using a knife and fork.
- I find it hard to concentrate.
- Sometimes I just want to be left alone.
- I find it difficult to walk very far.
- I try to avoid shaking hands with people.
- I often get depressed.
- I'm unable to join in activities with my family or friends.
- I have problems taking a bath or shower.
- I sometimes have a good cry because of my condition.
- My condition limits the places I can go.
- I feel tired whatever I do.
- I feel dependent on others.
- My condition is always on my mind.
- I often get angry with myself.
- It's too much effort to go out and see people.
- I sleep badly at night.
- I find it difficult to take care of the people I am close to.
- I feel that I'm unable to control my condition.
- I avoid physical contact.
- I'm limited in the clothes I can wear.

Further evaluation in Europe is proceeding.

Visual Analogue Scales (VAS) (Huskisson, 1982) are another widely utilised but rather subjective instrument which can indicate levels of particular disease features, e.g. pain/stiffness/disability/frustration (see Chapter 4).

Objective Measures

Various scales and measurement tools exist to enable the clinician to quantify the severity of the patients' RA. These tend to be numerical measures which facilitate the use of the material for research purposes either currently or at a later date and also assist the audit process. In addition as a serial index, disease activity can be monitored and efficacy of therapy assessed. Work is proceeding to develop further

the existing scales and items mentioned here may thus be superseded rapidly.

The Ritchie Index (Ritchie *et al.*, 1968)

This is an established method of recording joint tenderness and is widely used. Pressure is applied around the joint margin of every joint, except for the hips, cervical spine, talocalcaneal and midtarsal joints, where tenderness is assessed by passive movement. The MCPs and PIPs are scored as 1 joint. As the index is calculated by the patient's response to palpation, it is important that the same operator is used for the same patient on each assessment since inter-observer agreement is low and observers vary in the amount of pressure they use (Thompson *et al.*, 1991).

Figure 8.3 shows a Ritchie articular index chart: the joints are scored 0 for no reaction; 1 for a complaint of pain; 2 for a complaint of pain and a wince; score of 3 for wincing and withdrawing the limb. The total score is the sum of the individual joint scores.

It can be easily appreciated that operator pressure and patient reaction to this is variable and that the grading of reaction is fairly coarse. The Ritchie index has been found to have an insignificant correlation with CRP levels (Thompson *et al.*, 1987); this study found that weighting for joint surface area improved correlation with CRP.

Thompson/Kirwan Articular Index

This is a weighted scoring system that also indicates the presence of swelling (Figure 8.4). Weighting depends on the size of the joint and thus the amount of inflammed synovium. The knee, if swollen and tender, scores 95 and the ankle joint scores 32 (Thompson *et al.*, 1987). It was agreed that for good correlation with measures of the inflammatory state certain joints could be omitted, but simultaneous tenderness and swelling must be included.

It can be appreciated that the inclusion of joint counts within an objective assessment by the physiotherapist will add time to the procedure, but it will also contribute increased validity and reproducibility. The extra time required has been estimated at 13 minutes per patient (Bell *et al.*, 1990). In addition, scores and counts can be plotted visually to aid evidence of therapy efficacy and to help evaluation of management protocols.

Recognising the significance of these measurement trends could be used as a teaching tool for receptive patients to attempt to evaluate their own joints and disease activity.

Joint Assessment

In addition to the holistic recording of active joints within the body, the physiotherapist will require an accurate documentation of the range of motion, muscle power, ligamentous laxity, deformity and function at each joint including those apparently not affected by the current flare-up. It is important in patients with chronic progressive conditions like RA that regular assessments are undertaken, and therapy regimes updated and progressed to incorporate fresh problems. Results can be recorded on serial data charts and trends can thus be simply identified. It is useful to measure the patient at the same time of day each visit to account for diurnal variations.

Range of Movement

This can be measured using a goniometer (Figure 8.5), or by eye in the experienced therapist. Video recorders are useful, as are methods using tape measurement between bony points. Active and passive range of movement (ROM) with sensitive application of over pressure must be recorded.

Assessment of the end feel of the joint is important, as this will help to predict the likely success of physiotherapeutic measures and assist in identifying limiting features which may benefit from therapeutic intervention.

Muscle Power

The Oxford scale of muscle power is currently the objective measure of choice for rheumatoid patients. It does however have many limitations concerning accuracy and sensitivity,

joints examined		not tender (0)	tender (+1)	tender and winced (+2)	tender, winced and withdrew (+3)	joint score
temporomandibular						
cervical spine*						
acromioclavicular						
sternoclavicular						
shoulders	L					
	R					
elbows	L					
	R					
wrists	L					
	R					
MCP	L					
	R					
PIP	L					
	R					
hips*	L					
	R					
knees	L					
	R					
ankles	L					
	R					
talocalcaneal*	L					
	R					
midtarsal*	L					
	R					
metatarsals	L					
	R					
* passive movement					total =	

Figure 8.3 **Ritchie Articular Index chart.**

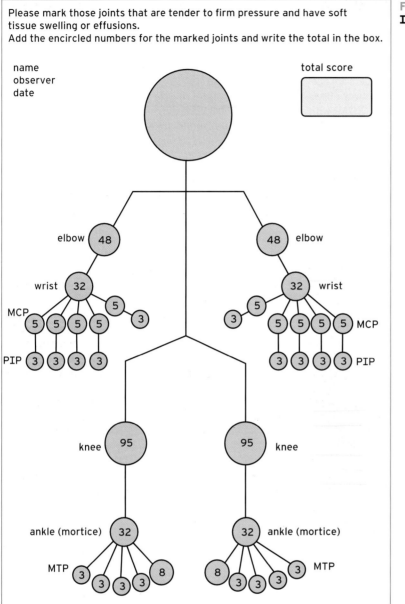

Please mark those joints that are tender to firm pressure and have soft tissue swelling or effusions.
Add the encircled numbers for the marked joints and write the total in the box.

name
observer
date

total score

elbow 48 · 48 elbow

wrist 32 · 32 wrist

MCP 5 5 5 5 5 · 5 5 5 5 5 MCP

PIP 3 3 3 3 · 3 3 3 3 PIP

knee 95 · 95 knee

ankle (mortice) 32 · 32 ankle (mortice)

MTP 3 3 3 3 8 · 8 3 3 3 3 MTP

Figure 8.4 Thompson/Kirwan Index chart.

and involves a high degree of subjectivity on the part of the examiner. Power should be tested at different points within the available range, avoiding provocation of pain if possible. Hand held dynamometers are used in some departments to assess strength with greater accuracy; they have been little evaluated currently and are not in widespread use.

Various finely tuned technologically advanced computerised machines are now available to record both isotonic and isometric muscle power. However, while these confer a high degree of measurement accuracy, they may not be appropriate for the regular rheumatoid patient. Rehabilitation in these patients is geared towards gross function, since it is unlikely that they will regain full ROM or muscle power due to the structural changes in the joints previously mentioned. However, these sophisticated machines are used widely in research and will ultimately become available for the assessor of the rheumatoid patient.

Deformity
All deformities should be recorded since they require regular monitoring to assess change (Figure 8.6 shows a rheumatoid knee). Degree of deformity and whether a fixed position has been acquired or whether the abnormality is correctable are also relevant statistics since they will assist the management programme. Further assessment will then reveal any change and indicate an alteration in strategy.

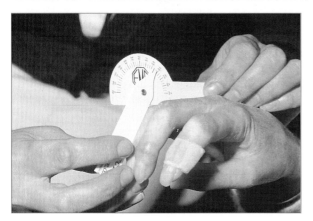

Figure 8.5 **Goniometry of hands.**

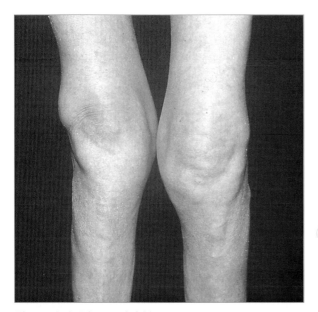

Figure 8.6 **Rheumatoid knee.**

Ligamentous Laxity

All relevant ligaments particularly those of weight bearing joints must be stressed to assess their integrity. Measures such as increasing muscle power and provision of supporting splints may be required to protect these structures.

Function

Patients will often volunteer information regarding their functional capabilities during the subjective interview. It is vital, however, that activities are checked by the physiotherapist or the occupational therapist to assess quality of movement, possible stress on lax ligaments and to verify the patient's report. Furthermore, it may be possible to suggest easier ways to achieve the same outcome, enabling the patient to conserve energy and protect their joints. Functional tasks are often more appropriate outcome measures for rheumatoid patients than some finer measure which will have little significance for the patient's activities.

The physiotherapist can decide which functional measures should be considered following evaluation of the subjective and objective examinations. This task may be undertaken in consultation with the occupational therapist and can include items such as:

- Ability to put on a cardigan unaided in 5 seconds.
- Brushing the whole head of hair.
- Writing one's name.
- Putting on shoes and socks.
- Sitting to standing—how many times in 1 minute.
- Step ups—how many times in 1 minute.

PHYSIOTHERAPY INTERVENTIONS

The role of the physiotherapist in caring for the patient with RA is paramount. In some units, the physiotherapists run clinics of their own to assess new patients and to monitor their progress and will then co-ordinate their therapy. In other areas the physiotherapist attends the rheumatology clinic and discusses possible management strategies with the consultant and the patient following diagnosis, indicating possible modes of delivery.

Alternatively there may be no specialised physiotherapy service available and the patient will be referred from the out-patient clinic to the physiotherapy department for management. However, in any management structure communication between members of the team is vital for efficient use of scarce resources.

The physiotherapist will use the available tools following an accurate assessment to subjectively and objectively identify the presenting problems (Stewart 1996).

Ice

The use of cryotherapy in the management of chronic inflammatory conditions has long been a tradition. There is however little objective evidence to reinforce this. Ice packs applied to the affected joint cool the skin temperature which is possibly elevated from the inflammation. Cooling will diminish the rate of swelling and production of irritants and so alleviate some of the pain (Low & Reed, 1990). Many studies have supported the theory that cold therapy can help to reduce pain (Benson & Copp, 1974). Contra-indications to the application of this modality should of course be strictly observed, particularly when there is the potential of vasculitis or Raynaud's. Ice can be applied regularly (possibly twice each day if the skin condition allows); it can also be indicated as a treatment at home when frozen peas can be substituted for the flaked ice which is usually available in physiotherapy departments. Commercial cold packs can be used in addition but lack the 'mouldability' of a pack of frozen peas.

Heat

The application of heat to an inflamed joint is not recommended since it may serve to further increase the inflammation already present within the joint. However, during disease remissions and for chronic rather than acutely inflamed joints heat is much appreciated by patients. It reduces pain attributed to muscle spasm, has a sedative effect on sensory nerve endings and may activate the pain gate (Low & Reed, 1990). Mild superficial heat may facilitate stretching of rheumatoid joints as increased collagen extensibility occurs at elevated temperatures (Lehman *et al.*, 1970). Heat can be applied in the form of a hot water bottle, infra red lamp, wax bath or a commercially available electrically heated pad. There are in addition further advantages in the use of wax therapy as a heat treatment, as the oils in the paraffin wax may help to moisturise dry skin. The wax can also be used as a form of resisted exercise therapy following removal from the joint!

It could probably be said that the use of heat in the rheumatoid patient is in order to prepare the joint for exercise.

Exercise

This is probably one of the most important areas for physiotherapists to use their skill, imagination and expertise. Therapeutic exercise is recognised as one of the main self management strategies for the patient with RA. The prescription of the exercise programme will vary with the purpose of the exercise, the activity of the disease, the non-articular manifestations and the facilities available.

Patients may be treated in a gym, an exercise area, a hydrotherapy pool (or a swimming pool!), a hospital ward and their own home. The programme should be versatile and adaptable; it must be mentioned to the patient that though accuracy in the starting position is important, there are several ways to perform an exercise to achieve similar effects.

While muscle strength, endurance and aerobic capacity are decreased in the rheumatoid patient (Ekdahl & Brown, 1992), exercise may lead to improvement in disease status, e.g. reduction in joint pain, swelling and EMS (Minor & Brown, 1993). Range of movement exercise may also aid joint metabolism and blood flow, consequently reducing oedema and stiffness (Gerber, 1990). There is some evidence that patients undergoing moderate conditioning exercise have some immunological gains (Hoffman-Goetze & Klarlund, 1994) and improvement of psychological well-being (Perlman *et al.*, 1990). It has been suggested that functional performance in the rheumatoid hand correlates with strength (Hoenig *et al.*, 1993), the conclusion of this study indicating that a scheme of hand exercises performed for 10–20 minutes twice daily improves grip strength.

Training for gains in strength should involve careful application of resistance to avoid damage to already stretched ligaments. Patients will require regular review to ensure progression in strength, function and endurance. Correct performance should also be monitored.

Gait and Function

Gait re-education is one of the areas of involvement for the physiotherapist treating the patient with RA. The intervention required will depend on the roles of the physiotherapist and the occupational therapist within that team.

Walking aids must be chosen with regard to the state of the upper limb joints, since these will be taking some of the patient's weight. Sticks and elbow crutches are available with moulded handles which alter the weight bearing areas of the hand for those patients unable to use conventional grips. If the patient has painful or restricted wrists it may be preferable to take the weight through the forearms and shoulders using a gutter frame. Gait re-education must be functional and directed at the patient's objectives.

Electrotherapy

It is not proposed to discuss electrotherapy in depth here; its use is indicated along basic principles, and is discussed in the relevant texts. Laser has been found to be useful in pain management (Colov *et al.*, 1987) and in the improvement of hand function (Goldman *et al.*, 1980). Pulsed short-wave can also be used beneficially since it is known to reduce inflammation and swelling (Low & Reed, 1990).

Hydrotherapy

Exercise in water is used widely in the management of patients with RA, although there is little objective evaluation of its therapeutic properties. It is an ancient panacea and one surrounded by much mystique; in addition it is an expensive modality so the physiotherapist must ensure the intervention is appropriate.

The use and effects of hydrotherapy have been discussed in various texts, e.g. Hall *et al.*, 1990, Golland 1981; it is helpful as buoyancy greatly assists the rheumatoid patient who has difficulty mobilising due to weightbearing through painful and unstable joints. The temperature of the water, normally around 36°C, helps to relax superficial muscle spasm and relieves pain. Exercises can be graded using turbulence and buoyancy to strengthen weakened muscles gradually without stressing the joints.

Contra-indications for immersing patients in water must be observed and their safety considered at all times, particularly those who are immuno-suppressed and those with systemic manifestations of their disease. Instability of the cervical spine should be considered a precaution rather than a contra-indication. Additionally there are also people who are hydrophobic; for this group exercise on land would be a more suitable alternative.

However, for the rheumatoid patient who enjoys water and for whom EMS is a major problem a morning hydrotherapy session is the best way to start the day! It provides warmth, movement, increases confidence, improves range of movement and muscle tone and starts the endorphins circulating. Furthermore, it is an excellent precursor to exercise performance.

Education

This is documented and well supported as a major contribution to the overall management of the patient with RA, both individually and in groups. See Chapter 1.

Splinting

Although there is little documented support for this method of intervention it is in widespread use, and is covered in Chapters 6 and 17.

CASE HISTORY OF MR B

Mr B was 52 years old when RA was diagnosed in 1988. He had worked first as a miner, then, following redundancy, as a bus driver. The patient was not in employment when first seen by the rheumatology department in March 1993 after transferring from another hospital. Medical history was quite eventful and included:

- 1959 Closed fracture of scaphoid complicated by non-union and pseudoarthrosis.
- 1970 Lumbar disc degeneration.
- 1973 Knee injury (unspecified).
- 1974 Fracture of phalanges of hand. Gall bladder calculi, exploratory laparotomy.
- 1986 OA in hands noted; carpal tunnel release later that year.
- 1987 Morton's metatarsalgia.
- 1988 RA diagnosed.
- 1990 Ptosis of eyelid, due to D-penicillamine-induced myasthenia gravis.
- 1991 Surgery for haemorrhoids.

March 1993 First admission to this hospital. Medication at this time was diclofenac and co-proxamol; the patient had found salazopyrin ineffective, and had a rash with gold. Main joints affected were the R shoulder, R wrist, R ankle and both knees. The patient responded well to daily hydrotherapy and the ward exercise class, and was started on methotrexate. The diclofenac was changed to a diclofenac/misoprostol combination.

In October the patient had a chest infection, and continued with intermittent sore throats until February 1994. In May a chest X-ray revealed nodular shadowing upper bases, and occasional night sweats were reported; investigations for tuberculosis were negative. The diagnosis was presumed pneumonitis, and methotrexate was stopped.

In the meantime, the patient had a course of out-patient physiotherapy aimed at increasing muscle power around his R knee, which had previously required aspiration of a large effusion and instillation of steroid. Ultrasound was administered to painful MTP joints, and the patient was provided with a Fischer stick to aid mobilisation. Hydrotherapy was also helpful for the L shoulder and elbow pain. The occupational therapy department was involved in the provision of splints for night and day time, in addition to a bath board and toilet seat raise. Social services arranged for the installation of a stair rail and an armchair of suitable height.

July 1994 Methotrexate was restarted briefly. A short time later, Mr B was admitted as an emergency with pericarditis, swollen tonsils and elevated white cell count, an ESR of 78 and a CRP165. Platelets were 480, dropping over the next few days to 23. The patient was diagnosed with auto-immune thrombocytopaenia and possible systemic lupus erythematosus (SLE); methotrexate was stopped again, and he was started on 60 mg prednisolone. The patient's platelet count recovered within days, and the ESR also dropped to 17. During this admission Mr B was assessed by the physiotherapist and it was felt that the patient's medical condition contra-indicated much active physiotherapy. The patient's joints however benefited from the high dose of steroid; it proved extremely difficult to reduce the dose. In August Mr B was readmitted with deep vein thrombosis (DVT) and possible pulmonary embolus. Warfarin was commenced.

In April 1995 azathioprine was started, but had to be stopped in July due to proteinuria. Nephrotic syndrome was diagnosed and Mr B was prescribed an increased dose of steroid. A rectal biopsy at this time showed no evidence of amyloid. Mr B's RF showed a weakly positive result. It had previously been negative, which was surprising in someone with such clinically active disease (and confirms the idea that the patient is treated rather than the blood tests). In September Mr B's bone mineral density was measured and found to be decreased; he was started on alendronate.

Mr B was referred to the ear, nose and throat department in February 1996 complaining of difficulty in swallowing. Nothing abnormal was detected on laryngoscopy, so it was suggested that RA could be affecting the cricoarytenoid joints. Raynaud's and Sjögren's syndromes were also diagnosed on this occasion. In March Mr B was admitted again, this time for knee injections and physiotherapy. The patient had a markedly reduced ROM in his wrist joints, with only a quarter range of flexion and extension. Shoulders were also reduced with flexion of 120^0. The patient's R knee had $0-115^0$ movement and L knee $5-120^0$. Muscle power was globally decreased and the patient was having increasing difficulty coping at home. Mr B's wife was the main carer. The patient's HAQ scores were dropping (from 1.75 to 1.5), reflecting disease activity and increasing dependence.

By August 1996 the patient's prednisolone had been reduced to 7 mg daily. Consequently disease activity increased (ESR 82, CRP 114), so the patient was commenced on cyclosporin.

When last seen in April 1997, Mr B was readmitted. He had been generally unwell since December with several episodes of feeling faint; the CRP was 150 and ESR was 79. Mr B had an attack of pain and swelling in R hallux but uric acid was within normal range. The patient's disease was starting to become out of control again, so prednisolone was increased once more and the patient was admitted for joint injections.

This history illustrates the role of the multidisciplinary team in the management of the patient with RA which is difficult to control. It also shows the constant necessity to manipulate the drug therapy to reduce side effects whilst attempting to moderate the activity of the condition. The physiotherapist works as a key member of the team monitoring the musculoskeletal aspects of the condition, and liaising with other team members to promote the optimum intervention for the patient.

Conclusion

The patient with RA is a huge challenge. The disease fluctuates both in its systemic and its articular manifestations and constantly presents fresh and stimulating questions.

A broad, holistic and functional approach is necessary along with developed communication skills, a sense of humour and well-consolidated core skills. A thorough knowledge of the disease and its likely progressions is essential for the physiotherapist to assess and evaluate the necessary interventions and contra-indications.

Regular assessment and periodic review of therapy will be required and whilst these patients may well achieve their outcome measures they are rarely discharged from care, although many can be maintained on a review basis. Succinct and appropriate case management is desirable to ensure efficient use of resources.

REFERENCES

Akil M, Amos RS. Rheumatoid arthritis -1: clinical features and diagnosis. *BMJ* 1995, **310**:587-590.

Arnett FC, Edworth SM, Bloch DA *et al*. The American Rheumatism Association 1987 revised criteria for the classification of RA. *Arth Rheum* 1988, **31**:315-324.

Barnes CG. Rheumatoid arthritis. In: Currey HLF ed., Mason and Currey's *Clinical Rheumatology*. Bath: Pitman Books Ltd; 1980.

Beck TA, Steer RA, Garbin MG. Psychometric properties of the Beck depression inventory: twenty five years of evaluation. *Clin Psychol Rev* 1988, **8**:77-100.

Belch JJF. *Raynaud's phenomenon*. ARC Reports on Rheumatic Diseases; May 1987.

Bell MJ, Bombardier C, Tugwell P. Measurement of functional status, quality of life, and utility in rheumatoid arthritis. *Arthritis Rheum* 1990, **33**:591-601.

Bennett PH, Burch TA. New York Symposium on population studies in the rheumatic diseases: new diagnostic criteria. *Bull Rheum Dis* 1967, **17**:453-458.

Benson TP, Copp EP. The effects of therapeutic forms of heat and ice on the pain threshold of the normal shoulder. *Rheumatol Rehab* 1974, **13**:101-104.

Bowling A. *Measuring disease*. Buckingham: Open University Press; 1995.

Breedveld FC. Vasculitis associated with connective tissue disease. In: Yazici H, Husby G, eds. Baillières *Clin Rheumatol: Vasculitis* 1997, **11**:2315-2334.

Brennan P, Silman A. Are hormonal associations with rheumatoid arthritis due to HLA DR4 status? *Br J Rheum* 1996, **35**:228 (abstract).

Brower AC. Rheumatoid arthritis: imaging. In: Klippel JH, Dieppe PA eds. *Rheumatology*. London: Mosby; 1995, 2:6.1-6.8.

Buchanan WM, Keen WF. Articular and systemic manifestations of rheumatoid arthritis. In: Scott JT ed. *Copemans textbook of rheumatic diseases*. Edinburgh: Churchill Livingstone; 1986:653-705.

Butler RC. Rheumatoid arthritis and juvenile chronic arthritis. In: Tidswell ME ed. *Cash's textbook of orthopaedics and rheumatology for physiotherapists, 2nd edition*. London: Mosby; 1990:214-248.

Campion G, Maddison PJ. *Felty's syndrome*. ARC Reports on Rheumatic diseases; May 1986.

Caplan A. Rheumatoid disease and pneumoconiosis (Caplan's syndrome). *Proc R Soc Med* 1953, **52**:1111.

Carpenter DF, Golden A, Roberts WC. Quadrivalvular rheumatoid heart disease associated with left bundle branch block. *Am J Med* 1967, **43**:922.

Carson-Dick W. *An introduction to clinical rheumatology*. Edinburgh, Churchill Livingstone;1972.

Chakravarty K. Vasculitis by organ systems. In: Yazici H, Husby G eds, Baillières *Clin Rheumatol: Vasculitis* 1997, **11**:2357-2393.

Colov HC, Palmgren N, Jensen GF *et al*. Convincing clinical improvement of rheumatoid arthritis by soft laser therapy. *Lasers Surg Med* 1987, **7**:77.

De Jong Z, Van der Heijde D, McKenna SP *et al*. The reliability and construct validity of the RAQoL: a rheumatoid arthritis specific quality of life instrument. *Br J Rheum* 1997, **36**:878-883.

Dieppe PA, Doherty M, Macfarlane DG *etal*. *Rheumatological Medicine*. London: Churchill Livingstone; 1985.

Ekdahl C, Brown G. Muscle strength, endurance and aerobic capacity in rheumatoid arthritis: a comparative study with healthy subjects. *Ann Rheum Dis* 1992, **51**:35-40.

Emery P. The optimal management of early rheumatoid disease: the key to preventing disability. *Br J Rheum* 1994, **33**:765-768.

Emery P, Salmon M. Early rheumatoid arthritis: time to aim for remission? *Ann Rh Dis* 1995, **54**:944-947.

Gardner DL. Pathology of rheumatoid arthritis. In: Scott JT ed. *Copemans textbook of rheumatic diseases*. Edinburgh: Churchill Livingstone; 1986:604-653.

Gerber LH. Exercise and arthritis. *Bull Rheum Dis* 1990, **39**:1-9.

Goldman JA, Chiapella J, Casey H. Laser therapy on rheumatoid arthritis. *Lasers Surg Med* 1980, **1**:93-101.

Golding DN. Management of rheumatoid arthritis. In: Golding DN ed. *A synopsis of rheumatic diseases, 5th edition*. London: Wright; 1988:78-79.

Golland A. Basic hydrotherapy. *Physiotherapy* 1981, **67**:258-268.

Hall J, Bisson D, O'Hare P. The physiology of immersion. *Physiotherapy* 1990, **76**:517-520.

Hara KS, Ballard DJ, Ilstrum DM *et al*. Rheumatoid pericarditis: clinical features and survival. *Medicine* 1990, **69**:81.

Hickling P, Golding JR. *An outline of rheumatology*. Bristol: John Wright and Sons; 1984.

Hochberg MC, Chang RW, Dwosh I *et al*. The American College of Rheumatology 1991 revised criteria for the classification of global functional status in rheumatoid arthritis. *Arthritis Rheum* 1992, **35**:498-502.

Hoenig H, Groff G, Pratt K, Goldberg E, Franck W. A randomised controlled trial of home exercise on the rheumatoid hand. *J Rheumatol* 1993, **32**:392-395.

Hoffman-Goetze L, Klarlund PB. Exercise and the immune system: a model of the stress response? *Immunol Today* 1994, **15**:382-387.

Hurley MV, Newham DJ. The influence of arthrogenous muscle inhibition on quadriceps rehabilitation on patients with early osteoarthritic knees. *Br J Rheumatol* 1993, **32**:127-131.

Huskisson EC. Measurement of pain. *J Rheumatol* 1982, **9**:768-769.

Kidd BL. Problems with pain: is the messenger to blame? *Ann Rheum Dis* 1996, **55**:275.

Kidd BL, Morris VH, Urban L. Pathophysiology of joint pain. *Ann Rheum Dis* 1996, **55**:276-283.

Kirwan JR, Reeback JS. Stanford health assessment questionnaire modified to assess disability in British patients with rheumatoid arthritis. *Br J Rheum* 1986, **25**:206-209.

Lehman JF, Masock AJ, Warren CG *et al*. Effect of therapeutic temperatures on tendon extensibility. *Arch Phys Med Rehab* 1970, **51**:481.

Low J, Reed A. *Electrotherapy explained: principles and practice*. Oxford: Butterworth-Heinemann; 1990.

Marks R. Peripheral mechanisms in pain production in osteoarthritis. *Aust J Physiother* 1992, **38**:289-298.

Matteson EL, Cohen MD, Conn DL. Clinical features of rheumatoid arthritis: systemic involvement. In: Klippel JH, Dieppe PA eds. *Practical rheumatology*. London: Times Mirror; 1995.

Maycock JA. Role of health professionals in patient education. *Ann Rheum Dis* 1991, **50**:429-434.

McEwen J. The Nottingham health profile. In: Walker S, Rosser R eds. *Quality of life assessment; key issues in the 1990s*. Dordrecht: Kluwer; 1993:111-130.

Meenan RF, Mason JH, Anderson JJ *et al*. AIMS2: The content and properties of a revised and expanded Arthritis Impact Measurement Scales Health Status Questionnaire. *Arthritis Rheum* 1992, **35** (1):1-10.

Minor MA, Brown JD. Exercise maintenance of persons with arthritis after participation in a class experience. *Health Educ Q* 1993, **20**:83-95.

Panayi GS. The aetiopathogenesis of rheumatoid arthritis. In: Scott JT ed. *Copemans textbook of rheumatic diseases*. Edinburgh: Churchill Livingstone; 1986:595-604.

Perlman SG, Connell KJ, Clark A *et al*. Dance based aerobic exercise for rheumatoid arthritis. *Arth Care Res* 1990, **3**:29-35.

Ritchie DM, Boyle JA, McInnes JM *et al*. Clinical Studies with an articular index for the assessment of joint tenderness in patients with rheumatoid arthritis. *Quart J Med* 1968, **37**:393-406.

Schaible H-G. Why does inflammation in the joint hurt? *Br J Rheum* 1996, **35**:405-406.

Schaible H-G, Grubb BD. Afferent and spinal mechanisms of joint pain. *Pain* 1993, **55**:5-54.

Shipley M. Pain in the hand and wrist. *BMJ* 1995, **310**:239-243.

Soar J, Handel J. A safe airway in rheumatoid arthritis? *Br J Hospital Med* 1995, **53**:214.

Sokoloff L. The heart in rheumatoid arthritis. *Am Heart J* 1953, **45**:635.

Spector TD, Brennan P, Harris P, Studd JWN, Silman A. Does oestrogen replacement therapy protect against rheumatoid arthritis? *J Rheumatol* 1991, **18**:1473-1476.

Steinbrocker O, Traeger CH, Batterman RC. Therapeutic criteria in rheumatoid arthritis. *J Am Med Assoc* 1949, **140**:659-662.

Stewart M. Researches into the effectiveness of physiotherapy in rheumatoid arthritis of the hand. *Physiotherapy* 1996, **82**:666-672.

Symmons D. Quantifying progress in rheumatoid arthritis. In: Butler RC, Jayson MIV, eds. *Collected Reports on the Rheumatic Diseases*. ARC; 1994.

Thompson PW, Silman AJ, Kirwan JR *et al*. Articular indices of joint inflammation in rheumatoid arthritis. *Arth Rheum* 1987, **3**:618-623.

Thompson PW, Hart LE, Goldsmith CH *et al*. Comparison of four articular indices for use in clinical trials in rheumatoid arthritis: patient, order and observer variation. *J Rheum* 1991, **18**:661-665.

Tucker M, Kirwan JR. Does patient education in rheumatoid arthritis have therapeutic potential? *Ann Rheum Dis* 1991, **50**:422-428.

Turnbull A. *Anaemia in RA - does it matter?* Collected reports on rheumatic diseases ARC; 1995.

Walker DJ. *Rheumatoid arthritis*. Collected reports on rheumatic diseases ARC; 1995.

Ware J, Sherbourne C. The MOS 36-item short form health survey (SF-36). *Med Care* 1992, **30**:473-483.

Whalley D, McKenna SP, De Jong Z *et al*. Quality of life in rheumatoid arthritis. *Br J Rheum* 1997, **36**:884-888.

Zigmond AS, Snaith RP. The hospital anxiety and depression scale. *Acta Psychiat Scand* 1983, **67**:361-370.

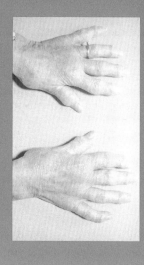

9

A Chadwick

OSTEOARTHRITIS

CHAPTER OUTLINE

- Incidence, aetiology, prognosis
- Pathology
- Clinical features
- Diagnosis/Special tests
- Medical management
- Surgical management
- Physiotherapy management
- Involvement of other multidisciplinary team members
- Outcome measures
- Case histories

INTRODUCTION

Osteoarthritis (OA) is one of the most common conditions treated by physiotherapists. In this chapter the multi-disciplinary assessment and management of OA will be detailed. The aetiology, pathology and diagnostic tests will be discussed and examples of case histories given.

Definitions of OA vary, but it is considered to be a chronic, degenerative and progressive condition affecting synovial joints. It is characterised by pain, limitation of range of movement and possible deformity in the later stages. Cartilage and bone are involved before peri-articular structures. It has been thought to be a condition where the normal repair response to every day joint damage is absent. However, there is now a growing belief that OA may be the result of several different processes leading to symptomatic articular disease (Altman, 1986).

CRITERIA FOR DIAGNOSIS OF OSTEOARTHRITIS

Criteria for diagnosis of OA are also varied but tend to be broad, referring to the history of joint pain, early morning stiffness (EMS) of short duration, the presence of radio-graphical changes and normal serology (Altman, 1986).

Classification of Osteoarthritis

Classification is various and often dependent on several factors:

- Number of joints involved i.e. mono-, oligo- or poly-articular.
- The type of OA described, e.g.

  Inflammatory—there is obvious inflammation in many joints.

  Erosive OA—typically an aggressive polyarticular OA which mainly affects the interphalangeal joints of the hand, progresses rapidly and is accompanied by radio-graphically detectable bony destruction. Often a rapidly progressive OA is one in which joint space decreases by 2 mm or more in a 6-month period.

  Generalised OA (GOA)—affecting many joints, usually in women aged 45–64 (Cooper et al., 1996).

- The site of OA, e.g. nodular OA, often inflammatory OA involving the joints of the hand (Cooper, 1994).

Others classify OA as primary idiopathic or secondary to another known pathology—this will be discussed later. Terminology can be confusing, but it is accepted that OA and osteoarthrosis are interchangeable terms describing degenerative changes in synovial joints. Spondylosis describes degenerative changes in cartilaginous intervertebral joints, including the disc.

INCIDENCE, AETIOLOGY, PROGNOSIS

INCIDENCE

Osteoarthritis is a very common condition, with 44–70% of people over the age of 55 having radiological evidence (Fisher et al., 1991) while in the over 75 age group this figure rises to 85% (Moskowitz, 1987). The peak onset for development of OA is between 50 and 60. It is estimated amongst the population over 65, about 12% are likely to have symptomatic OA.

The incidence of symptomatic OA increases with age and weight. The knee, distal interphalangeal (DIP), carpometacarpal (CMC) and facet joints are most commonly affected. OA of the hip has a definite correlation with age and is almost three times more common in men. Women, however, tend to have more severe polyarticular disease which frequently affects the hands and knees (Hirsch, 1996). Age, genetics and the presence of other local articular pathologies will all affect biomechanical structures in joints and influence both the site and severity of development of OA in the joint.

Interestingly, professional athletes without previous injuries do not have any increased incidence of OA and high mileage runners have comparable prevalence of OA with non-running controls. However, fair weather or seasonal athletes will be more at risk of injury (Lane et al., 1993). Premature development of OA in lower limb joints is likely to occur in regularly exercising subjects who have ligamentous instability from a prior injury or condition.

Studies have shown an inverse relationship between osteoporosis and OA involving large joints (Sambrook & Naganathan, 1997).

AETIOLOGY

There are many theories regarding the aetiology of OA. Primary OA is essentially still a condition of unknown aetiology. Studies are ongoing regarding a potential genetic link relating to the development of OA of the hands and knees, especially common in females.

Primary Osteoarthritis

This is typically found in women of menopausal age who have multiple joint involvement often of knees, hands and hips. Bouchard's and Heberden's nodes are forms of osteophytosis which may be seen at the proximal and distal interphalangeal (IP) joints respectively. Axial involvement mainly affects the lower cervical and lumbar regions. These are areas of large amplitude movement and repetitive stresses in the spine. The least affected joints are the ankle, wrist, elbow and shoulder.

Secondary Osteoarthritis

Traumatic Osteoarthritis

Abnormal biomechanics following trauma, with or without repeated high impact joint loading, obesity or restriction of normal joint range of movement, will cause an alteration in the stresses on different portions of articular cartilage. The flow of synovial fluid to articular surface margins will be restricted and precipitate the onset of OA.

Anatomical

Conditions such as congenital dislocation of the hip or hypermobility syndrome will all cause disproportionate stress on articular cartilage.

Inflammatory

Joint disease, e.g. rheumatoid arthritis, septic arthritis. When inflammation is present it is thought that free radicals may be produced causing the breakdown of hyaluranon (hyaluronic acid), a protein found in cartilage. This breakdown causes changes in the viscosity of tissue fluid and the elasticity of cartilage needed for shock absorbency. It also has a detrimental effect on the pseudo-plasticity needed to minimise friction at shearing surfaces of articular cartilage (Lotts et al., 1987).

Metabolic

Conditions secondary to endocrine dysfunction such as Paget's disease or crystal deposition diseases such as gout lead to altered biomechanics and joint degeneration (Apley & Solomon, 1994).

Neuropathic

Diabetic patients, amongst others, may get peripheral neuropathies with impaired pain perception and proprioception. This can lead to joint subluxation and chronic instability creating destructive intra-articular changes.

Haemophiliac

Joint degeneration is a sequel to repeated bleeding. Chronic synovitis is followed by cartilage degeneration (Apley & Solomon, 1994).

PROGNOSIS

The prognosis of OA is variable and individual. Most people experience a slow evolution of symptoms which then wax and wane. Flares of symptoms may last for days or months. Prognostically OA is not a life threatening condition though it can affect quality of life considerably and tends to be progressive. It should be noted, however, that some studies have shown that after exercise programmes are initiated and attempts made to improve biomechanical factors, function can improve and objective improvement on X-ray is demonstrated with improved joint space and evidence of bone end remodelling (Bland, 1994). The risk factors associated with a poorer prognosis are obesity and multiple joint involvement at early stages.

Studies currently underway are suggestive of an improved prognosis in patients with high Vitamin C intake, which may decrease risk of cartilage loss and disease progression in subjects with OA of the knee (McAlindon et al., 1996).

PATHOLOGY

It has been established that OA is a multi-factorial, meta-bolically active process usually beginning in middle age. Until recently it was thought to be only degenerative, but is now recognised also to have reparative features. The activity and behaviour of chondrocytes provide the key to the progressive nature of cartilage and joint degeneration in secondary OA.

Biochemical Changes

The water content of the articular cartilage is increased in an osteoarthritic joint. There are also changes in the quality of collagen fibres, which increase in diameter and disrupt the collagen bundles. At a molecular level there is also a loss of proteoglycans in the cartilage, and the severity of lesions appears to be proportional to this (Lotts *et al.*, 1987).

Metabolic Changes

Initially there are subtle alterations in hyaline cartilage metabolism. The cartilage matrix is made up of chondro-cytes, collagenous and elastic fibres. Gradually collagen is broken down resulting in a loss of matrix integrity and surface continuity. This usually occurs in central areas of articular cartilage where soft patches of fibrillation or fray-ing occurs and pitted areas form. As the fibrillation pro-gresses loose bodies of flakes of cartilage may form and create a secondary synovitis.

There are four zones of cartilage: superficial, middle, deep and a calcified layer adjacent to the bone. It is now recognised that metabolic processes vary between the dif-ferent layers of cartilage. Recent studies indicate that the most superficial layers of human articular cartilage are the most susceptible to damage and that these chondrocytes are also less responsive to therapeutic measures (Häuselmann *et al.*, 1996). Cartilage has no nerve endings, with the exception of the outer third of the intervertebral disc, and pain receptors are absent from subchondral bone, so at this stage the arthritis can be asymptomatic (Lotts *et al.*, 1987).

It should be noted that the cartilaginous fibrillation of OA is progressive and occurs at weightbearing sites, where-as fibrillation that occurs with ageing is not progressive and is found at non-weightbearing sites (Bland, 1994).

The Role of Osteoblasts

As articular cartilage is lost, there is a marked increase in the activity of underlying bone. This is detectable on iso-tope scans which demonstrate increased blood flow at OA sites, probably due to increased metabolic activity in cartilage and bone. Underlying bone becomes hardened (sclerotic).

Early Osteophyte Formation

Osteophyte and chondrophyte (bony and cartilaginous out-growths respectively) form at the margins of the joint with related synovial hyperplasia. The patient may experience early symptoms of pain and be protective of the joint at this stage. However, chondrocytes need mechanical stimula-tion to survive (Bland, 1994) and so patients should continue to exercise gently in weightbearing positions.

Reparation Phase

Increased chondrocyte activity follows in an attempt to repair the cartilage matrix. Some healing does occur but it is a combination of fibro cartilage and hyaline cartilage which reforms (McKeag, 1992). Fibro cartilage is not as resilient as hyaline cartilage. The chondrocytes clone by mitosis and there is a marked increase in the rate of type II collagen synthesis and levels of proteoglycan enzymes which are identifiable in the tissues and joint fluid.

Remodelling

Increased hyaline cartilage synthesis leads to increased stiffness and decreased compliance of peri-articular tissues. It is suggested that this may lead to micro-fractures in the trabecular articular surface of subchondral bone (Bland, 1994). This catalyses a hypertrophic reaction. Increased osteoblastic activity occurs and the bone end is remodelled. This creates an increased load-bearing capacity at the joint surface and helps compensate for increased biomechanical stresses which are secondary to the incon-gruity of the altered articular surface. Subchondral cysts may be found in the trabecular bone and marginal osteo-phytes form to help compensate for the functional insta-bility of the joint.

Bony Eburnation

As degenerative changes progress sub-articular bone is exposed and appears polished as there is complete loss of articular cartilage.

Soft Tissue

Hypertrophy of the capsule, tendons and ligaments decreases joint range of movement. There may also be an associated deterioration in the synovial membrane which can become fibrotic and possibly atrophic.

The inflammatory reaction initiated in response to intra-articular disruption and synovial changes can cause a 50% reduction in tensile strength of tissue. This may lead to overstretch or tearing of ligaments and the joint capsule (Kannus, 1988). Pain and effusions may inhibit surround-ing muscles, leading in turn to muscle atrophy and further loss of joint stability.

CLINICAL FEATURES

There are several interrelated features common to osteoarthritic joints.

PAIN

Pain is often of most immediate importance to the patient, who will describe it as being worse at night due to raised pressure in subchondral bone (Pinals, 1996), and after rest. Pain is often eased by movement. Many structures may give rise to pain in OA:

- Peri-articular soft tissue—capsular or ligamentous strains in an unstable joint.
- Periosteal elevation secondary to raised intraosseous pressure.
- Muscular pain and weakness.
- Referred pain—from spinal nerve roots, or may be referred distally from joints themselves.
- Inflamed and overstretched synovium.
- Inability to cope (Van Baar *et al.*, 1998).

There is also some evidence that physiological changes occur in the wide dynamic range neurones, which are related to nociception. When normal movement and subsequent normal afferent input ceases the receptors and their membranes change and stop responding to excitatory or inhibitory stimuli or pharmacological therapies, but start to activate spontaneously and pain is perceived by the patient. This would suggest immobilisation of a joint should be avoided wherever possible (Bogduk, 1994).

STIFFNESS
The stiffness a patient experiences is probably also linked with deprivation of normal movement in affected tissue. There is a reduction in compliance of soft tissue as the degenerative and secondary inflammatory processes occur. In addition, as the subchondral micro-fractures heal and callus forms this causes a loss of joint mobility and stiffness follows. In OA, EMS of up to 30 minutes is common and is relieved by movement. Stiffness lasting for more than this time should be investigated to exclude primary inflammatory processes.

INFLAMMATION AND EFFUSION
This is not always present unless a joint is undergoing an exacerbation, which may be related to overactivity. Signs and symptoms may include heat, erythema, tenderness, effusion, discomfort and pain. Many patients have intermittent effusions; some may be chronic, especially in the knee, metacarpophalangeal (MCP) or IP joints of the hand.

LOSS OF RANGE OF MOVEMENT
The combination of joint pain, stiffness and possible effusion will often cause patients to limit their activities, and a consequent loss of end of range movement is common. This is usually correctable with appropriate instruction, but as the osteophytosis progresses a residual permanent lack of range may develop. Certain joints may develop capsular patterns with restriction in certain ranges of movement.

Capsular Patterns
- Hip—adduction contractures—due to increased forces in the lateral margin of acetabulum.
- Knee—flexion contractures. 75% medial compartment involvement, 25% lateral, 48% patello-femoral.
- Ankle—increased valgus forces—limited inversion and supination.
- Great toe—hallux valgus—restricted abduction.

- Shoulder—adhesive capsulitis may develop—restricted abduction, lateral and medial rotation.
- Hands—the small joints of the fingers are often involved.
- DIP involvement—typically Heberden's nodes—in 70% of patients with hand OA.
- Proximal interphalangeal (PIP) joints with Bouchard's nodes—in 35%.
- MCPs—in 10%.
- CMCs—in 60%.

MUSCLE INHIBITION AND ATROPHY
Effusions will inhibit the surrounding muscles of a joint. This may in part be a safety mechanism as the intra-articular pressure becomes relatively positive. If for example the quadriceps muscle was contracted, this could lead to the rupture of the knee joint capsule (Bland, 1994). Chronic muscle inhibition is often linked to chronic pain and will lead to atrophy and ensuing muscle weakness.

JOINT INSTABILITY
As the surrounding muscles weaken, possibly unequally, a muscle imbalance may develop. Pain episodes may be variable and unpredictable, causing the joint to give way. These processes, together with chronic stretching of soft tissue secondary to joint effusion and osteophytes, will alter the joint alignment leading to instability and possibly subluxation.

DEFORMITIES
It is thought that osteophyte development helps to compensate for reduced joint stability by increasing the peripheral articular surface area. Such deformities are most pronounced in established OA (Figure 9.1), but may not develop equally at medial and lateral joint margins. This may contribute to valgus or varus deformities. Together with soft tissue laxity this will alter the joint biomechanics.

REDUCED FUNCTION
All of the clinical features described above can result in functional difficulty, but this is variable. Patients with OA may describe such problems as walking a distance, climbing stairs, getting out of chairs, writing or opening jars.

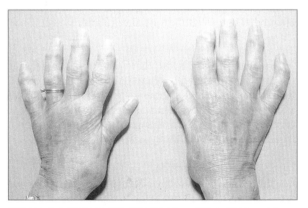

Figure 9.1 Osteoarthritic hands with evidence of Heberdens and Bouchards nodes.

Most people compensate subconsciously and try alternative ways of achieving a task if they are in pain, have lost joint range of movement or are no longer strong enough to carry out an activity. Most patients will be able to return to their previous capabilities by being taught to modify the task, manage their symptoms and retrain their muscles. Figure 9.2 highlights the inter-relationship between signs and symptoms in OA.

OSTEOARTHRITIS OF THE SPINE

It is thought the inter-vertebral disc may act as a catalyst for degenerative changes within the inter-vertebral joint complex. The elasticity and water-binding capacity of the disc lessens with age. Nuclear material can bulge out creating increased pressure on the annulus fibrosus laterally. Fragmentation and disc degeneration can then occur with a resultant reduction in disc height. This causes approximation of the vertebral end plates, which can be seen on a lateral X-ray. Apophyseal (facet joint) osteoarthritic changes and uncovertebral joint degeneration then occur.

Schmorl's nodes may also be seen on X-ray. This is where a disc may herniate into an adjacent vertebral body. Peri-articular sclerosis may also be seen. As the disc height reduces the surrounding ligaments slacken and may become dissected away from periosteal attachments by extruded disc material, which in itself may initiate a local inflammatory reaction. The disc material will subsequently be replaced by fibrous tissue calcification and osteophytes may form causing further narrowing at the facet joint space. Subsequent malalignment will cause an encroachment of the intervertebral foramina, with a resulting nerve root irritation often exacerbated by movements of the spine.

DIAGNOSIS/SPECIAL TESTS

Specific classification of OA for different joints, e.g. hip and knee, have evolved over recent years, but there are still no definitive criteria for the diagnosis of generalised OA. Diagnosis tends to be based on history, X-ray changes and an absence of inflammatory markers in the blood.

The history often described by the patient will be discussed later, in the section on Physiotherapy Management.

RADIOLOGY

In 1957 Kellegren & Lawrence established a grading system of severity of OA when seen radiologically (Figure 9.3) and it is still used today, mainly for research purposes.
0—no evidence on X-ray.
1—doubtful, but possible.
2—minimal severity, but identifiable.
3—moderate severity.
4—severe osteoarthritic changes.

Three criteria are used:
• Formation of osteophytes.
• Narrowing of joint space.
• Sclerosis of subchondral bone.

Joint alignment, subchondral cysts and loose bodies should also be noted. Capsular thickening and joint effusions may also be seen. When reading X-rays it is also wise to check if they were taken in a weightbearing position to assess joint stability. Spinal X-rays may also reveal spondylolisthesis, which is often associated with advanced OA of facet joints combined with lumbar disc disease.

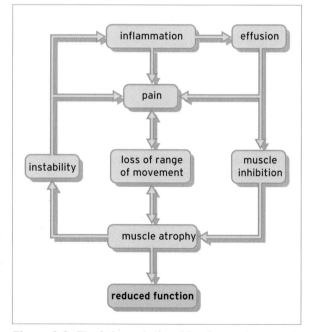

Figure 9.2 **The inter-relationship of symptoms and signs in osteoarthritis.**

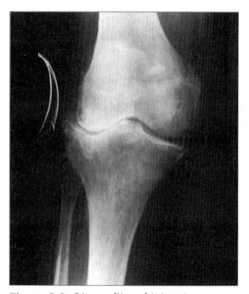

Figure 9.3 **Stress film of lateral compartment knee joint osteoarthritis.**

However, radiography is not useful in assessing the severity of symptoms because there is frequently a marked discrepancy between symptoms, clinical features seen and evidence of OA found on X-rays.

LABORATORY INVESTIGATIONS

There are no specific laboratory tests for OA. Haematological, biochemical and serological tests are usually within normal limits, but may be useful to exclude other pathologies, eg. gout, septic arthritis and hypothyroidism. Synovial fluid will typically be viscous, clear and straw-coloured with a low cell count. It may contain fragments of cartilage.

OTHER INVESTIGATIONS

Arthroscopy may be used to detect local changes in the joint and may be used therapeutically as a lavage.
- Arthrography using radio-opaque agents may carry an increased risk of sepsis.
- Computerised tomography (CT) scan may be useful for imaging facet joints but cannot identify hyaline cartilage.
- Magnetic resonance imaging (MRI) is a more sophisticated and detailed scan for soft tissue, but it is expensive and not always available.
- Ultrasound may be used to detect effusions.
- Thermography can be useful to determine temperature alterations and measure superficial blood flow when there is extensive soft tissue involvement.

MEDICAL MANAGEMENT

Team work amongst the disciplines is needed for effective care. The patient's first point of contact will usually be the general practitioner (GP), who may prescribe medication, reassure and educate the patient, and then refer on to other team members. The patient will often initially complain of pain of gradual onset, which limits function and disturbs sleep. The GP may also give simple advice to reduce weight (and thus joint loading), spacing out activities and treating the joints with heat or cold. This will be discussed in depth later.

MEDICATION

The GP will often advise a simple analgesia, e.g. paracetamol, or prescribe a non-steroidal anti-inflammatory drug (NSAID), e.g. ibuprofen or diclofenac. Effects and side effects of NSAIDs and other drugs are to be found in Chapter 3.

The appropriate use of NSAIDs in OA patients is debatable. Muncie (1986) demonstrated an 80% improvement in symptoms and 36% of subjects experiencing no pain at 3 months, but others suggest that there is little support for the use of NSAIDs in OA. The long-term effect of NSAIDs on cartilage is unknown, but some may even hasten joint destruction by deleteriously affecting cartilage metabolism.

Glucosamine sulphate occurs naturally in the body and acts as a building block for glycosaminoglycans in the extracellular matrix. It is thought to help promote cartilage repair (Lozada & Altman, 1997). Some studies report fewer side effects than with NSAIDS (Anon, 1994). Some patients in chronic pain may benefit from antidepressants. These may promote sleep and enhance compliance with other therapies, especially exercise.

Topical NSAIDs, such as ibuprofen cream or piroxicam gel, are administered locally on sites of soft tissue inflammation. They are popular but may not be of great value, and should not be used long-term. Capsaicin cream has been shown to cause a 30% decrease in OA knee pain, but side effects of skin allergy and burning are common in topical preparations (Deal et al., 1991).

Occasionally intra-articular steroid injections are given, most frequently to knees or CMC joints which are not responding to other therapy. However, the long-term effects are not yet clear in osteoarthritic patients. It is advised that such injections should not be given more frequently than 3 monthly to any joint (McAlindon & Dieppe, 1990). Persistently effused and painful osteoarthritic joints may benefit from mini-arthroscopies and tidal lavage provided medical regimes are stabilised. These can relieve pain for many months.

Other treatments under investigation attempt to restore the joint. They involve cartilage transplant and the injection of certain cytokines into joints to stimulate the host cells to form cartilage and produce new tissue. Future research will clarify whether these drugs can stimulate the formation of tissue which duplicates the structure, composition, mechanical properties and durability of articular cartilage (Mankin & Buckwalter, 1996).

SURGICAL MANAGEMENT

Surgical measures attempt to restore the joint, unlike most medical treatments which address the symptoms. A patient may require surgery if experiencing significant functional difficulties and pain which is uncontrolled by conservative measures. The various types of surgery and their rationale are discussed in greater depth in Chapter 7.

OSTEOTOMIES

Osteotomies reduce pain and can lead to the formation of new articular cartilage. They are used to correct abnormal biomechanics, e.g. genu varus deformity, where a femoral lateral wedge osteotomy may be performed.

ARTHROPLASTIES

Arthroplasties replace the joint structure and decrease pain as well as improve function. Hip and knee arthroplasties are usually very successful, provided the patient's compliance is gained and it is fully understood that intensive post-operative rehabilitation is vital for a successful outcome.

Excision arthroplasty may be very successful. In the Kellers' operation the proximal end of the phalanx of the great toe is excised. This often results in pain relief although it may not be long-standing. Excision arthroplasty is now rarely used for failed hip replacement surgery. A 'Girdlestone' procedure is performed, but can lead to severe functional limitation.

In the thumb, trapezio-metacarpal and trapezium-scaphoid joints are commonly involved. Grasping objects can become difficult and painful but can be considerably improved with surgery to excise the trapezium or introduce a silastic implant in the joint.

ARTHRODESES

Arthrodeses or surgical fusions of hips, knees or ankles are uncommon, but are performed primarily to relieve pain and restore joint stability. Function may be considerably restricted due to the subsequent reduction in range and mobility, but compensatory movements are often learnt.

Foot surgery may involve hind foot arthrodesis of sub-talar and mid-tarsal joints. Secondary OA often arises in these joints following fractures of the calcaneum. Osteotomies and arthroplasty may be performed in the forefoot.

The orthotist's opinion will often be requested by the medical team, both prior and subsequent to lower limb surgery. Additional biomechanical assessments may be of value from podiatrists and physiotherapists.

PHYSIOTHERAPY MANAGEMENT

Patients with OA are rarely admitted to hospital unless requiring surgery. Most will be seen as outpatients or in their homes. In all cases physiotherapy management will centre on regaining function and mobility through exercise, pain relieving measures and advice. The physiotherapist will attempt to minimise future disability while maximising function. In the short-term, assessment and management are based on the individual's symptoms and level of ability, but the long-term focus is on educating patients to manage their condition independently.

ASSESSMENT OF OSTEOARTHRITIC PATIENTS

History

As there is a poor correlation between symptoms related by the patient and radiological changes, the history from the patient is very important. They will tend to complain of pain, stiffness, swelling, creaking and decreased range of movement at a joint. They may present with possible deformities, typically of hands, feet and knees, and may complain of feelings of instability in a joint. Previous physiotherapy and other therapies, exacerbating and relieving factors should be documented.

The problems arising because of the patient's condition should be translated into functional goals which could be achieved through physiotherapy or referral to other disciplines. Occupational and social difficulties should be included and sport/leisure activities discussed as well as ergonomic issues. The patient's expectation from treatment and knowledge about the condition should be investigated.

Pain and Early Morning Stiffness

The use of a body chart to document pain, paraesthesia and anaesthesia can serve as a useful speedy reminder of some problems. Pain should be measured using a validated tool such as the visual analogue scale (VAS) (Waterfield & Sim, 1996) and length of duration noted if EMS is present. In OA pain at rest and at night is usually most pronounced and relieved with movement (Adler, 1985). Sleep disturbance due to pain often affects patients with large joint OA of the lower limbs.

Palpation

Note should be taken of any effusion, any increase in temperature or active synovitis when palpating the joints. In the knee a Baker's cyst may also be present. Tenderness may be felt around the greater trochanter and pes anserinus insertion. Tenosynovitis in the hand may be palpated as crepitus in the flexor tendons which may cause finger triggering. Ligamentous laxity should be noted, especially of the medial and lateral collateral ligaments of the knee and the CMC joint of the thumb.

Joint Stability and Proprioception

If joints are unstable, poor afferent information is fed back to the central nervous system (CNS) and this will greatly accelerate joint degeneration (Hurley & Newham, 1993). In such cases proprioception may be tested, initially in a non-weightbearing position, progressing to weightbearing with less support and no visual clues. This can highlight lack of proprioception in the ankle and other lower limb joints, which is often a problem after trauma. These tests can be timed and used as a treatment, progressing to take patients in and out of their base of support through movement whilst maintaining their balance.

Range of Movement

An experienced clinician can often measure range of movement as accurately by eye as with a goniometer (Williams & Callaghan, 1990). Limitation of movement should always be related to functional tasks. Active and passive ranges of movement including those proximal and distal to the affected joints should be noted, with the end of range feel and reason for lack of further range documented. Contractures may be present in the chronic degenerative joint which may also be inflamed. Perry *et al.* (1975) established that even a 10° flexion contracture at the knee will produce some degree of handicap by causing a compensatory increase in hip flexion and an increased lumbar lordosis. This facilitates more knee extension and maintains the centre of gravity, but will increase the loading at the hip extensors. The foot may then compensate by trying to remain fixed on the floor, thus increasing the load on the plantar flexors. Such a compensatory posture attempts to decrease the load at the quadriceps and maintain mobility.

Certain minimum ranges of movement are necessary to perform daily tasks with normal biomechanical movement patterns. In order to climb and descend the stairs the minimum knee flexion needed is 110°. To tie shoe laces, a hip range of movement between 30–120° is needed while in order to comb hair, shoulder abduction of 40° and wrist extension of 40° are needed (Badley *et al.*, 1984). Compensatory movement patterns should be noted.

Neurological Assessment

A neurological assessment may be needed to investigate and exclude spinal pathology. An in-depth assessment will assist diagnosis of the structures giving rise to symptoms. Adherence and dysfunctional problems may need further attention, as may symptoms of carpal tunnel syndrome or adverse mechanical tension.

Posture

An evaluation of the patient's static and dynamic postures will often highlight individual adaptation and compensatory posture, with resulting imbalance of muscle function. Muscles may be inhibited by pain and subsequently atrophy, or conversely they may be over-used, e.g. upper fibres of Trapezius in the presence of abnormal biomechanics in the shoulder girdle or glenohumeral joint.

Muscle Power

Assessing muscle strength of individual or groups of muscles can be of value if also related to function. The method of measuring muscle power is under considerable debate (Oldham & Howe, 1995). In clinical practice the Oxford scale (0–5) of manual muscle testing is often still used, though not considered reliable. An evaluation of relevant individual muscle groups often highlights an imbalance of muscle activity around the pelvic or shoulder girdle, leading to instability which may in turn exacerbate symptoms. Both static and dynamic, eccentric and concentric testing may be necessary, and can be accurately measured using isokinetic machines.

Alternatively hand-held dynamometers can assess more accurately isometric muscle strength, whereas isometric dynamometers can estimate torque at a given velocity. A strain gauge device is often cheaper and more practical. Electromyographic (EMG) analysis may be necessary.

In patients with osteoarthritic knees the ratio of quadriceps to hamstrings is often relatively weaker at 1.43, whereas in the unaffected population the ratio is 2.0 (Hayes, 1992). This may need to be addressed. The value of measuring quadriceps bulk is now doubtful. Research shows there is no correlation between the knee joint and mid thigh circumferential measurements. In women there is considerable inaccuracy compared with men and it is also impossible to measure the percentage of fat relative to muscle (Dovey, 1987).

Function

A functional assessment for the osteoarthritic patient is vital and this should be specific for the individual, depending on joints involved, and should involve static as well as dynamic tests. In addition a functional scoring method can be used via a questionnaire of the patient's ability, e.g. SF36 (Ware & Sherbourne, 1992). Function should be assessed and be relevant to the individual's daily lifestyle, e.g. upper limb, dressing, washing and personal care should be assessed.

Gait Analysis

The gait of patients with lower limb conditions can be assessed using a timed walk over a set distance, which is therefore reproducible (Badley *et al.*, 1984). When gait analysis is undertaken footwear and insoles should also be taken into consideration. Biomechanics of the joints should also be considered dynamically. A video camera can be of great value giving immediate and sequential feedback to the patient. Further data can be obtained if used in conjunction with a personal computer (Wall & Crosbie, 1997). Transfers, quality of movement and postural awareness should be investigated.

With the lower limb, gait and transfers with or without relevant aids should be checked. These tasks can be timed to gain a baseline objective measure and documented using an appropriate VAS.

Exercise Tolerance

Exercise tolerance may also be relevant and be documented in terms of timed distance walked/run with an associated heart rate/respiratory rate (HR/RR), which patients can be taught to measure themselves. Osteoarthritic patients in chronic pain will often have a reduced aerobic capacity, reduced mobility when lower limb joints are affected and reduced ability to carry out activities of daily living. In addition, they will have lost confidence in their ability to get fitter and may be frightened of exacerbating their pain through exercise.

Psychological Factors

The patient's understanding of their condition and its management should also be discussed. Depressive symptoms may accompany high levels of pain and disability. An awareness of the psychosocial aspects of the patient's condition may also be valuable, e.g. erosion of self image, an increase in social isolation accompanying decreased mobility and possible alteration in family roles, which may accompany the disease process (Krick, 1986).

It is accepted that those who exert more control over their behaviour have fewer anxiety and depressive symptoms and are better able to manage their disease (De Forge, 1986). Passive treatments should therefore be combined with active treatments.

JOINTLY AGREED OBJECTIVES OF TREATMENT

At the end of the assessment when a working diagnosis is made and explained to the patient, joint aims of treatment can be agreed and an informal contract of care negotiated. The emphasis should be on self-management, as with most chronic conditions. This can only follow after the patient understands realistically about his or her condition and its prognosis. Attendance early on at an OA education group run by professionals is frequently invaluable for gaining patient compliance and can be cost-effective.

Part of the physiotherapist's role is to reassure the patient and give simple advice, e.g. changing activities regularly, exercising 'little and often', taking a bath/shower in the mornings to minimise EMS, advising on posture/seating in the car, at work or at home or correct positioning of pillows. All of this can enhance the patient's quality of life. Specific treatments may also be necessary.

TREATMENT TECHNIQUES

The treatment techniques used in OA patients are numerous and mostly unresearched to date. However, appropriate management relies upon applying knowledge gained from research in other areas of musculoskeletal therapy and focuses on the problems identified at the first interview. Reassessment at every treatment session is useful to evaluate progress and amend treatment as appropriate.

Management of the Acutely Inflamed Joint

When treating the acutely inflamed joint, which is often a weightbearing joint, a period of partial weightbearing and the use of a mobility aid may be useful. Long periods of non-weightbearing should be avoided however, and a balance sought between rest and exercise. Prolonged immobilisation can adversely affect articular cartilage and will often exacerbate the pain and stiffness (Ytterberg, 1994). If joint effusions are present this will increase the intra-articular pressure. If the effusion is large anoxia may occur in surrounding tissues. It is useful to remember, therefore, that if the joint cannot be aspirated, heat should be avoided for fear of accentuating and accelerating hypoxia in the tissues. Ice therapy can be of more benefit, both subjectively to decrease pain and also in objectively reducing the effusion, albeit temporarily. Ice can also be used independently at home. During this time it is important to maintain joint range of movement through simple daily mobilising exercises of the affected and surrounding joints. These should be performed slowly and with few repetitions. Static quads contractions in an effused knee joint will further increase the intra-articular pressure. Maintaining strength and tone in mid-range via auto-resisted quadriceps and hamstring exercises in prone or sitting would be a more valuable exercise.

REST AND EXERCISE

Rest should not be totally discouraged because it will help to suppress the inflammatory response. However, daily exercises through the available range are necessary, even with only minimal repetitions to maintain range of movement and avoid atrophy and contractures. It should also be remembered that chondrocytes need mechanical stimulation to survive. It has been shown that with prolonged immobilisation a proliferation of fibro-fatty tissue occurs, which may eventually fill the joint. It appears like pannus in RA, ultimately eroding the cartilage by enzymatic degradation (Enneking & Horowitz, 1972). Even slight movement of a joint will slow this process, which is thought to be reversible if mechanical stimulation is restarted.

PAIN RELIEVING MODALITIES

There are several methods of pain relief available to the physiotherapist. Research is scarce and has mainly focused on patients with osteoarthritic knees; however, these findings can often be applied to other joints. Traditionally pain relief has been a primary focus with OA patients and this has tended to involve a passive treatment. Function is now considered to be a more appropriate focus, with an increased emphasis on self-management and active involvement by the patient.

Clarke (1974) investigated the perceived benefits of ice therapy versus pulsed short wave diathermy (PSWD) or placebo PSWD. At 3 weeks the ice packs provided most benefit, but at 3 months there was no difference. Though the placebo effect cannot be ignored the therapist must also justify treatments which should be cost-effective.

Ultrasound (US) has been more recently evaluated against placebo US. Both groups also received exercise programmes, but there was no statistical difference on conclusion; both had increased range of movement and decreased pain with improved gait (Falconer et al., 1992).

Transcutaneous electrical nerve stimulation (TENS) can play a valuable role in the management of osteoarthritic joints at home. It can be used on most joints, does not interfere with function and can usually be self-administered. It is also a relatively cheap treatment with minimal side effects.

Another effective and cheap method of pain relief for OA of a patella-femoral joint has proven to be taping the patella medially. The tape can be self-administered after tuition, is safe and simple, and functions to improve the patella tracking and thus function of the quadriceps mechanism. Often the lateral facet of the patello-femoral joint is degenerate and this method relieves the compression and thus affords significant pain relief. Taping should be administered with concurrent strengthening exercises to enhance patella tracking. Strengthening of vastus medialis obliquus may be especially valuable (Cushnaghan, 1994).

Acupuncture is now used in many physiotherapy departments. It has been found to have a pain relieving effect in some studies of patients with OA knees (Han & Terenius, 1982). It is believed this is following an increased production of endorphins and enkephalins and the stimulation of afferent pathways. However, not all studies have conclusively shown the benefits from acupuncture (Takeda & Wessel, 1994).

EXERCISE THERAPY

Exercise and education together is the most effective way to regain function. Back education groups are particularly effective when used in combination with a comprehensive rehabilitation programme and based on education specific to the work site (Ross, 1997). Exercises for patients with OA should aim to be in a joint loading position to help preserve the integrity of articular cartilage and maintain bone mineralisation. This may have the effect of temporarily increasing the inflammatory response, but long-term will improve the activities of daily living.

Although many studies currently focus on the inflammatory markers of erythrocyte sedimentation rate (ESR) and C-reactive protein (CRP), functionally orientated outcome measures are becoming deservedly more important in research.

Aims of Exercise Therapy

Increase/Maintain Range of Movement

This can be achieved in many ways, for instance through free active exercises, auto-assisted exercises or hydrotherapy. Passive stretches and active contraction of the antagonist muscle group can be included in a treatment programme to decrease stiffness in joints and maintain range of movement. Studies on animals have shown that sustained stretches for 15 minutes a day are sufficient to retard substantially losses of range of movement and for 30 minutes completely prevent loss of range of movement (Williams, 1990). Sustained stretching is considered to be more effective in clinical practice, although there is some debate about the length of time that is most beneficial (Light *et al.*, 1984). Using heat prior to stretching may also be of benefit. Flowtron can be used to reduce flexion contractures, especially in knees and elbows (Figure 9.4).

Increase Muscle Power

This can be achieved through free active exercises against gravity, eccentrically and concentrically, auto-resisted exercises, hydrotherapy, or use of theraband or weights. Isokinetic machines can also give a graduated resistance with computer feedback on performance.

Increase Endurance

Functional exercises in weightbearing, if able—many slow repetitions, e.g. slow step-ups, eccentric and concentric activity.

Increase Aerobic Capacity

Warm up and cool down periods are essential. An increase in heart and respiratory rate can be encouraged through a controlled progression of exercises in a circuit, such as static bike, treadmill, step-ups, sitting to standing, or in hydrotherapy.

Increase Activites of Daily Living (ADL) Capacity

Practising functional tasks relevant to the individual under the supervision of trained staff.

Physiological Effects of Exercise

Exercise will improve blood pressure, decrease the risk of cardiovascular (CV) disease and induce the secretion of endorphins (Carr *et al.*, 1981). It would be anticipated that exercise should facilitate weight loss and for all these reasons also help to reduce pain levels. Studies have also indicated that after 3 months' aerobic activities there is a reduction in levels of depression and anxiety (Minor *et al.*, 1989). Certainly there is a cross-training effect amongst isometric, isotonic and isokinetic exercise techniques and it is advisable to design programmes that incorporate endurance as well as strength of specific muscle groups and address fitness levels.

Aerobic activity should be calculated at 60–80% of predicted maximum HR (maximum HR = 220 minus patient's age). Even low impact aerobics can provide a significant increase in CV fitness. See Chapter 14 for more details.

Signs and Symptoms of Excessive Exercise

Patients should be alert to the following, and taught how to modify their regime accordingly:
- Increased joint swelling.
- Significant fatigue.
- Persistent muscle soreness.
- Post exercise pain lasting more than 2 hours (Hicks, 1990).

HYDROTHERAPY

Hydrotherapy is often of great subjective benefit and may be valuable in reducing pain, using the effect of buoyancy and controlled loading in an acutely painful stage. It can also be used very differently for strengthening purposes using the effects of turbulence etc. for patients with chronic non-inflamed osteoarthritic joints (Palomski *et al.*, 1980). Strengthening exercises must be designed specifically for the individual patient and aim to maximise joint stability through the functional range.

Patients describe improved function, decreased pain and increased life satisfaction. This was so with both groups of patients with OA of the hip in a trial of hydrotherapy and exercise versus SWD and exercise. However, objective measures of gait and range of movement remained static in both groups (Sylvester, 1990). Other studies have shown that home exercises are as effective as outpatient hydrotherapy for osteoarthritic hip (Green *et al.*, 1993). Perhaps the enjoyment factor of hydrotherapy helps to make it a more socially therapeutic modality. Therapists should be aware of this and use it to their advantage, to encourage not only improved fitness levels but also progression to local pool facilities and independent management.

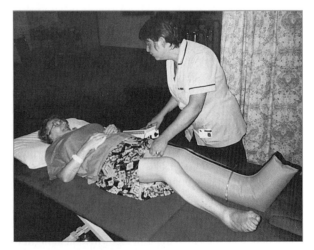

Figure 9.4 Flowtron.

ROLE OF POSTURE

Re-education of posture will be relevant for most patients, who should be assessed and advised in static, dynamic and functional positions. The use of a pressure biofeedback device (Figure 9.5) can be valuable in retraining postural muscles and the patient can be trained to use this independently.

Management of OA of the Spine

When treating spinal OA the aim is to improve sequential alignment and thereby restore normal movement patterns and reduce pain. This should be achieved by:

- Obtaining optional loading and mobility of the joints through exercise, thus nourishing and minimising forces through the joints.
- Gaining balanced muscle activity with appropriate agonist, antagonist and synergist muscle action—using the principles of muscle imbalance.
- Ensuring adequate mobility of neuromeningeal structures—assessing adverse mechanical tension (AMT) components.

Generally, patients with OA in facet joints respond to a programme of exercises avoiding extension and patients with disc degeneration and derangement avoiding flexion activities. Patients with spinal OA should strengthen their postural and primary agonist muscles (e.g. abdominals). In addition, proprioceptive retraining of joints should be incorporated into their exercise programme and performed in positions which do not aggravate their symptoms.

PATIENT COMPLIANCE

Studies have shown that compliance with exercise programmes for patients with arthritis varies between 50–95% (Hicks, 1990). In order to maximise compliance, educational leaflets should accompany the exercises and the therapist should ensure that the specific exercises are written or drawn for the individual patient. Guidelines will also be

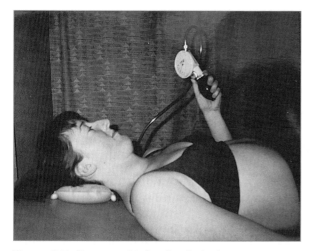

Figure 9.5 **Pressure biofeedback device.**

useful, indicating when to progress or stop exercises as well as recognise fatigue. It is important exercises are supervised and followed up, even if only by telephone, and that exercises are progressed. Using record sheets to document activity and completion of exercises can also assist compliance. If exercises can be made fun and relevant to the individual this will also improve the patient's co-operation and facilitate a successful outcome (Minor *et al.*, 1989).

INVOLVEMENT OF OTHER MULTI-DISCIPLINARY TEAM MEMBERS

Referral to other multidisciplinary team (MDT) members may be appropriate. All have a role as health educators. The occupational therapist (OT) will assess and advise the patient on devices to assist ADL function at home or work and can supply equipment as necessary. The OT is best skilled to assess for adaptations to the home and may also have expertise in hand function and be able to supply custom-made or off the shelf splints to protect the joint, e.g. thumb splint to support an osteoarthritic CMC joint. OTs may also be able to help with relaxation techniques and coping strategies in conjunction with a clinical psychologist, who can help the patient to manage chronic pain.

A podiatrist/chiropodist may make wedged insoles to decrease medial compartment loading in osteoarthritic knee patients, or alter other abnormal biomechanics of the lower limb as well as provide foot care advice. Advice may be given regarding shock absorbent insoles or the wearing of appropriate footwear which is both supportive and aesthetically acceptable, e.g. trainers.

A dietician may be necessary to advise on weight reduction. Studies indicate there is a positive correlation with obesity and pain experienced in OA. As yet there are no scientific data to identify specific nutrients having a role in the aetiology or management of OA, but a well balanced diet is advisable (White O'Connor, 1986).

Homeopathy may have a valuable place in the management of OA. Studies have shown that in conjunction with physiotherapy a significant decrease in joint stiffness can ensue, along with decreased number of subsequent consultations required and a reduction in the number of re-referrals. Effects are rapid and seem to be long-lasting (Pires-Mesquita, 1987). At present this is not commonly available through the National Health Service.

Finally the patient may benefit from peer support and attendance at local Arthritis Care groups, which are run nation-wide. Staff can put patients in contact with their local branch.

OUTCOME MEASURES

Serial reassessment is necessary to identify trends of improvement or deterioration. There are several self-administered functional assessment questionnaires designed for patients with arthritis which can be valuable, such as:

- Modified Health Assessment Questionnaire (HAQ) (Kirwan & Reeback, 1986).
- SF 36—(Ware & Sherbourne, 1992).
- Arthritis Impact Measurement Scales (AIMS) (Meenan, 1992).
- Nottingham Health Profile (Hunt *et al.*, 1981).

MEASURES USED IN CLINICAL PRACTICE

Other measures used in everyday clinical practice include:
- Pain—VAS at rest—at night (Waterfield & Sim, 1996).
- Range of movement:
  Goniometer.
  Tape Measure.
- Muscle Power:
  Oxford scale.
  Isokinetic analysis.
  Pressure biofeedback.
- Function:
  Video feedback—quality of movement, gait analysis.
  Timed walk/run/stairs.

CASE HISTORIES

CASE 1

A 54-year-old woman was admitted to hospital with a 5-year history of OA of the knees. Knee pain was rated by VAS as 8/10, and the patient described decreased mobility over the previous few months. On examination the patient had effusions bilaterally, and flexion contractures of 50° in the right knee and 35° in the left. She also had shortening of the right tendo-achilles (TA). Quadriceps and glutei were weak bilaterally, as were the abdominal muscles. The patient's posture was kyphotic, and she walked with flexed hips and knees using two sticks. The patient took 42 seconds to walk 10 metres.

The patient was taught the use of ice, taught stretches of her TA, quadriceps and hip flexors and advised to lie prone daily. Flowtron was applied to her knees for 20 minutes twice daily. The patient also attended hydrotherapy to increase knee extension and increase muscle power of the hip flexors, abductors and quadriceps—flippers were used in the pool to facilitate this. She was advised on gait and posture and the correct way to climb stairs.

As the effusions reduced, ice was used less frequently. The patient used TENS to manage discomfort, and applied it half an hour before intensive exercise sessions and as required during the day. Exercises were made more challenging with the use of 1 kg weights on ankle—inner, outer and through ranges of quadriceps and hamstrings. The patient attended the gym working on the static bike to improve her exercise tolerance, and controlled eccentric sitting to standing exercises.

On discharge 10 days later the patient was able to walk with one stick for up to 10 minutes with rests and her knee pain was 3/10. Her flexion contractures had reduced to 20° on the right and 15° on the left. A bony block was felt at the end of range. A 10 metre walk test was reduced to 16 seconds. The patient was discharged with a home exercise programme.

CASE 2

A 40-year-old female teacher was diagnosed with OA of right CMC joint, complaining of gradual onset of pain which increased both with writing and with gripping.

On examination, pain was reproduced on compression of the joint, especially on extension and mid range abduction of the thumb. Pain, rated by VAS as 6/10, was localised to the CMC joint and first metacarpal. Grip strength was measurably reduced and the patient had difficulty with handwriting. All movements of the right thumb were reduced because of pain.

The patient was given home exercises to maintain range of movement of the thumb, wrist, MCP and IP joints. The thumb was strapped for activities at work and writing reports. Initially the patient was treated with pulsed US and after three treatments reported 60% less pain. Maitland postero-anterior grade II mobilisations of the right CMC joint in thumb extension, together with added compression, further reduced the patient's pain.

After a further three treatments the patient was painfree and had full range of movement restored. She was taught isometric strengthening exercises of the thumb flexors, extensors and abductors to maintain stability of the CMC joint and progressed to resisted exercises through the available range using elastic resistive material. The patient was advised to pace herself when correcting assignments and was discharged with improved handwriting and only occasional 1/10 pain when gripping.

CASE 3

A 72-year-old man with cervical and lumbar spondylosis complained of pain rated by VAS as 6/10 and 8/10 respectively. The patient complained of several years' history of general aches in the cervical spine but no referred pain or headaches.

When examined the patient had a protracted cervical spine, exaggerated in sitting and complained of increased pain on all cervical spine movements. On palpation C5, 6 and 7 were especially tender and the upper fibres of Trapezius were in spasm. In the lumbar spine the patient demonstrated some rotational instability of the pelvis, was hyperlordotic in standing and had underactive abdominals. The man's gait was antalgic, leaning to the left, and he used a stick to alleviate his back pain. The patient complained of pain at the end of range of lumbar extension. On palpation L3/4 were tender and L1/2 were stiff but painfree. Cervical and lumbar spine neurology was normal.

The patient was taught mobilising exercises for cervical spine, shoulder girdle and glenohumeral joints, as well as hips and lumbar spine. Following a course of hydrotherapy to facilitate increased range of movement, he was advised to continue these exercises little and often throughout the day. The patient found heat beneficial and used hot packs to reduce the trapezius spasm at home. The patient was advised not to wear a collar as this exaggerated his poor posture. He was given advice on the use of pillows and how to correct his posture. The patient was taught exercises to improve the activity of abdominal and gluteal muscles and thus improve standing and walking posture. Using a mirror, he could observe his asymmetrical gait and could then correct this independently. The patient was provided with an Arthritis Research Campaign (ARC) leaflet on OA and its management.

When the patient returned a month later for review he had improved cervical spine movements and minimal pain, rated at 1/10 through range. The patient was using hot packs occasionally and had reduced low back pain of 2/10, experienced after walking for 20 minutes, and his posture had improved. Proprioceptive strapping was applied, which his wife agreed to continue at home, and he was taught to use the pressure biofeedback machine. This was used to enhance his awareness of his hyperlordotic posture and encourage further abdominal muscle control. The patient also attended the OA Education group to gain further understanding of the condition.

At a further review appointment 1 month later, the patient reported minimal pain and was independently mobilising without a stick. The patient continued to exercise independently and attended the local Arthritis Care hydrotherapy sessions.

ACKNOWLEDGEMENTS

Staff at Medical Library Services—Walsgrave Hospitals NHS Trust, Coventry, Warwickshire.
Secretariat—especially Debbie Dabbs and Sharon Murphy. Cannock Rheumatology Centre, Cannock Chase Hospital, Mid-Staffordshire District General Hospitals NHS Trust, Staffordshire.

REFERENCES

Adler S. Self care in the management of the degenerative knee joint. *Physiotherapy* 1985, **71**:58-60.

Anon. Glucosamine sulphate: effective osteoarthritis treatmnent. *Am J of Natural Medicine* 1994, **1(1)**:10-14.

Apley G, Solomon L. *Concise system of orthopaedics and fractures, 2nd edition.* Oxford: Butterworth-Heinemann; 1994:36-41.

Altman R. Development of criteria for classification and reporting of osteoarthritis. *Arthritis Rheum* 1986, **29**:1039-1049.

Badley EM, Wagstaff S, Wood PHN. Measures of functional ability (disability) in arthritis in relation to impairment of range of movement. *Ann Rheum Dis* 1984, **43**:563-569.

Bland JH. Mechanism of adaptation in the joint. In: Crosbie J, McConnell J eds. *Key issues in musculo-skeletal physiotherapy*. Oxford: Butterworth-Heinemann; 1994:88-113.

Bogduk. N. The anatomy and physiology of nociception. In: Crosbie J, McConnell J eds. *Key issues in musculo-skeletal physiotherapy*. Oxford: Butterworth-Heinemann; 1994:48-87.

Carr D, Bullen B, Skinar G *et al*. Physical conditioning facilitates the exercise induced secretion of beta-endorphin and beta-lipotropin in women. *N Engl J Med* 1981, **305**:560-563.

Clarke G, Willis L, Stenner L, Nicholls P. Evaluation of physiotherapy in the treatment of knee osteoarthritis. *Rheumatol Rehab* 1974, **13**:190-197.

Cooper C. Osteoarthritis. In: Klippel JH, Dieppe P eds. *Rheumatology*. London: Mosby; 1994:2.1-11.1.

Cooper C, Egger P, Coggon D. Generalised osteoarthritis in women: pattern of joint involvement and approaches to definition for epidemiological studies. *J Rheumatol* 1996, **23(11)**:1938-1942.

Cushnaghan J. Taping the patella medially–a new treatment for osteoarthritis of the knee joint? *BMJ* 1994, **308**:753-755.

Deal C, Schnitzer T, Lipstein E *et al*. Treatment of arthritis with topical capsaicin–a double blind trial. *Clin Ther* 1991, **13**:383-395.

De Forge B. Psychological evaluation of well being in multidisciplinary assessment of osteoarthritis. *Clin Ther* 1986, **9**:52-61.

Dovey G. Assessment of quadriceps bulk with girth measurements in subjects with patella-femoral pain. *J Ortho Sp Phys Ther* 1987, **9**:177-183.

Enneking WF, Horowitz M. The intra-articular effects of immobilisation of the human knee joint. *J Bone Jt Surg* 1972, **54A**:973.

Falconer J, Hayes KW, Chang RW. Effect of ultrasound on mobility of osteoarthritic knees. *Arthritis Care Res* 1992, **5**:29-35.

Fisher N, Pendergast DR, Gresham GE *et al*. Muscle rehabilitation–its effect on muscular and functional performance of patients with osteoarthritis of the knees. *Arch Phys Med Rehab* 1991, **72**:367-374.

Green J, McKenna F, Redfern EJ, Chamberlain MA. Home exercises are as effective as outpatient hydrotherapy for osteoarthritis of the hip. *Br J Rheum* 1993, **32**:812-815.

Han J, Terenius L. Neurochemical basis of acupuncture analgesia. *Ann Rev Pharmacol Toxicol* 1982, **22**:193-220.

Häuselmann HJ, Flechtenmacher L, Michal J *et al*. The superficial layer of human articular cartilage is more susceptible to Interleukin-1 induced damage than the deeper layers. *Arthritis Rheum* 1996, **39**:478-488.

Hayes KW. Differential muscle decline in osteoarthritis of the knee. *Arthr Care Res* 1992, **5**:24-27.

Hicks J. Exercise in patients with inflammatory arthritis and connective tissue disease. *Rheum Dis Clin North America* 1990, **16(4)**:845-870.

Hirsch R. Association of hand and knee osteoarthritis: evidence for a polyarticular subset. *Ann Rheum Dis* 1996, **55**:25-29.

Hunt S, McKenna SP, McEwen J *et al*. The Nottingham health profile. *Social Sci. Med* 1981, **15A**:221-229.

Hurley M, Newham DJ. Influence of arthrogenous muscle inhibition in joints on quadriceps rehabilitation of patients with early unilateral osteoarthritis of the knee. *Br J Rheum* 1993, **32**:127-131.

Kannus P. Knee flexor and extensor strength ratios with deficiency of lateral collateral ligament. *Arch Phys Med Rehab* 1988, **69**:928-931.

Kellegren J, Lawrence J. Radiological assessment of osteoarthritis. *Ann Rheum Dis* 1957, **16**:494-502.

Kirwan J, Reeback J. Stanford health assessment questionnaire modified to assess disability in British patients with rheumatoid arthritis. *Br J Rheum* 1986, **25**:206-209.

Krick J. Psychosocial aspects of multidisciplinary assessment of osteoarthritis. *Clin Ther* 1986, **9**:43-52.

Lane NE, Micheli B, Bjorkengren A *et al*. The risk of OA with running and aging: a 5 year longitudinal study. *J Rheumatol* 1993, **20(3)**:461-468.

Light KE, Nuzik S, Personius W *et al*. Low load prolonged stretch versus high load brief stretch in treating knee contractures. *Phys Ther* 1984, **64(3)**:330-333.

Lotts DJ, Jasani MK, Birdwood GFB. *Studies in osteoarthrosis: pathogenesis intervention and assessment*. Chichester, New York: Wiley Medical Publications; 1987.

Lozada CJ, Altman RD. Chondroprotection in osteoarthritis. *Bull Rheum Dis* 1997, **46(7)**:5-7.

Mankin H, Buckwalter J. Restoration of the osteoarthrotic joint. *J Bone Jt Surgery* 1996, **78A**:1.

McAlindon T, Dieppe P. The medical management of osteoarthritis of the knee–an inflammatory issue? *Br J Rheum* 1990, **29**:471-473.

McAlindon T, Jacques P, Zhang Y *et al*. Do antioxidant micronutrients protect against the development and progression of knee osteoarthritis. *Arthritis Rheum* 1996, **39**:648-656?

McKeag D. The relationship of osteoarthritis and exercise. *Clinics Sports Med* 1992, **11**:471-487.

Meenan R. Content and Properties of a revised and expanded AIMS health status questionnaire. *Arthritis Rheum* 1992, **35**:1-10.

Minor M, Hewitt J, Webel R *et al*. Efficiency of physical conditioning exercise in patients with rheumatoid arthritis and osteoarthritis. *Arthritis Rheum* 1989, **32**:1396-1405.

Moskowitz R. Primary osteoarthritis, epidemiology, clinical aspects and general management. *Am J Med* 1987, **83**:5.

Muncie HL. Medical aspects of multidisciplinary assessment and management of osteoarthritis. *Clin Ther* 1986, **9B**:5-13.

Oldham JA, Howe TE. Reliability of isometric quadriceps muscle strength testing in young subjects and elderly osteoarthritic subjects. *Physiotherapy* 1995, **81**:399-404.

Palomski M, Colyer R, Brandt K. Joint motion in the absence of normal loading does not maintain normal articular cartilage. *Arthritis Rheum* 1980, **23**:325-334.

Perry J, Antonelli D, Ford W. Analysis of knee joint forces during flexed knee stance. *J Bone Joint Surgery* 1975, **57A**:961-967.

Pinals RS. Mechanisms of joint destruction, pain and disability in osteoarthritis. *Drugs* 1996, **52(3)**:14-20.

Pires-Mesquita L. Homeopathy and physiotherapy, with specific references to osteoarthropathy. *Br Homeopathic J* 1987, **76**:16-18.

Ross M. Manipulation and back school in the treatment of low back pain. *Physiotherapy* 1997, **83**:181-183.

Sambrook P, Naganthan V. What is the relationship between osteoarthritis and osteoporosis? *Ballière's Clinical Rheumatology* 1997, **11(4)**:695-710.

Sylvester KL. An investigation into the effect of hydrotherapy in treatment of osteoarthritis of the hips. *Clin Rehab* 1990, **4**:223-228.

Takeda W, Wessel J. Acupuncture for treatment of pain of osteoarthritis of the knees. *Arthritis Care Res* 1994, **7**:118-122.

Van Baar ME, Dekker J, Lemmens JA. Pain and disability in patients with osteoarthritis of the hip or knee: the relationship with articular, kinesiological and psychological characteristics. *J Rheumatol* 1998, **25(1)**:125-133.

Wall JC, Crosbie J. Temporal gait analysis using slow motion video and a personal computer. *Physiotherapy* 1997, **83**:109-115.

Ware J, Sherbourne CD. The MOS 36 Item Short Form Health Survey (SF-36). *Med Care* 1992, **30**:473-483.

Waterfield J, Sim J. Clinical assessment of pain by the visual analogue scale. *Br J Ther Rehab* 1996, **3**:94-97.

White O'Connor B. Nutritional intake and obesity in the multidisciplinary assessment of osteoarthritis. *Clin Ther* 1986, **9**: 52-61.

Williams JG, Callaghan M. Comparison of visual estimation and goniometry in determination of shoulder joint angle. *Physiotherapy* 1990, **76**:655-657.

Williams P. The use of intermittent stretch in the prevention of serial sarcomere loss in immobilized muscle. *Ann Rheum Dis* 1990, **49(5)**:316-317.

Ytterberg S. Exercise for arthritis. *Ballière's Clinical Rheumatology* 1994, **8(1)**:161-189.

GENERAL READING

Brandt KD. *Diagnosis and non-surgical management of osteoarthritis*. Caddo, OK: Professional Communications Inc; 1996.

Bates A, Hanson N. *Aquatic exercise therapy*. Philadelphia: WB Saunders; 1996.

Fries J. Measurement of patient outcome in arthritis. *Arthritis Rheum* 1980, **23**:137-145.

Kendall FP, McCreary EK, Provance PG. *Muscle testing and function, 4th edition*. Baltimore: Williams and Wilkins; 1993.serologic status for HIV 1. *Biofeedback Self Regul* 1990, **15**:229-242.

La Pierriere A, Antoni M. Exercise intervention alternates emotional distress and natural killer cell decrements following notification of positive

Low J, Reed A. *Electrotherapy explained - principles and practice*. Oxford: Butterworth-Heinemann; 1994.

Norkin C, Levangie P. *Joint structure and function in the vertebral column - a comprehensive analysis, 2nd edition*. Philadelphia: FA Davis Co; 1992:57-86, 125-170.

The Disability Information Trust. *Arthritis - an equipment guide*. Oxford; 1991.

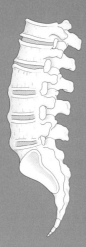

10 K Dziedzic
ANKYLOSING SPONDYLITIS

CHAPTER OUTLINE

- Aetiology, incidence and prevalence
- Prognosis
- Diagnosis and special tests
- Radiographic and pathological signs and features

- Assessment
- Medical management including surgery
- Physiotherapy management
- Case histories

INTRODUCTION

Ankylosing spondylitis (AS) is an inflammatory systemic disease predominantly affecting the axial skeleton in genetically predisposed individuals. It is probably induced by environmental factors. Peripheral joint disease and extra-articular manifestations, for example in the eye, heart and lung, may also precede its onset or complicate its course (Dougados *et al.*, 1988; Landewe & Goei The, 1989).

AS is an ancient disease, with evidence to be found in human remains from a couple of thousand years BC. Bernard O'Connor (1666–1698), an Irish physician, was the first author of a report on AS in the medical literature. The nomenclature is derived from the Greek words 'ankylos' meaning stiffening and 'spondylos' meaning vertebra, and describes inflammation of the spine which can lead to fusion of the bones.

Inflammation at the sites of attachment to bone of tendon, ligament or joint capsule (enthesitis) is a characteristic of AS (Ball, 1971). Bilateral bony fusion of the sacroiliac joints is a hallmark of this condition, which on progression may ascend to involve ligamentous and disco-genic attachments of the spine (Dudley Hart, 1985).

Individuals with AS commonly report problems of pain, stiffness, fatigue, loss of movement and function, and often find that physiotherapy plays an important role in the management of their disease (Gall, 1994).

This chapter details the clinical and non-clinical aspects of this seronegative spondyloarthropathy.

AETIOLOGY, INCIDENCE AND PREVALENCE

There are two thoughts on the causes of AS. The first is that an infectious agent is the initiating factor (e.g. *Klebsiella pneumoniae*) and the second is that people have an inherited susceptibility to develop a spondyloarthropathy (O'Mahony *et al.*, 1992; Inman & Scofield, 1994). Its prevalence in Great Britain has been reported as 1–3 cases per 1000 population, which is similar to the USA (Rigby, 1991).

Human leukocyte antigen (HLA) B27 and AS show the strongest association of all the rheumatic diseases. The MHC (major histocompatability complex) is found on chromosome 6 and is comprised of three classes of genes: class I, class II and class III. The MHC class I genes are HLA A, B and C. They present on all nucleated cells. Of all AS patients 95% are B27 positive compared to around 10% of healthy controls (Albert & Scholz, 1987).

Traditionally AS has been described as a rare disease affecting young men. However, the prevalence of HLA B27 is reported as equal in both sexes (Kidd *et al.*, 1988), and the sex ratio of sacroiliitis (inflammation of the sacroiliac joints alone) is now considered almost equal (Pal, 1987). The male:female ratio for AS was previously described as 10:1 (Bellamy, 1985), but is now thought to be between 2.5 and 4:1 (Kennedy *et al.*, 1993a). In fact there may well be fewer male AS patients in the total population than is reflected in hospital records and hospital based studies (Gran & Husby, 1984).

Women are believed to experience milder and atypical disease which may be unrecognised for years (Calabro, 1983; Barlow *et al.*, 1991) although women are reported to have now caught up with men in their speed of diagnosis. Until 1974, median diagnosis delay was 9 years in women and 6 years in men (Calin *et al.*, 1988).

In the black African and Japanese people AS is very rare, possibly due to the lack of inherited HLA B27 gene in their population (<4%) (Burgos-Vargas *et al.*, 1989).

There are a number of suggestions as to how HLA B27 is involved in AS. Rats which are able to express the HLA B27 (transgenic rats) are susceptible to a disease similar to human spondyloarthropathies (MacLean, 1992). In the future, HLA B27 may well provide the answers to questions surrounding disease expression.

PROGNOSIS

Mau *et al.* (1988) studying the prognosis of patients in a 10-year follow up found that the development of AS was characterised by a prolonged course and that 78% of patients maintained good or adequate function, indicating a good functional prognosis. Sturrock (1991) has followed up 63 AS patients over a number of years. Over a 5-year period they remained stable. Chest expansion increased, while peripheral joint disease and iritis decreased over time. This suggests that AS does not progress rapidly in the majority of patients although it may not eliminate a small subgroup of patients with a progressive, disabling disease. Smoking has been associated with a worse outcome (Averns *et al.*, 1996a).

It is generally accepted that the overall functional outcome of AS patients is good in the long-term, but patients will continue to be episodically symptomatic and that 'burn out' of the disease is rare (Thomson & Chalmers, 1993). Most severe pain is thought to be experienced earlier in the disease although Kennedy *et al.* (1993b) found disease activity to be worse in older patients in a two-year study, and concluded that:
• Less than 1% of patients 'burn out'.
• 20% of patients will develop active disease 2 years later.
• Prognosis of those with active disease is poor.

Donnelly *et al.* (1994) found that changes in clinical measures of range of movement occur only slowly, may initially improve with treatment, and require 4 or more years to reflect in the loss of function. The prognosis regarding employment suggests that 29% of patients with AS become unemployed prior to the age of 65 with the majority of patients working well into their fifties (Jones *et al.*, 1994).

Cervical spine fractures continue to be a high cause of mortality and morbidity in AS patients. The most frequent fracture site is at C6/7 (Khan, 1993). Early studies of mortality were complicated by deaths caused by treatment with irradiation. Respiratory disease, cardiovascular disease and amyloidosis are the most noted causes of death but considering the fair functional outcome of most patients it is often more appropriate to discuss morbidity rather than mortality (Rigby, 1991, Thomson & Chalmers, 1993).

DIAGNOSIS AND SPECIAL TESTS

Diagnostic criteria were first proposed in Rome in 1961 (Kellgren *et al.*, 1963) and later in New York in 1966 (Bennett & Burch, 1968). The New York criteria have now been modified (Table 10.1) (Cats *et al.*, 1987). Although such criteria are useful for epidemiological studies and research in defining a homogeneous patient population, in clinical practice careful consideration of all presenting features is needed when diagnosing individual patients. Secondary AS is diagnosed if it coexists with psoriatic arthritis, Reiter's syndrome and inflammatory bowel disease (Calin, 1993).

HLA B27 testing in patients is expensive and its usefulness is evaluated in each individual case. Khan & Khan (1982) suggested that if the clinical diagnosis of AS was 50%, then knowing that the patient was HLA B27 positive would increase the probability of AS to 90%, and if negative would reduce it to about 10%. Family history may be crucial in ascertaining a diagnosis and pattern of disease in different family members may be variable.

Those in whom a definite diagnosis cannot be determined will benefit from being managed as possible AS patients. Those patients who, with the passage of time, are found not to have AS but a simple mechanical back problem should not be disadvantaged, as the management of back pain with dynamic exercises has now become more established (Frost *et al.*, 1995). Referral to a rheumatologist at this early stage is desirable. Patients may subsequently be managed in the primary care setting but this will depend upon the individual case.

RADIOGRAPHIC AND PATHOLOGICAL SIGNS AND FEATURES

AXIAL SKELETON
General

Spontaneous bilateral inflammation in the iliac portion of the sacroiliac joints, followed by erosion and sclerosis and subsequent reactive bone formation bridging the sacroiliac joint (from the ilium to the sacrum), is the frequent mode of onset in AS. From here it may progress and ascend the spine with the erosion, sclerosis and reactive bone formation producing syndesmophytes (or enthesophytes) (Figure 10.1). A syndesmophyte is a bridge of bone from the margin of one vertebral body to another. In the zygoapophyseal joints for example, enthesophyte formation at the site of the joint capsule may grow to encapsulate the joint which may then undergo secondary ossification (Figure 10.2) (Resnick & Niwayama, 1988).

Discovertebral Junction

At the discovertebral junction, syndesmophytes may form at lesions around the attachment of the annulus fibrosus. Subsequent bridging of the disc space to the adjacent vertebra can then occur. Ligamentous calcification may ascend the anterior longitudinal ligament, posterior longitudinal ligament, and the inferior and superior interspinous ligaments. The pattern of this calcification is predominantly symmetrical (Resnick & Niwayama, 1988). The involvement of the discovertebral junction can be divided into 5 categories:
• Osteitis.
• Syndesmophytosis.
• Erosions/destruction.
• Discal calcification.
• Osteoporosis.

Osteitis
Osteitis is seen as bony erosions on the anterior corners of the vertebral body (Romanus lesion) or healed lesions ('shiny corner sign').

Syndesmophytosis
Syndesmophytosis is the ossification of the outer fibres of the annulus fibrosis, anterior longitudinal ligament and paravertebral connective tissue. This can be evident before gross sacroiliac joint changes and a 'Bamboo' spine (where fusion can occur throughout the length of the vertebral column) is possible in the later stages.

Erosions and Destruction
Erosions and destruction (Andersson lesions) can be:
• Localised centrally and associated with disc displacement into the vertebral body (Schmorl's nodes).
• Localised peripherally with anterior collapse similar to that in thoracic kyphosis.
• Occurring together (pseudoarthrosis).

Modified New York criteria for ankylosing spondylitis			
Diagnosis			
Clinical criteria			**Grading**
Low back pain >3 months, exercise eases, rest aggravates	Limitation of the lumbar spine in frontal and sagittal planes	Limitation of chest expansion (age/sex related)	Definite – X-ray plus 1 clinical criteria Probable – 3 clinical criteria
X-ray criteria			**Grading**
Sacroiliitis ≥ grade 2 bilaterally or grade 3–4 unilaterally			Definite – X-ray plus 1 clinical criteria Probable – X-ray criteria

Table 10.1 **Modified New York criteria for ankylosing spondylitis.**

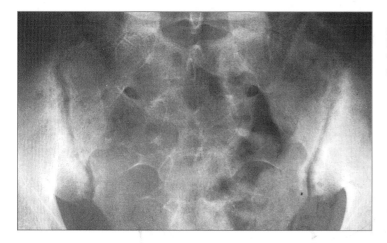

Figure 10.1 **Spontaneous bilateral inflammation in the iliac portion of the sacroiliac joints, followed by erosion, is a frequent mode of onset in ankylosing spondylitis.**

Discal Calcification

Discal calcification may be caused by immobilisation of a segment and subsequent poor nutrition (Resnick & Niwayama, 1988).

Osteoporosis

Osteoporosis is probably due to reduced bone turnover (Edmunds, 1990), diminished trabecular density (Rubinstein, 1991) or the systemic effect of the disease (Calin, 1991).

Cervical Spine

In the atlantoaxial joint, inflammation of the synovium and ligament leads to erosion of the dens which may disappear entirely. Atlantoaxial subluxation is a rare complication of AS but the joint may re-ankylose in the subluxed position affording it some stability. Spinal fractures in AS are predominantly found in the cervical spine and subsequent paralysis is always a danger (Resnick & Niwayama, 1988). A pseudoarthrosis is also to be suspected in an established patient with sudden onset of acute spinal pain or with a history of injury.

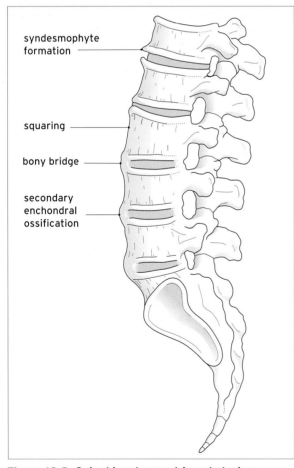

Figure 10.2 **Spinal involvement in ankylosing spondylitis.**

Bony Ankylosis

Bony ankylosis can ascend to involve the whole spine. On a frontal X-ray, three lines of ossification can be detected (known as the 'trolley-track sign'), two ascending the apophyseal joints laterally and one centrally ascending line following the supraspinous and interspinous ligaments. Costovertebral joint ankylosis functionally limits chest expansion and respiratory function. On the posterior ligamentous attachments, evidence of ossification of interspinous and supraspinous ligaments can be seen as a single line on X-ray ('dagger sign') (Resnick & Niwayama, 1988).

PERIPHERAL JOINT DISEASE

Peripheral joint disease may precede onset of AS or present during its course (Landewe & Goei The, 1989). 20% of patients initially present with a peripheral arthritis and 35% may experience it at some time during their disease (Bellamy, 1985). Concurrent peripheral joint disease and AS is also associated with a poor outcome. Juvenile AS patients show greater hip involvement and late onset AS patients greater involvement of the glenohumeral joints (Calin et al., 1990). In a teenager, especially male, the insidious onset of a single joint arthritis (oligoarthritis) can be the presenting feature, for example a knee effusion. Even the temporomandibular joint (TMJ) can be a site of stiffness and discomfort in some patients. Not only are synovial articulations involved, cartilaginous joints can also be affected, e.g. sternocostal joints.

EXTRASKELETAL

Ringsdal & Andreasen (1989) found that 51% of women and 30% of men had experienced extra-articular disease. In the eye iritis occurs in 25% of patients (Bellamy, 1985); 33% of women and 15% of men had iritis before the diagnosis of AS was established (Ringsdal & Andreasen, 1989). Patients should seek immediate medical treatment for iritis, either through their general practitioner or Eye Accident and Emergency Department, to prevent chronicity and damage to sight.

In the heart, symptomatic involvement occurs in approximately 5% of AS patients. Problems can be associated with aortic insufficiency from inflammation of the aortic valve, conduction defects, cardiomyopathy and fibrosis, cardiac enlargement, pericarditis and aortic aneurysms (O'Neill & Bresnihan, 1992). The lung involvement is similar to tuberculosis with apical pulmonary fibrosis and cavitation. Pleuritis can be another feature, while amyloidosis is a potentially fatal problem for patients (Bellamy 1985). The main organ involved in spondyloarthropathy is the bowel with subclinical, low grade involvement having all been observed. Inflammatory bowel disease (IBD), Crohn's disease and ulcerative colitis are linked with AS (Calin, 1993). Muscle fibrosis found on postmortem assessment of the heart of AS patients (Marshall, 1991) is in keeping with abnormalities reported on biopsy of the paraspinal muscles (Cooper et al., 1991).

ENTHESITIS

One of the histopathological characteristics of AS is enthesitis. An enthesis is the site of attachment to bone of tendon, ligament or joint capsule (Ball, 1971) and the presence of enthesitis is regarded as important in classification of spondyloarthropathies by the European Spondylo arthropathy Study Group (Burgos-Vargas & Pineda, 1991).

An enthesis, for example a tendon or ligament, comprises four zones. Zone 1 consists of the bands of collagen fibres which provide strength and resistance to traction. Zone 2 is unmineralised fibrocartilage with chondrocytes. An abrupt transition occurs at Zone 3, with mineralised fibrocartilage directly adjacent to the bone. Zone 4 is the bone matrix. Tendon fibres become compact, then cartilaginous (Sharpey's fibres) and then calcified. Entheses are found in synovial joints, cartilaginous joints, syndesmoses and in extra-articular regions (Schweitzer & Resnick, 1994).

Common sites for enthesitis include the insertions of the Achilles tendon and plantar fascia in the calcaneum. Other areas have been considered as entheses, for example interosseous ligaments, symphysis pubis, manubriosternum and intervertebral discs. The annulus fibrosus is a classic site of enthesitis with its attachment to the margin of the vertebral body, and the fibres around the nucleus pulposum being equivalent to the cells found between tendon fibres (Fournie, 1993).

Enthesopathy is not specific to AS, occurring in other conditions such as osteoarthritis (OA) and diabetes mellitus either acutely or chronically, or following trauma (Niepel & Sit'aj, 1979). Enthesopathy, either isolated or combined with peripheral arthropathy, was found to be very common in Mexican juvenile AS patients, 47% showing involvement of enthesopathies following 1 year of onset of the disease and in some it preceded onset of sacroiliitis (Burgos-Vargas & Clark, 1989, Khan, 1989). Although multiple sites of peripheral enthesitis are affected in AS, the tarsal region accounts for 83–89% of juvenile and 27–44% of adult onset AS (Burgos-Vargas, 1990).

In a study of human entheses the presence of type II collagen has been demonstrated, which significantly occurs in cartilage, the nucleus pulposus and vitreous body (Fener *et al.*, 1992). The aortitis seen in some AS patients may also be due to this selective tissue inflammation (Jacobs, 1983).

ASSESSMENT

Assessment is possibly one of the most important roles of physiotherapists in the multidisciplinary management of AS patients, given their knowledge of physical therapies, movement and musculoskeletal evaluation. In the established patient, assessment is important in monitoring the disease. Patients stable in their condition would ideally be assessed at yearly intervals by the rheumatology team. This may be the prime responsibility of the physiotherapist in an extended role as a clinical specialist. Patients with more severe disease would be monitored more frequently with regular intervention by the rheumatologist (e.g. drug management, assessment of extra-articular manifestations). A system of emergency appointments through self-referral can enhance the follow-up process.

Clinical assessment is comprised of subjective, objective and semi-objective measurements. It is important to consider prior to assessment the potential clinical signs and symptoms that may be expressed by AS patients.

CLINICAL SIGNS AND SYMPTOMS

Pain and stiffness are the two most common problems reported by AS patients (Brown *et al.*, 1987). Pain in AS as described by Good (1986) can be divided into three stages which may overlap.

Stage 1

Isolated sacroiliac 'inflammatory' pain is often described as 'hip pain' by the patient and is experienced on the outer quadrant of the buttock. It may alternate from side to side, occasionally with referral into the thigh as far as the knee. and is often mislabelled as 'sciatica' (Figure 10.3). 'Pure' sacroiliac pain is mild and nagging, wakening the patient at night. Getting up, sitting and walking eases the pain. A few patients experience transient, sharp and severe pain exacerbated by jarring or vigorous activity. Episodes may be followed by extended asymptomatic periods.

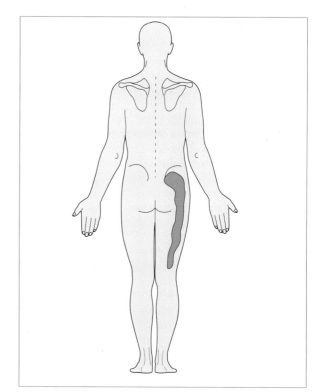

Figure 10.3 **Body chart illustration of pseudo-sciatica.**

Stage 2

The initial pain is limited to the lumbar segment but patients can experience simultaneous or even exclusive interscapular or low cervical pain. Pain is now largely not relieved by rest or immobility. Crippling pain and stiffness is frequently described immediately after getting up in the morning, only to disappear as the stiffness resolves within 30–90 minutes, and can break through again by mid-afternoon. Anterior chest pain is another feature; non-anginal and 'mechanical', typically a sharp, jabbing pain encircling the hemithorax precipitated by coughing or laughing. It can be localised or may coexist with thoracic spine pain.

Stage 3

A nagging interscapular, cervical or even lumbar pain is experienced. When excruciating focal pain appears abruptly in patients with late or dormant AS a pseudoarthrosis should be suspected. Most of these patients have ankylosed thoracic and lumbar segments which finally give way, usually at a fulcrum in the lower dorsal spine. Severe pain resolves only with immobilisation and natural reankylosis (Good, 1986). Costovertebral joint pain may be experienced locally or may radiate along the course of a nerve root, and may be due to an enthesitis and associated with more severe disease (Dawes *et al.*, 1988). In rare instances, this pain is intractable (Tsai & Eastmond, 1987).

Pain may vary in nature and frequency, be a dull constant or an intermittent pain with sharp, excruciating episodes. Patients may also present with an acute discitis or a fractured syndesmophyte with localised lumbar pain which is aggravated by exercise. Paraspinal muscle fibrosis, a specific pathological component of AS, may contribute to back stiffness and weakness (Cooper *et al.*, 1991). Local spinal complications can cause severe, crippling backache and a person with a fixed spine is predisposed to symptoms (Dunn *et al.*, 1985). Cauda Equina Syndrome is probably due to early arachnoiditis with subsequent loss of meningeal elasticity and expansion of the dural sac. It is of gradual onset, the most disabling symptoms being genitourinary and radicular pain in the legs and feet (Milde *et al.*, 1977).

Inflammatory spinal pain has features distinguishing it from mechanical pain. Inflammatory pain is charcterised by:
• Frequently insidious onset.
• Family and medical history.
• Younger individual (under 40 years of age).
• Affects sleep.
• Worse in the mornings.
• Better with exercise and worse with rest.
• Diffuse radiation of pain (rarely below the knee).
• Normal straight leg raise test.
• Diffuse local tenderness and muscle spasm.
• Other signs and symptoms (perhaps hip or other symmetrical joint involvement).

Conversely, mechanical spinal pain is characterised by:
• Acute onset.

• Striking any age.
• Worse with exercise and relieved with rest.
• Radiation of pain which may go below the knee.
• Sensory and motor symptoms.
• Reduced straight leg raise and neurological signs (Calin, 1993).

Dudley Hart (1955) explored the initial presenting symptom of patients: 73.4% experienced pain and/or stiffness in the lower back and buttocks as the initial symptom, as compared with 24% in whom the initial symptom lay in the periphery. Spinal complications, for example cysts in the dura of the spinal cord, can also be a cause of pain.

After pain and stiffness, one of the most important complaints of patients with AS is disability (Dougados *et al.*, 1988). AS patients rate highly in the inability to do everyday tasks when compared with patients with rheumatoid arthritis (RA) and OA. This is not surprising given the well known axial and peripheral effects of the disease (Brown *et al.*, 1987).

All rheumatic diseases affect the whole system and attention to the locomotor system in clinical practice and research can often detract from extra-articular manifestations and symptoms, e.g. fatigue (Toivanen & Toivanen, 1994). Calin *et al.* (1993) have suggested that fatigue should be considered a major problem in AS.

Barlow *et al.* (1992) studied psychosocial factors associated with AS, in particular looking at patients who attended a National AS Society (NASS) self-help group and those who did not, and demonstrated that these were important factors to consider. One-third of people with AS report high levels of depression, women being affected more than men (Barlow *et al.*, 1993). AS patients seem to adjust over a period of years to changes in lifestyle and possibly patients choose not to approach the clinician with problems with certain functional activities, for example sexual difficulties (Wright, 1991).

Sexual problems for the patient can include lack of desire, pain on approach and stiff or immobile hips. For the partner it can mean fear of hurting the patient and uncertainty over duration of symptoms. This can obviously lead to a strain on the relationship (Calin & Elswood, 1989).

Nemes (1991) reported on psychosocial and physical problems in AS as a result of questionnaire and telephone interviews of members of the American sister group of NASS. Problems fell into three categories: physical, relationship and individual. In relationships, AS patients may feel misunderstood or unsupported by their spouse and isolated from their previous social group. Fatigue may prevent participation in social activity and sport. Sexual activity may be reduced. Diminished body image may lead to embarrassment in existing family relationships and prospective relationships. Often patients struggle to work in an unaccommodating environment. The problems of control of the disease and the failure to cope can cause the onset of 'learned helplessness' where the patient stops trying anything (Nemes, 1991).

The top nine rated physical problems were: difficulty sleeping on the stomach, stiffness on waking, standing for long periods, prolonged sitting, bending, being a spectator rather than participating in activities, increased pain with increased stress, tiredness on waking and limitation on leisure activities. The physical problems could be grouped into four areas:

- The neck, for example in driving, reaching, hugging.
- Sexual function.
- Pain aggravated by rest, for example if someone had a problem with sleep it would lead to tiredness.
- Low back dysfunction, for example putting on shoes and socks (Nemes, 1991).

Table 10.2 provides a summary of the clinical features in AS.

SUBJECTIVE ASSESSMENT

Frequently recorded baseline and follow-up data can include demographic details, social history, family history, past and present medical history (including treatment, general health, length of diagnosis and length of symptoms). Pain, stiffness, fatigue, disability and psychological well-being are also addressed in various forms in clinical practice (Chartered Society of Physiotherapy, Standards of Practice in Ankylosing Spondylitis).

An example of a sociodemographic assessment is detailed in Table 10.3.

Pain

Visual Analogue Scales

Assessment of pain in AS patients is routinely performed with a visual analogue scale (VAS) or a 5-point descriptive scale (Garrett *et al.*, 1994). A commonly used method of evaluating clinical pain, VAS consists of a line, normally 10 cm long, which is anchored at each end by verbal descriptors. The verbal descriptor may be any word or phrase which can be used to describe pain (e.g. 'no pain' to 'intolerable pain'). Subjects are asked to place a mark on the line at a point which they feel represents their pain. VAS scores constitute a method of evaluating pain which is valid and sensitive and has a reasonable degree of reproducibility (Dixon & Bird, 1981).

Pain can be evaluated singularly on a VAS, for example when assessing present pain or night pain, or it can be evaluated as a part of an index as in the Bath AS Disease Activity Index (BASDAI) (Garrett *et al.*, 1994). Others suggest the use of a 4-point scale or listing the number of times a patient is woken by pain for evaluation of night pain (Van der Linden and Van der Heijde, 1995). Although a VAS can be used vertically or horizontally, the vertical line can be mistaken for a representation of the spine in AS patients (Bird and Dixon, 1987).

Most clinical measures of pain in AS are unidimensional in nature and concentrate on severity rather than the multi-dimensional aspects of the pain experience.

Table 10.2 **Summary of clinical features.**

Summary of clinical features	
Presentation and summary of clinical features in ankylosing spondylitis	
Systemic disease Bilateral sacroiliitis Predominantly axial skeleton HLA B27 positive 95% patients Insidious onset Family history Usually < 40 years of age Males and females	
Affects sleep Pain (especially night) Stiffness (especially morning) Better with exercise, worse with rest Diffuse radiation of pain Local tenderness Muscle spasm Pseudosciatica, rarely below knee Hip pain Oligoarthritis Enthesitis Chest pain Fatigue Loss of normal range of movement Disability Depression	Possible additional involvement Eye, heart, lung Peripheral joints Inflammatory bowel disease

The Body Chart

Pain drawings are used by physiotherapists to assess pain in patients by location and distribution of symptoms. Pain mapping on a body chart has been used to differentiate between different types of rheumatic disease (RA, OA and fibromyalgia) where patients were asked to draw a body map of their painful areas and score each painful area using a simple descriptive scale (Nolli *et al.*, 1988).

The use of a body chart for the assessment of pain in patients with AS has been validated (Dziedzic *et al.*, 1995). Patients shade in areas of pain on the chart and then score each area of pain as mild =1, moderate =2, severe =3 or very severe =4. The body chart score is the sum of the individual pain intensity scores.

Stiffness

Stiffness has a strong association with AS and is cited in the diagnostic criteria as one of the clinical symptoms important in the disease (Calin, 1987). Duration of morning stiffness or assessment on a VAS are commonly used methods of measurement.

Disability

Assessment of function in the patient with AS is often approached in a similar way to RA. In RA, assessments such as the Stanford Health Assessment Questionnaire (HAQ) (Fries *et al.*, 1980, Kirwan & Reeback, 1986) is used.

Disability is often specific for each rheumatic disease. For example, because most patients with RA have involvement of the small joints of the hands, many questions comprising these indices are biased towards limb function, i.e. the capacity to open a door, lift a cup to drink with one hand etc. An AS assessment questionnaire (HAQ-S) has been developed to include five additional questions which encompass the assessment of problems specific to patients with spondyloarthropathies (Daltroy *et al.*, 1990). Others have also modified the HAQ score (Guillemin *et al.*, 1990; Nemeth *et al.*, 1990).

Pain and functional capacity have been assessed using the AS Assessment questionnaire (ASAQ) and a modified Arthritis Impact Measurement Scales (AIMS) questionnaire (Meenan *et al.*, 1980; Calin & Elswood, 1989).

Dougados *et al.* (1988) introduced a tool which has been widely used. Patients rate their ability to perform 20 functional tasks such as: put on shoes, pull on trousers/tights, get into a bath, remain standing for 10 minutes, run, sit down, crouch, turn in bed, cough or sneeze, etc.

Calin *et al.* (1994) have developed the Bath AS Functional Index (BASFI) as a way of evaluating functional ability. The index consists of 10 questions relating to everyday function and each question is reported on a 10 cm VAS with 0 as easy and 10 as impossible. It is designed to be quick and simple for patients to administer themselves.

Abbott *et al.* (1994) published work with a new self-administered questionnaire for assessment of specific disability in AS. It covers four areas of difficulty for AS

Table 10.3 An example of a sociodemographic assessment.

An example of a sociodemographic assessment
Name: Hospital Number:
Consultant: GP: Date of birth: Age: Sex: Address: Tel no:
Occupation: Hobbies/Sports:
Family (history of condition):
Past medical history (iritis/chest pain/trauma):
Past treatments (medication/admissions/therapy/surgery):
General health (bowel/skin/smoker):
Diagnosis: Length of diagnosis: Length of symptoms:
HLA B27: positive: negative: unknown:
Date: Clinician:

patients (mobility, bending down, reaching up and neck movements) and is an adaptation of the HAQ. The questions are similar to the Functional Index by Dougados but include questioning the ability to 'wipe yourself after using the toilet' which is often glossed over in clinical practice.

Fatigue

Fatigue is a disabling symptom of AS (Calin *et al.*, 1993). It has been recognised in the literature and is now incorporated into the assessment of AS (Garrett *et al.*, 1994). Fatigue is commonly reported on a VAS, and can be anchored by verbal descriptors of 'none' at one end and 'worst possible' at the other.

Psychosocial Factors

Measures of psychosocial features of AS are not universally addressed in clinical practice, although this area is gaining importance (Calin, 1994). Barlow *et al.* (1992) have used several measures in their work in this area: The Centre for Epidemiological Studies-Depression (CES-D) scale, the Multi-Dimensional Health Locus of Control (MHLC) Scales and the Social Support Scale (SSS). Other tools, for example the Hospital Anxiety and Depression Scale (HAD) (Zigmond & Snaith, 1983), have also been used in AS.

'Coping with disease' and 'quality of life' will have an important place as outcome measures in the future evaluation of therapy intervention.

OBJECTIVE ASSESSMENT

In an attempt to quantify onset and progress of disease, methods of objective assessment continue to form a battery of clinical and diagnostic measurement.

Radiographic Investigations

The diagnostic criteria state the value of X-ray evaluation in AS, changes in the sacroiliac joints being the hallmark of the disease. Such changes can be graded and high quality radiographs of sacroiliac joints are often sufficient for diagnosis (Calin, 1993).

Radionuclide techniques (scintigraphy), computerised tomography (CT), magnetic resonance imaging (MRI) and ultrasonography may be useful in early or late stages in the disease and in enthesopathy to examine areas of disease activity, severity and damage (Taylor *et al.*, 1991a).

Range of Movement Measures

Range of movement measures (see Table 10.4) are useful in monitoring disease over time and have been shown to

Examples of the range of movement measures used in the assessment of ankylosing spondylitis		
Measurement	**Method**	**Reference**
Tragus to wall	Patient standing against a wall, heels and hips touching wall, distance in cm from tragus to wall	Jenkinson *et al.*, 1994
Chest expansion	Hands on the back of the head, arms flexed in the frontal plane, measure at level of nipple line, or in women at level of 4th intercostal space. Record difference between full inspiration and expiration. <2.5 cm indicates restriction	Moll & Wright, 1972
Finger tip to floor distance	Patient stands erect, knees straight and feet shoulder width apart. Measure the vertical distance between middle finger tip and floor (cm)	Fitzgerald *et al.*, 1983
Lateral lumbar flexion	As above but patient bends sideways. Repeat to opposite side (cm)	Pile *et al.*, 1991
Modified Schober flexion	Patient standing, mark the spinal intersection of a line joining the dimples of Venus. Mark two points, 5 cm below and 10 cm above this level. The increase in distance is measured when the patient bends forwards. <4–6 cm increase can indicate restriction	Schober, 1937; Macrae & Wright, 1969; Moll & Wright, 1973
Neck rotation-1	Patient rotates head as far as possible. Measure with a tape measure from the tip of the nose to the opposite acromio-clavicular joint. Repeat to opposite side (cm)	modification of Pile *et al.*, 1991
Neck rotation-2	Simple inclinometer secured to the head	Klaber Moffett *et al.*, 1989
Intermalleolar distance	Patient supine, measure intermalleolar distance when patient abducts legs apart as far as possible (cm)	Jenkinson *et al.*, 1994

Table 10.4 **Examples of range of movement measures used in the assessment of ankylosing spondylitis.**

correlate well with X-ray scores (Kennedy *et al.*, 1995, Viitanen *et al.*, 1995, Averns *et al.*, 1996b).

Many assessments are performed with crude instruments such as goniometers, inclinometers and tape measures. In the future, the use of electromagnetic tracking systems to measure dynamic movement may be widely available for use in the clinical setting. These systems (e.g. Isotrak, Fastrak) allow real-time recording of dynamic movement or 'virtual reality' (Russell *et al.*, 1993, Saleh *et al.*, 1994).

Enthesitis Index

AS patients may experience pain at sites of entheses on palpation. Enthesitis indices are used as a clinical measure of AS and are suitable for the assessment of therapy, a positive enthesitis score being associated with more severe disease (Dawes *et al.*, 1987, Mander *et al.*, 1987). An example of an enthesitis index is illustrated in Table 10.5. This has been modified from the Haywood Hospital Enthesitis Index (Zukovskis *et al.*, 1991). Observer training helps to improve the standardisation of the degree of pressure required in the palpation of different sites.

ASSESSING DISEASE ACTIVITY

In AS, there is no satisfactory measure of disease activity which can demonstrate improvement after therapy. Disease activity is usually described in terms of pain, early morning stiffness, range of movement and mobility, peripheral joint disease, iritis, erythrocyte sedimentation rate (ESR) and C-reactive protein (CRP) (Scott *et al.*, 1981). If the disease is active ESR and CRP may be raised, although there are limitations in assessing disease activity with laboratory investigations (Nashel *et al.*, 1986; Sheehan *et al.*, 1986; Taylor *et al.*, 1993).

Disease activity is often associated with iritis and the presence of peripheral joint disease but using these in axial disease may not be helpful (Taylor *et al.*, 1991b). Enthesitis has been another attempt to develop a clinical measure of disease, assessing severity of tenderness in entheses. It has been found to correlate with pain and stiffness (Dawes *et al.*, 1987) and be sensitive to change (Mander *et al.*, 1987). The relationship between disease activity and prognosis has yet to be determined.

There is no simple relationship between disease activity and disability, highlighting the fact that disability needs to be investigated as the end product of a process of adaptation (McFarlane & Brooks, 1988). Furthermore, disease activity has to be distinguished from functional disability (Calin, 1994). However, the importance of defining disease status and impact of illness in AS patients is recognised (Calin, 1995).

OUTCOME MEASUREMENT

Fries *et al.* (1980) started the ball rolling in terms of patient outcome in arthritis where outcome was described in terms of the five 'D's: death, discomfort, disability, drug toxicity and dollar costs. A definition of outcome in patient terms could be that 'their requirements from the health care system are to remain alive as long as possible, be free of symptoms, have no functional disability, no adverse effects from therapy, and all this at a reasonable cost to themselves or society' (Fries, 1993).

Outcome measurement in rheumatic disease encompasses two aspects: the disease outcome and the patient outcome. The patient aims to be pain free and fully functional whereas the clinician searches for a combination of inflammatory markers (laboratory tests) and damage indicators (X-ray). Different categories of measure assess

Table 10.5 **The modified Haywood Enthesitis Index.**

The modified Haywood Enthesitis Index		
	Right	**Left**
Achilles tendon		
Insertion of plantar fascia		
Greater trochanter		
Hip adductor origin		
Iliac crest (superior and anterior borders)		
Sterno-costal		
Sterno-clavicular		
C7/T1		
Total score:		
0 = no pain 1 = discomfort 2 = definite pain 3 = withdrawal		

disease characteristics (classification, diagnosis, status), activity (the effect of treatment, side effects) and damage (prognosis) (Symmons, 1995).

The Wessex Region Physiotherapy Audit Project is an example of outcomes-based clinical audit. Patients were categorised into four groups. Patients with AS were classified in the third group, described as 'conditions where persistent disability or degenerative disease prevents physiotherapy from "curing" the patient. Short-term, regular courses of maintenance are indicated. Outcome measures need to be individually tailored in each episode of treatment' (Barnard, 1995). Although this approach was not condition specific, the recommendations for outcome measures for patients falling into this category were meaningful in AS. They conclude that:

- Objective measures may be a better indicator of disease process rather than physiotherapy intervention.
- Use of VAS for pain and fatigue, for example, may be an indicator of coping with disease.
- The patients' understanding of their condition, management and coping strategies could be indicators of a positive effect of physiotherapy intervention.

MEDICAL MANAGEMENT INCLUDING SURGERY

DRUG TREATMENT

Currently there are three categories of drug therapy in use with AS patients: drugs influencing the disease process, e.g. sulphasalazine; non steroidal anti-inflammatory drugs (NSAIDs) suppressing the inflammation without influencing the disease process; and analgesics and muscle relaxants (Gran & Husby, 1992).

Drug management will vary between patients. Most will be maintained on intermittent or continuous doses of NSAIDs, although many patients prefer not to take medication because of the potential side effects. During periods of high disease activity, NSAIDs can be used selectively. A drug will be used at the appropriate dose until it is shown to be ineffective. A high dose of NSAIDs before bedtime or pre- and post-operatively may be efficacious. The benefits of being able to move free from pain and stiffness and to continue normal activities of daily life cannot be underestimated. In some instances the use of a maintenance dose of NSAIDs can be essential, e.g. Diclofenac, Indomethacin and Naproxen. Sulphasalazine can be useful in suppressing disease and may be used in patients with high disease activity, peripheral arthritis and with a short disease duration (Gran & Husby, 1992).

Methotrexate can be advantageous for use in AS patients with psoriasis, while peripheral arthritis may be treated with local injections of corticosteroids as may enthesopathy. In resistant enthesopathy local radiotherapy will be considered. Total body radiotherapy for aggressive disease is rare. Specialist drug counselling clinics are available for patients who need monitoring and counselling.

Further reading on the role of medication in inflammatory conditions can be found in Chapter 3.

SURGERY

Hip joint replacement, and more rarely shoulder joint replacement, may be beneficial. Highly specialised spinal surgery for AS patients would normally be carried out at specialist centres. A retrospective study of patient outcome following surgical correction of fixed kyphotic deformities of the spine in AS has demonstrated excellent improvement in health status using the Modified AIMS (Halm et al., 1995).

Spinal fractures (traumatic or pseudoarthrosis), progressive spinal deformity, rotary instability (secondary to atlanto-occipital or atlanto-axial subluxation) and spinal stenosis (with associated neurological deficit, pain or spinal instability) are the most common indications for spinal surgery (Fox et al., 1993). Spinal anaesthesia may be used as an alternative to a general anaesthetic in AS patients undergoing lower limb surgery (Schelew & Vaghadia, 1996).

PHYSIOTHERAPY MANAGEMENT

Ideally the rheumatology team would help patients cope with their disease and empower them to pursue an improved quality of life. Physiotherapy is recognised as being a vital part of any management programme in AS (Gall, 1994, Viitanen & Suni, 1995).

Patients firstly need to receive advice and education about the condition. They need to be prepared for events that may present during the course of their disease so that patients are able to seek assistance at the appropriate time. A physiotherapist should be prepared to listen to the patient and to counsel when appropriate. Patient focussed management will be enhanced by shared goal setting between therapist and patient.

Seeking to maintain a patient's maximal potential movement is paramount to the management process, along with prevention of postural deformities. It has been suggested that inflammation in the zygoapophyseal joints encourages patients to adopt pain-relieving postures like flattening the lumbar spine or increasing a lumbar kyphosis. As a response to this change in spinal posture the patient may then develop a poking chin as they protract their cervical spine, leading to the question-mark posture which is frequently seen in a patient with classic AS.

Symptoms have been discussed previously. Although pain and stiffness are most commonly reported, surprisingly few patients should need individual 'pain-relieving' physiotherapy treatments. Transcutaneous Electrical Nerve Stimulation (TENS) may be useful for self-management of pain in some AS patients. Exercise is preferable to any treatment which reduces the active participation of the patient, and hydrotherapy may be helpful to patients in considerable discomfort.

EXERCISE

Exercise is one of the main treatment approaches for AS patients (Wordsworth et al., 1984, Pearcy et al., 1985, Tomlinson et al., 1986, Hidding et al., 1993, Kraag et al., 1994, Helliwell et al., 1996) and this will take many forms, depending on patients' capabilities and the approach of the team caring for them; 'keep moving to prevent fusing'.

Many patients are self caring and are well motivated to perform a routine home programme of exercises and/or are able to participate in sport and leisure activities suited to their ability. Swimming is to be encouraged but the dangers in continuing to participate in contact sports need to be stated.

Group exercises in a physiotherapy department gym may facilitate compliance. Some rheumatology departments may offer regular hospital outpatient classes of exercises and hydrotherapy whilst others offer inpatient stays for 2 to 3 weeks for intensive physiotherapy, either as a routine procedure for all patients or for the individual patient with problems. Admitting a patient for a 2-week course of intensive treatment at a time of need, for review of drug treatment, daily hydrotherapy (Figure 10.4), supervised exercise programmes and group work, is of great value.

Patients should be encouraged to join self-help groups in their area run through the NASS, who provide a supportive environment enabling patients to share their experiences and participate in exercise programmes. A visit to a NASS group to meet patients and observe supervised exercise classes would be very beneficial to therapists new to this field looking to develop their own exercise programmes and wanting to know the limits to which patients

can be pushed. Tables 10.6 and 10.7 illustrate some examples of exercises commonly used by AS patients.

Dangers and Precautions

- Atlanto-occipital/atlanto-axial subluxation.
- Pseudoarthrosis.
- Osteoporosis.
- Heart abnormalities.
- Joint replacements, e.g. hip and shoulder.
- Severely restricted breathing.

Standard fitness testing of patients prior to exercise prescription or recruitment to an exercise class (Jones & Barker, 1996, Buckley *at al.*, 1998) is probably overlooked by many physiotherapists who lack experience in this, and yet it would appear essential to the management of patients with AS. Future research in this field may well open up this area of need. Regular follow-ups in a measurement clinic can allow the physiotherapist to motivate and facilitate patients in achieving their goals. Self-help groups can become another mechanism through which patients manage their own disease with guidance and counselling.

Patients with increasing disability may be referred to the occupational therapist for advice on driving and aids to daily living. The headquarters of NASS is also an invaluable source of information and support for patients.

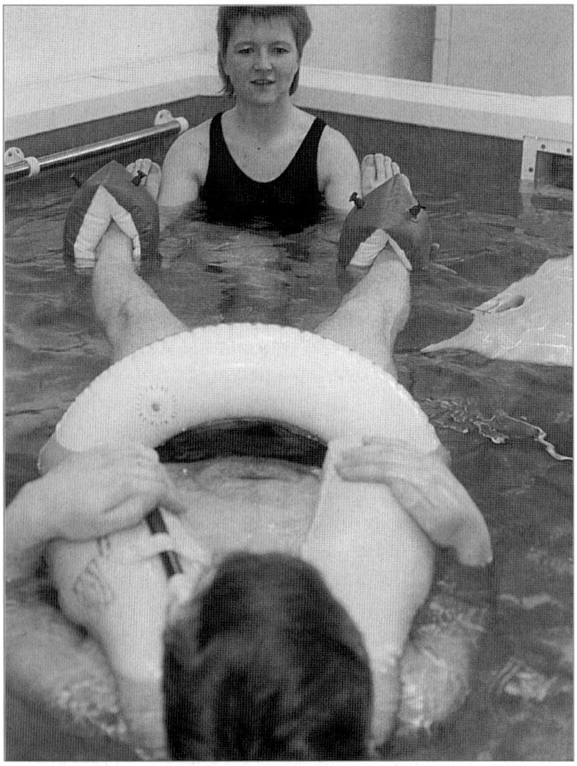

Figure 10.4 **Example of supervised individual hydrotherapy exercises for an ankylosing spondylitis patient.**

Examples of types of exercise performed by ankylosing spondylitis patients	
Exercise type	**Examples**
Warm up (5 minutes)	Step-ups on a bench
Stretches	Upper or lower limb (e.g. pectorals, hamstrings)
Mobilising exercises	Neck rotation and side flexion in sitting
Strengthening	Back extensions over a bench
Aerobic activities	Star jumps
Endurance	Basket ball
Flexibility	Trunk side flexion (sitting or standing)
Balance, co-ordination, proprioception	Competitive team games with a ball
Function	Trunk rotation in sitting
Open kinetic chain	Leg or arm circumduction exercises
Closed kinetic chain	Press-ups
Warm down (5 minutes)	Deep breathing exercises

Table 10.6 **Examples of types of exercise performed by ankylosing spondylitis patients.**

Examples of exercises categorised by the patient's starting position	
Starting position	**Examples**
Sitting in a chair	Hands behind head/back
Standing	Pelvic circling
Supine	Neck retractions
Crook lying	Bridging
Prone kneeling	Arching and hollowing the spine
Prone lying	Passive lumbar extension
Half lying	Sit and reach
Side lying	Leg and shoulder raising
Additional activities	
Games	Basket ball, volley ball
Hydrotherapy	Free, with floats, assisted/resisted exercises
Activities in pairs	Paired stretching
Gymnastic ball	Press-ups with feet balanced on a gym ball
Resistance exercises	Theraband, arm weights, leg weights

CASE HISTORIES

CASE 1

Mr HB was a new patient assessed in the AS measurement clinic by the physiotherapist. The sociodemographic details can be seen in Table 10.8 and location of symptoms in Figure 10.5. All ranges of movement and posture were within normal limits.

Following assessment, HB was seen in the physiotherapy department for advice and education on the disease on a one-to-one basis. The session lasted approximately 40 minutes and included the role of exercise and NSAIDs, advice on pain relief, and demonstration of the distribution of joint/muscle/ligament/extra-articular involvement in AS using a skeleton. At the end of this session the patient was issued a NASS patient information booklet and a home exercise programme to view prior to the next individual session.

On the second visit, HB arrived appropriately dressed to work through a home exercise programme under the instruction of the physiotherapist. This second session lasted approximately 60 minutes allowing the patient time to practise the exercises independently but having the

opportunity to refer back to the physiotherapist if in difficulty. HB was then encouraged to continue a 15-minute daily exercise programme at home, varying the exercises from the original routine as required. It was recommended the patient also participate in all his usual sporting activities (walking and cycling) and be encouraged to go swimming. HB was informed about the weekly gym exercise classes and hydrotherapy sessions running in the hospital for AS patients. Ideally HB would attend this on a regular basis for the first month and then on a drop-in basis as work commitments allowed.

Follow-up

A weekly, evening NASS group also meets at the hospital and HB was encouraged to make this a regular visit. After 3 months following the initial assessment HB will attend the AS measurement clinic again for a review, and if he is coping well he will be reviewed annually thereafter unless he needs to be seen sooner.

Case 1: Demographic assessment

Name: HB   Hospital Number:
Consultant: GP: Date of birth: Age: 29 years   Sex: M Address: Tel no:
Occupation: Conservation work. Was a gardener. Now organising > labouring Hobbies/Sports: cycling, walking, tennis when time allows
Family (history of condition): Great Aunt? Ankylosing spondylitis
Past medical history (iritis X/chest pain √/trauma X): Symptoms since 16 years old. Hip pain. Injected with cortisone. Years later 'stiffened up' with sore ribs - difficulty breathing. Stiffness in the lumbar spine, thoracic spine and variable morning stiffness. One occasion of heel pain. Aged 22 years diagnosed with ankylosing spondylitis by orthopaedic team. Moved house last year and new GP referred him to rheumatology
Past treatments (medication √/admissions X/therapy √/surgery X): Past: Diclofenac, now Naproxen. Physiotherapy: prior to diagnosis – mainly exercise therapy
General health (bowel X/skin X/smoker X):

Diagnosis: ankylosing spondylitis
Length of diagnosis: 7 years   Length of symptoms: 13 years
HLA B27:   positive: √
                       negative:
                       unknown:

Date: Clinician:

Table 10.8 **Case 1: Demographic assessment.**

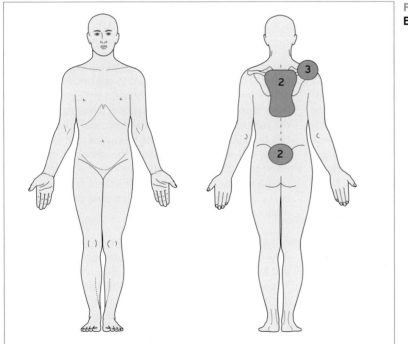

Figure 10.5 **Case 1. Body chart score of 7.**

CASE 2

AT is a 52-year-old lady with severe, long-standing, active AS involving peripheral joints. She has been taking sulphasalazine for a number of years along with paracetamol and has recently been transferred to methotrexate. The patient has bilateral hip joint replacements and walks with two sticks. She is very conscious of her stooped posture and attends a weekly ladies hydrotherapy class which is held for rheumatology patients during the day.

AT does not attend the local NASS group and has always refused inpatient treatment. Table 10.9 details her measurements taken by a single observer over a number of years. By offering on-going, weekly, outpatient hydrotherapy, this lady remains mobile and is enabled to cope with her condition.

Case 2: Longitudinal assessment									
Name AT						**Hospital number**			
Date	8.92	11.92	4.93	6.93	10.93	10.94	8.95	2.96	5.96
Drugs	sulpha-salazine	→	→	→	→	DNA	sulpha-salazine	→	methotrexate
Physio	new	hydro	→	→	→		nil	hydro	→
Problems			wrists	iritis	eating		peripheral joint disease	getting out of bed	feet
Body chart score	40	8	18	13	20		28	17	17
Visual analogue scales pain	1	0	0	0.5	0		0	3	5
Visual analogue scales night pain	0	2	4.5	2	2		2	3	3
Visual analogue scales stiffness	9	9	9.5	8.5	9		9.5	8	8
Erythrocyte sedimentation rate							92	92	
C-reactive protein							113	122	
Tragus to wall	33	30.5	31.5	31	31		32	34	30.5
Chest expansion	1	1.5	2	3	2		0.5	1.5	not determined
Finger-floor	36.5	33.5	31	33.5	34		35	34.5	32
Modified Schober	15	15.5	15.5	16.5	15		16	16	16
Neck rotation cm R	27	27	27	27.5	28		26	26	26
Neck rotation cm L	23	23	24	24	23		23	22.5	22
Hip Abduction	35	28	33.5	35.5	38		33	30	31
Modified Enthesitis Index	9	2	2	0	5		2	6	7

Table 10.9 **Case 2: Longitudinal assessment.**

ACKNOWLEDGEMENTS

I would like to thank the RCACP Editorial board for their helpful comments and criticisms; patients and staff from the Staffordshire Rheumatology Centre, Haywood Hospital, Stoke on Trent; Fergus Rogers, Director of the National AS Society; and the Physiotherapy Departments of the North Staffs Hospitals Trusts and Keele University.

Much of this work has been submitted to Keele University in part fulfillment of a PhD by research.

REFERENCES

Abbott CA, Helliwell PS, Chamberlain MA. Functional assessment in ankylosing spondylitis: evaluation of a new self-administered questionnaire and correlation with anthropometric variables. *Br J Rheum* 1994, **33**:1060-1066.

Albert E, Scholz S. Immunogenetics and rheumatic disease. *Clin Exp Rheumatol* 1987, **5**:S30-S31.

Averns HL, Oxtoby J, Taylor HG, Jones PW, Dziedzic K, Dawes PT. Smoking and outcome in ankylosing spondylitis. *Scand J Rheum* 1996a, **25**:138-142.

Averns HL, Oxtoby J, Taylor HG, Jones PW, Dziedzic K, Dawes PT. Radiological outcome in ankylosing spondylitis: use of the Stoke Ankylosing Spondylitis Spine Score (SASSS). *Br J Rheum* 1996b, **35**:373-376.

Ball J. Enthesopathy of rheumatoid and ankylosing spondylitis. *Ann Rheum Dis* 1971, **30**:213-223.

Barlow JH, Macey SJ, Struthers G. Psychosocial factors and self-help in ankylosing spondylitis patients. *Clin Rheumat* 1992, **11**:220-225.

Barlow JH, Macey SJ, Struthers GR. Sex differences and depression in ankylosing spondylitis patients: do women with AS fit the stereotype of a typical AS patient? *NASS Newsletter* 1991, Aut/Win:5-7.

Barlow JH, Macey SJ, Struthers GR. Gender, depression and ankylosing spondylitis. *Arth Care Res* 1993, **6**:45-51.

Barnard S. Wessex Region Physiotherapy Audit Project: models for intervention audit. *Physiotherapy* 1995, **81**:202-207.

Bellamy N, ed. Seronegative spondyloarthropathies. In: *Colour atlas of clinical rheumatology*. MTP Press Ltd; 1985:81-87.

Bennett PH, Burch TA. *Population studies of the rheumatic diseases*. Amsterdam: Excerpta Medica Foundation; 1968:456-457.

Bird HA, Dixon JS. The Measurement of Pain. *Ballière's Clin Rheumatol, Int Practice Res* 1987, **1**:71-89.

Brown GMM, Dare CM, Smith PR, Meyers OL. Important problems identified by patients with chronic arthritis. *South African Med J* 1987, **72**:126-128.

Buckley J, Holmes J, Mapp G. *Exercise on prescription: cardiovascular activity for health*. Oxford: Butterworth-Heinemann (in press); 1998.

Burgos-Vargas, R. Isolated juvenile onset HLA-B27 associated peripheral enthesitis - reply. *J Rheum* 1990, **17**:568.

Burgos-Vargas R, Clark P. Axial involvement in the seronegative enthesopathy and arthropathy syndrome and its progression to ankylosing spondylitis. *J Rheum* 1989, **16**:192-197.

Burgos-Vargas R, Pineda C. New clinical and radiographic features of the seronegative spondyloarthropathies. *Curr Op Rheumatol* 1991, **3**:562-574.

Burgos-Vargas R, Naranjo A, Castillo J, Gabor K. Ankylosing Spondylitis in the Mexican Mestizo: patterns of disease according to age at onset. *J Rheum* 1989, **16**:186-191.

Calabro JJ. Clinical aspects of juvenile and adult ankylosing spondylitis. *Br J Rheum* 1983, **22**:104-109.

Calin A. The spondylarthropathies: clinical aspects. *Clin Exp Rheumatol* 1987, **5**:53-59.

Calin A. Osteoporosis and ankylosing spondylitis. *Br J Rheum* 1991, **30**:318-319.

Calin A. Ankylosing spondylitis. In: *Oxford textbook of rheumatology*. Maddison PJ, Isenberg DA, Woo P, Glass DN, eds. Oxford: Oxford Medical Publications; 1993:2:681-690.

Calin A. The Dunlop-Dottridge Lecture. Ankylosing spondylitis: defining disease status and the relationship between radiology, metrology, disease activity, function and outcome. *J Rheum* 1994, **22**:740-744.

Calin A. The individual with ankylosing spondylitis: defining disease status and impact of the illness. *Br J Rheum* 1995, **34**:663-672.

Calin A, Elswood J. Relative role of genetic and environmental factors in disease expression: sib pair analysis in ankylosing spondylitis. *Arth Rheum* 1989, **32**:77-81.

Calin A, Edmunds L, Kennedy LG. Fatigue in ankylosing spondylitis - why is it ignored? *J Rheum* 1993, **20**:991-995.

Calin A, Elswood J, Edmunds L. Late onset ankylosing spondylitis - a distinct disorder? (letter). *Br J Rheum* 1990, **30**:69-70.

Calin A, Elswood J, Rigg S, Skevington SM. Ankylosing spondylitis - an analytical review of 1500 patients: the changing pattern of disease. *J Rheum* 1988, **15**:1234-1238.

Calin A, Garrett S, Whitelock H, Kennedy LG, O'Hea J, Mallorie P, Jenkinson T. A new approach to defining functional ability in ankylosing spondylitis: the development of the Bath Ankylosing Spondylitis Functional Index. *J Rheum* 1994, **21**:2281-2285.

Cats A, Van der Linden SJ, Goei The HS, Khan MA. Proposals for diagnostic criteria of ankylosing spondylitis and allied disorders. *Clin Exp Rheumatol* 1987, **5**:167-171.

Chartered Society of Physiotherapy. *Standards of practice in ankylosing spondylitis*. CSP, 14 Bedford Row, London.

Cooper RG, Freemont AJ, Fitzmaurice R, Alani SM, Jayson MIV. Paraspinal muscle fibrosis: a specific pathological component in ankylosing spondylitis. *Ann Rheum Dis* 1991, **50**:755-759.

Daltroy LH, Larson MG, Roberts WN, Liang MH. A modification of the Health Assessment Questionnaire for the Spondyloarthropathies. *J Rheum* 1990, **17**:946-950.

Dawes PT, Sheeran TP, Hothersall TE. Chest pain - a common feature of ankylosing spondylitis. *Postgrad Med J* 1988, **64**:27-29.

Dawes PT, Sheeran TP, Beswick EJ, Hothersall TE. Enthesopathy index in Ankylosing Spondylitis (letter). *Ann Rheum Dis* 1987, **46**:717.

Dixon JS, Bird HA. Reproducibility along a 10cm vertical visual analogue scale. *Ann Rheum Dis* 1981, **40**:87-89.

Donnelly S, Mejia A, Denton A, Doyle DV. Which measures of ankylosing spondylitis best determine outcome? *Br J Rheum* 1994, **33**:27.

Dougados M, Gueguen A, Nakache J-P, Nguyen M, Mery C, Amor B. Evaluation of a Functional Index and Articular Index in Ankylosing Spondylitis. *J Rheum* 1988, **15**:302-307.

Dudley Hart F. Ankylosing spondylitis: a review of 184 cases. *Ann Rheum Dis* 1955, **14**:77-82.

Dudley Hart F. Ankylosing spondylitis. *Lancet* 1985, **2**:(8455)609 (letter).

Dunn N, Preston B, Jones KL. Unexplained acute backache in longstanding ankylosing spondylitis. *BMJ* 1985, **291**:(6509)1632-34.

Dziedzic K, Hay EM, Jackson SE, Jones PW, Dawes PT. *An assessment of the body chart in ankylosing spondylitis*. Abstract - Proceedings 12th International Congress of the WCPT, 1995. APTA:1008.

Edmunds L. Summary of the AS research at the RNHRD Bath. *NASS Newsletter* 1990, Spr/Sum:7-10.

Fener P, Ricard-Blum S, Gillet P, Netter P, Pourel J, Gaucher A. Human and bovine entheses contain type I and type II collagens. Br J Rheum 1992, **31**:69.

Fitzgerald GK, Wynveen KJ, Rheault W, Rothschild B. Objective assessment with establishment of normal values for lumbar spinal range of motion. Phys Ther 1983, **63**:1776-1781.

Fournie B. A broader concept of entheses (le territoire enthesique) and the hyperostosis-osteitis-periostitis (HOP) syndrome. A nosological radioclinical approach to inflammatory spondyloarthropathies. Rev Rheumatisme (English Edition) 1993, **60**:391-394.

Fox MW, Onofrio BM, Kilgore JE. Neurological complications of ankylosing spondylitis. J Neurosurg 1993, **78**:871-878.

Fries JF. The hierarchy of outcome assessment. J Rheum 1993, **20**:546-547.

Fries JF, Spitz PW, Kraines RG, Holman HR. Measurement of patient outcome in arthritis. Arth Rheum 1980, **23**:137-145.

Frost H, Klaber Moffett JA, Moser JS, Fairbank JCT. Randomised controlled trial for evaluation of fitness programme for patients with chronic low back pain. BMJ 1995, **310**:151-154.

Gall V. Exercise in the Spondyloarthropathies. Arth Care Res 1994, **7**:215-220.

Garrett S, Jenkinson T, Kennedy LG, Whitelock H, Gaisford P, Calin A. A new approach to defining disease status in ankylosing spondylitis: the Bath Ankylosing Spondylitis Disease Activity Index. J Rheum 1994, **21**:2286-2291.

Good AE. The pain of ankylosing spondylitis. Am J Med 1986, **80**:118-119.

Gran JT, Husby G. Ankylosing spondylitis: a comparative study of patients in an epidemiological survey, and those admitted to a department of rheumatology. J Rheum 1984, **11**:788-793.

Gran JT, Husby G. Ankylosing spondylitis - current drug treatment. Drugs 1992, **44**:585-603.

Guillemin F, Briancon S, Pourel J, Gaucher A. Long-term disability and prolonged sick leaves as outcome measurements in ankylosing spondylitis. Arth Rheum 1990, **33**:1001-1005.

Halm H, Metzstavenhagen P, Zielke K. Results of surgical-correction of kyphotic deformities of the spine in ankylosing spondylitis on the basis of the modified arthritis impact measurement scales. Spine 1995, **20**:1612-1619.

Helliwell PS, Abbott CA, Chamberlain MA. A randomised trial of three different physiotherapy regimes in ankylosing spondylitis. Physiotherapy 1996, **82**:85-90.

Hidding A, Van der Linden S, de Witte L. Therapeutic effects of individual physical therapy in ankylosing spondylitis related to duration of disease. Clin Rheumatol 1993, **12**:334-340.

Inman RD, Scofield RH. Etiopathogenesis of ankylosing spondylitis and reactive arthritis. Curr Opin Rheumatol 1994, **6**:360-370.

Jacobs JC. Spondyloarthritis and enthesopathy. Arch Int Med 1983, **143**:103-107.

Jenkinson TR, Mallorie PA, Whitelock HC, Kennedy LG, Garrett SL, Calin A. Defining spinal mobility in ankylosing spondylitis (AS) the Bath AS metrology index (BASMI). J Rheum 1994, **22**:1694-1698.

Jones K, Barker K. Exercise prescription. In: Jones K, Baker K. Human movement explained. Oxford: Butterworth- Heinemann Limited; 1996:120-158.

Jones SD, Koh WH, Garrett SL, Calin A. Risks and determinants of unemployment in ankylosing spondylitis (AS). Br J Rheum 1994, **33**:28.

Kellgren JH, Jeffrey MR, Ball J, eds. The epidemiology of chronic rheumatism. Oxford: Blackwell; 1963, 1:326.

Kennedy LG, Will R, Calin A. Sex ratio in the spondyloarthropathies and its relationship to phenotypic expression, mode of inheritance and age at onset. J Rheum 1993a, **20**:1900-1904.

Kennedy LG, Edmunds L, Calin A. The natural history of ankylosing spondylitis does it burn out? J Rheum 1993b, **20**:688-692.

Kennedy LG, Jenkinson TR, Mallorie PA, Whitelock HC, Garrett SL, Calin A. Ankylosing spondylitis 19; the correlation between a new metrology score and radiology. Br J Rheum 1995, **34**:767-770.

Khan MA, Khan MK. Diagnostic value of HLA-B27 testing in ankylosing spondylitis and Reiter's syndrome. Annals Internal Med 1982, **96**:70-76.

Khan MA. Newer clinical and radiographic features of seronegative spondyloarthropathies. Curr Opin Rheumatol 1989, **1**:139-143.

Khan MA. Spondyloarthropathies: editorial overview. Curr Opin Rheumatol 1993, **5**:405-407.

Kidd B, Mullee M, Frank A, Cawley M. Disease expression of ankylosing spondylitis in males and females. J Rheum 1988, **15**:1407-1409.

Kirwan JR, Reeback JS. Stanford health assessment questionnaire modified to assess disability in British patients with rheumatoid arthritis. Br J Rheum 1986, **25**:206-209.

Klaber Moffett JA, Hughes I, Griffiths P. Measurement of cervical spine movements using a simple inclinometer. Physiotherapy 1989, **75**:309-312.

Kraag G, Stokes B, Groh J, Helewa A, Goldsmith CH. The effects of comprehensive home physiotherapy supervision on patients with ankylosing spondylitis - an 8-month follow-up. J Rheum 1994, **21**:261-263.

Landewe RBM, Goei The HS. Ankylosing spondylitis and peripheral joint disease. Clin Rheumatol 1989, **8**:87-90.

MacLean L. HLA-B27 subtypes: implications for spondyloarthropathies. Ann Rheum Dis 1992, **51**:929-931.

Macrae IF, Wright V. Measurement of back movement. Ann Rheum Dis 1969, **28**:584-589.

Mander M, Simpson JM, McLellan A, Walker D, Goodacre JA, Carson Dick W. Studies with an enthesis index as a method of clinical assessment in ankylosing spondylitis. Ann Rheum Dis 1987, **46**:197-202.

Marshall D. The heart in ankylosing spondylitis. NASS Newsletter, 1991, Aust/Winter:12.

Mau W, Zeidler H, Mau R, Majewski A, Freyschmidt J, Stangel W, Deicher H. Clinical features and prognosis of patients with possible ankylosing spondylitis. Results of a 10-year follow up. J Rheum 1988, **15**:1109-1114.

McFarlane AC, Brooks PM. Determinants of disability in rheumatoid arthritis. Br J Rheum 1988, **27**:7-14.

Meenan RF, Gertman PM, Mason JH. Measuring health status in arthritis. Arth Rheum 1980, **23**:146-152.

Milde E-J, Aarli J, Larsen JL. Cauda equina lesions in ankylosing spondylitis. Scand J Rheum 1977, **6**:118-122.

Moll JMH, Wright V. An objective clinical study of chest expansion. Ann Rheum Dis 1972, **31**:1-8.

Moll JMH, Wright V. The pattern of chest and spinal mobility in ankylosing spondylitis. Rheumatol Rehabilitation 1973, **12**:115-134.

Nashel DJ, Petrone DL, Ulmer CC, Sliwinski AJ. C-reactive protein: a marker for disease activity in Ankylosing Spondylitis and Reiter's Syndrome. J Rheum 1986, **13**:364-367.

Nemes L. Psychosocial and physical problems in AS. NASS Newsletter 1991, Spr/Sum:8-10.

Nemeth R, Smith F, Elswood J, Calin A. Ankylosing spondylitis (AS) - an approach to measurement of severity and outcome: ankylosing spondylitis assessment questionnaire (ASAQ) - a controlled study (100). Br J Rheum Abstracts Autumn 1990, 69.

Niepel GA, Sit'aj S. Enthesopathy. Clin Rheum Dis 1979, **5**:857-872.

Nolli M, Ghirelli L, Ferraccioli GG. Pain language in fibromyalgia, rheumatoid arthritis and osteoarthritis. Clin Exp Rheumatol 1988, **6**:27-33.

O'Mahony S, Anderson N, Nuki G, Ferguson A. Systemic and mucosal antibodies to Klebsiella in patients with ankylosing spondylitis and Crohn's disease. Ann Rheum Dis 1992, **51**:1296-1300.

O'Neill TW, Bresnihan B. The heart in ankylosing spondylitis. Ann Rheum Dis 1992, **51**:705-706.

Pal B. Early diagnosis of ankylosing spondylitis. J Ind Med Assoc 1987, **85**:275-277.

Pearcy MJ, Wordsworth BP, Portek I, Mowat AG. Spinal movements in ankylosing spondylitis and the effect of treatment. Spine 1985, **10**:472-474.

Pile KD, Laurent MR, Salmond CE, Best MJ, Pyle EA, Moloney RO. Clinical assessment of ankylosing spondylitis: a study of observer variation in spinal measurements. Br J Rheum 1991, **30**:29-34.

Resnick D, Niwayama G, eds. Ankylosing spondylitis. In: Diagnosis of bone and joint disorders, 2nd edition. Philadelphia: W.B. Saunders Company; 1988, 32:1103-1170.

Rigby AS. Review of UK data on the rheumatic diseases-5. Ankylosing spondylitis. Br J Rheum 1991, **30**:50-53.

Ringsdal VS, Andreasen JJ. Ankylosing spondylitis - experience with a self administered questionnaire: an analytical study. Ann Rheum Dis 1989, **48**:924-927.

Rubinstein HM. Osteoporosis in ankylosing spondylitis. *Br J Rheum* 1991, **30**:2,160.

Russell P, Pearcy MJ, Unsworth A. Measurement of the range and coupled movements observed in the lumbar spine. *Br J Rheum* 1993, **32**:490-497.

Saleh J, Hassell AB, Rahmatalla A, Dziedzic K, Dove J, Dawes PT. The use of a new 3-dimensional tracking system (Fastrak) for assessment of cervical spine movement. *Br J Rheum Abstracts* 1994, **33**:113.

Schelew BL, Vaghadia H. Ankylosing spondylitis and neuraxial anesthesia – a 10 year review. *Can J Anaesth* 1996, **43**:65-68.

Schober P. The lumbar vertebral column and backache. *Munch Med Wschr* 1937, **84**:336.

Schweitzer ME, Resnick D. Spondyloarthropathies: enthesopathy. In: *Rheumatology*. Klippel JH, Dieppe PA, eds. London: Mosby International; 1994; 3:27.1-27.6.

Scott DGI, Ring EFJ, Bacon PA. Problems in the assessment of disease activity in Ankylosing Spondylitis. *Rheumatol Rehab* 1981; **20**:74-80.

Sheehan NJ, Slavin BM, Donovan MP, Mount JN, Mathews JA. Lack of correlation between clinical disease activity and erythrocyte sedimentation rate, acute phase proteins or protease inhibitors in ankylosing spondylitis. *Br J Rheum* 1986, **25**:171-174.

Sturrock R. Outcome in ankylosing spondylitis. *NASS Newsletter* 1991, Aut/Win: 15-16.

Symmons DPM. Disease assessment indices: activity, damage and severity. *Baillière's Clin Rheumatol* 1995, **9**:267-285.

Taylor HG, Gadd R, Beswick EJ, Venkateswaran M, Dawes PT. Quantitative radio-isotope scanning in ankylosing spondylitis: a clinical, laboratory and computerised tomographic study. *Scand J Rheum* 1991a, **20**:274-279.

Taylor HG, Wardle T, Beswick EJ, Dawes PT. The relationship of clinical and laboratory measurements to radiological changes in ankylosing spondylitis. *Br J Rheum* 1991b, **30**:330-335.

Taylor HG, Weiss JB, McLoughlin B, Dawes PT. Raised endothelial cell stimulating angiogenesis factor in ankylosing spondylitis. *Clin Exp Rheumatol* 1993, **11**:537-539.

Thomson GTD, Chalmers IM. Fiddling while Rome burns: burn out, remission and disease activity measurements in ankylosing spondylitis. *J Rheum* 1993, **20**:607-609.

Toivanen A, Toivanen P. Epidemiologic aspects, clinical features, and management of ankylosing spondylitis and reactive arthritis. *Curr Opin Rheumatol* 1994, **6**:354-359.

Tomlinson MJ, Barefoot J, Dixon AS. Intensive in-patient physiotherapy courses improve movement and posture in ankylosing spondylitis. *Physiotherapy* 1986, **72**:238-240.

Tsai HH, Eastmond CJ. Modified costotransversectomy in treatment of intractable costovertebral pain in ankylosing spondylitis (letter). *Br J Rheum* 1987, **26**:66-67.

Van der Linden S, Van der Heijde DM. Ankylosing spondylitis and other B27 related spondylarthropathies. *Baillière's Clin Rheumatol* 1995, **9**:355-373.

Viitanen JV, Suni S. Management principles of physiotherapy in ankylosing spondylitis – which treatments are effective? *Physiotherapy* 1995, **81**:322-329.

Viitanen JV, Kokko M-L, Lehtinen K, Suni J, Kautiainen H. Correlation between mobility restrictions and radiologic changes in ankylosing spondylitis. *Spine* 1995, **20**:492-496.

Wordsworth BP, Pearcy MJ, Mowat AG. In-patient regime for the treatment of ankylosing spondylitis: an appraisal of improvement in spinal mobility and the effects of corticotrophin. *Br J Rheum* 1984, **23**:39-43.

Wright V. Editorials: aspects of ankylosing spondylitis. *Br J Rheum* 1991, **30**:1-4.

Zigmond AS, Snaith RP. The hospital anxiety and depression scale. *Acta Psych Scand* 1983, **67**:361-370.

Zukovskis K, Taylor HG, Beswick EJ, Dawes PT, Jones P. Enthesitis as a measure of disease activity in ankylosing spondylitis (AS). *Br J Rheum Abstract* 1991, **30**:81.

SECTION 3

LESS COMMON CONDITIONS

Rheumatology (roo'mat'ol'o'je). Branch
of medicine which is concerned with the
diagnosis and treatment of rheumatic
disorders.

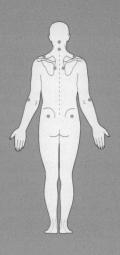

11 C Fenelon

SOFT TISSUE RHEUMATISM

CHAPTER OUTLINE

- **Adhesive capsulitis (frozen shoulder)**
- **Lateral epicondylitis (tennis elbow)**
- **Carpal tunnel syndrome**
- **Work-related upper limb disorder**
- **Complex regional pain syndrome**

- **Fibromyalgia**
- **Trochanteric bursitis**
- **Plantar fasciitis**
- **Hypermobility syndrome**

INTRODUCTION

As its name suggests, soft tissue rheumatism relates to the disease and dysfunction of structures such as joint capsules, tendons, bursae and entheses (for details on entheses, see Chapter 10).

ADHESIVE CAPSULITIS (FROZEN SHOULDER)

This term is a medical colloquialism rather than a diagnosis. It is characterised by gradually progressive pain and restriction of all glenohumeral movements, followed spontaneously by slow and often only partial recovery over 6 months to 2 years. Onset is most frequently in the sixth decade, and uncommon below 40 years of age. Rizk & Pinals (1982) found that the incidence is slightly greater in females.

CLINICAL FEATURES

The patient usually complains of generalised aching in the shoulder, radiating down the lateral aspect of the upper arm and sometimes to the forearm. The patient is often unable to sleep on the affected side (Rizk & Pinals, 1982).

Functional impairments include problems putting on a coat or reaching a high shelf and difficulty in combing hair. There is often a capsular pattern of movement restriction with lateral rotation being most restricted, followed by abduction and then medial rotation (Cyriax, 1984).

INVESTIGATIONS
Radiography
X-rays are normal in around 75% of cases; the remaining 25% have minor degenerative changes in the shoulder joint (Morris *et al.*, 1990).

Arthrography
Capsulitis leads to a marked reduction in joint volume. Neviaser (1989) stated that a reduced joint capacity and the absence of the axillary recess are diagnostic for adhesive capsulitis.

Arthroscopy
Arthroscopy may reveal the development of adhesions across the axillary recess onto the humeral head. The thickened synovium may vary in colour from red in the early stages to pink later on, as the synovitis diminishes (Neviaser, 1987).

Magnetic Resonance Imaging

Joint capsule and synovium thickness greater than 4 mm is a useful magnetic resonance imaging (MRI) criterion for the diagnosis of adhesive capsulitis. The volume of articular fluid seen on MRI is not significantly diminished in patients with the condition. This would seem to contradict arthrography findings— however, arthrography involves the distension of the joint with contrast material whereas MRI evaluates the shoulder with unaltered anatomy (Emig *et al.*, 1995).

AETIOLOGY

The pathogenesis of frozen shoulder is poorly understood. It is probably caused by inflammatory changes in the rotator cuff, biceps tendon and capsule following trauma or degeneration, leading to adhesions and capsular thickening (Simmonds, 1979). Cervical spine pathology may be associated with frozen shoulder, and some patients have demonstrated increased ranges of shoulder movement following cervical facet joint block (Schneider, 1989). One explanation for this may be autonomic dysfunction, but it is not clear whether sympathetic involvement is primary or secondary to the joint pain and pathology.

Diabetics have an increased incidence of adhesive capsulitis (Kingsley & Gibson, 1986) especially in younger individuals. It is also more often bilateral, and linked with microvascular disease and abnormalities of collagen repair.

MANAGEMENT

Management of frozen shoulder aims to relieve pain and restore range of movement. Since there are diverse opinions as to the cause there is no clear consensus as to treatment methods.

Drugs

Analgesics and non-steroidal anti-inflammatory drugs (NSAIDs) are commonly used, and antidepressants such as amitriptyline may be useful. Corticosteroid injections are of most benefit in the early stages of the condition (Bulgen *et al.*, 1984), although reports on the success of injections are extremely variable.

Manipulation Under Anaesthesia

Frequency of use of manipulation under anaesthesia (MUA) varies greatly between clinicians. Further evaluation is necessary to assess the efficacy of this procedure and also the part physiotherapy plays in the recovery process and outcome.

Arthroscopic Capsulotomy

In this procedure, structures are divided under direct vision and a more controlled release is possible than with MUA. This method of treatment also allows diagnosis and treatment of intra-articular disease (Segmullër *et al.*, 1995).

Physiotherapy

Useful treatment modalities include electrotherapy or ice for pain relief, mobilisations of the glenohumeral joint and passive stretching of the capsular structures. Acupuncture and transcutaneous electrical nerve stimulation (TENS) may also be helpful. The physiotherapist has a preventative role in recognising those conditions that may lead to frozen shoulder. These include any upper limb and cervical spine disorders that lead to protective restriction of shoulder movement. Advice regarding maintenance of mobility is important, and attention to the cervical and thoracic spine may also be useful in diagnosis and treatment.

PROGNOSIS

Shaffer *et al.* (1992) state that range of movement may be significantly restricted for several years despite significant reduction in pain, although this generally causes little functional impairment. Involvement of the second shoulder occurs in up to 17% of patients, usually after recovery of the shoulder initially involved (Rizk & Pinals, 1982).

LATERAL EPICONDYLITIS (TENNIS ELBOW)

Tennis elbow is a common, painful condition resulting from athletic or occupational activities. It affects around 3% of the population, most commonly between the ages of 40 and 60 years (Chard & Hazleman, 1989).

CLINICAL PICTURE

The patient complains of pain over the lateral aspect of the elbow, commonly radiating down the dorsum of the forearm. As well as tennis players it may affect those who have occupations in which they carry out resisted supination of the arm or dorsiflexion of the wrist.

PATHOLOGY AND TESTS

The primary pathology involves the origin of the extensor carpi radialis brevis and, less commonly, the extensor carpi radialis longus. The underlying lesion consists of small tears or microfibrillar degeneration within the tendons as a result of mechanical overload. The subsequent inflammation causes development of granulation tissue within the tendon (Thompson & Phelps, 1990).

The commonly used test for diagnosis of tennis elbow is Mills' sign. This test is carried out by flexing the elbow fully, pronating the forearm fully and flexing the wrist and fingers. The elbow is then extended, thus putting the extensors on full stretch. The test is positive when pain is felt in the region of the lateral epicondyle. If muscle wasting, refractory weakness or paraesthesia are present, neck radiographs and electromyographic studies may be needed to rule out cervical radiculopathy.

TREATMENT

Prompt treatment of tennis elbow is important as the condition becomes more difficult to treat with longer duration. The first step in treatment is to relieve pain and decrease inflammation. Corticosteroid injection into the spot of maximum tenderness may be helpful.

Various manipulative techniques have been advocated for the treatment of tennis elbow (Cyriax, 1984, Kushner &

Reid, 1986). Friction massage to the common extensor tendon is used to maintain the mobility of the soft tissue structures and to prevent adherent scars from forming. Friction may be used in isolation or in conjunction with ultrasound, laser, interferential (Stratford *et al.*, 1989) or acupuncture (Molsberger *et al.*, 1994). Ice may also be useful in relieving pain and inflammation.

The objective of treatment is the restoration of the integrity, mobility and length of the damaged tissues. Mobility should be maintained throughout the range of movement, but avoiding activity that strains the extensor origin and encourages the development of fibrosis through continued microtrauma. Mobilisation of neural tissues may also help to relieve symptoms. Clasps that apply pressure over extensor muscles may be useful in relieving pain in some cases.

As inflammation resolves and healing begins, specific exercise is important to strengthen and stretch the wrist musculature, paying attention to any biomechanical problems in the sport or the activity causing or exacerbating the problem. While clinical intuition and review of the existing literature suggest general guidelines for strength training of patients with lateral epicondylitis, there is virtually no research evidence for the efficacy of such approaches (Noteboom *et al.*, 1994).

Surgery
Up to 10% of patients with tennis elbow fail to respond to conservative measures and may need surgery, such as release of the epicondylar muscles and removal of granulation tissue from around the origin of the extensor carpi radialis brevis (Chop, 1989).

In conclusion, when treating this condition it is worth bearing in mind that its cause is often multifactorial and requires a global evaluation of the upper quadrant of the patient.

CARPAL TUNNEL SYNDROME

Carpal tunnel syndrome (CTS) is a painful wrist condition resulting from compression of the median nerve. Treatment at an early stage can bring a complete cure, but a delay in diagnosis and appropriate management may lead to irreversible damage to the nerve and permanent disability.

ANATOMY OF THE CARPAL TUNNEL AND PATHOPHYSIOLOGY
The carpal tunnel is formed by an arch of the carpal bones and the transverse carpal ligaments, and within it are located nine flexor tendons and the median nerve. Symptoms are caused by compression of the median nerve within the tunnel.

The causes of the syndrome are varied. In many cases there is tenosynovitis of the flexor tendons leading to eventual thickening of the tendon sheaths and then pressure on the median nerve. It is most common in those whose jobs or hobbies demand use of vibratory tools or repetitive wrist or hand movements (Sipos, 1995) but it may also be the presenting feature of rheumatoid arthritis (RA).

Carpal tunnel syndrome may also be associated with pregnancy, diabetes mellitus and hypothyroidism as well as gouty tenosynovitis, amyloidosis, sarcoidosis and malaligned fractures.

CLINICAL FEATURES
Initially, pressure on the median nerve leads to temporary symptoms of numbness, tingling and discomfort within the hand. Prolonged pressure may cause ischaemic changes leading to axonal death, muscular atrophy and pain. Sensory changes are found in the volar surfaces of the thumb, index and middle fingers and the radial half of the ring finger. Sensory changes are not found in the thenar region of the hand and part of the palm as the palmar branch of the nerve, which supplies this area, is not in the carpal tunnel (Whitley & McDonnel, 1995).

Symptoms frequently wake patients at night. As the condition worsens, burning pain may occur with thenar muscle wasting. In severe cases prognosis is poor despite treatment.

PHYSICAL EXAMINATION AND DIAGNOSTIC TESTING
The most common tests performed are the Phalen and Tinel tests (described by Sipos (1995)).

Phalen Test
The patient holds the wrists as shown in Figure 11.1 for 60 seconds. Numbness or burning in the median nerve distribution is a positive result for CTS.

Tinel Test
The transverse carpal ligament is tapped over the median nerve on the anterior aspect of the wrist. Tingling in the hand in the distribution of the median nerve is positive for CTS (Figure 11.2). Electromyography may also be used; the

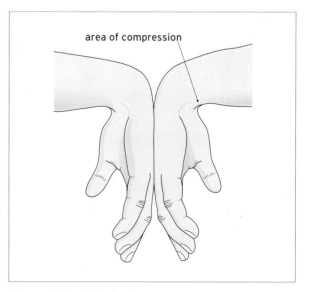

area of compression

Figure 11.1 **Phalen test.**

nerve is stimulated at forearm level and the amount of time recorded for the thumb muscles to react to the stimulus. X-rays may be taken to identify any bony pathology causing or contributing to the symptoms.

TREATMENT
Non-surgical
This includes avoidance of any precipitating activity, and splinting at night to maintain the wrist in a neutral position which maximises the diameter of the carpal tunnel. The best results from splinting have been demonstrated within the first 3 months of symptom onset (Kruger *et al.*, 1991). Sometimes, benefit is gained by the patient wearing a splint to protect the wrist from overstrain. Local steroid injection may also be helpful in some cases, as may NSAIDs and diuretics (Whitley & McDonnel, 1995).

Physiotherapy
In very early CTS electrotherapy such as ultrasound, pulsed short-wave and laser may be helpful in alleviating the problem, as may maintenance of brachial plexus and median nerve mobility (Totten & Hunter, 1991).

Surgical
If muscle atrophy and weakness are apparent, early referral for a surgical opinion and electromyography gives a better outcome than delayed referral. Median nerve decompression is usually achieved by transaction of the transverse carpal ligament. The success of surgery depends on the severity of the pre-operative symptoms. Recurrence of the problem is most commonly due to incomplete lysis of the transverse carpal ligament (Whitley & McDonnel, 1995).

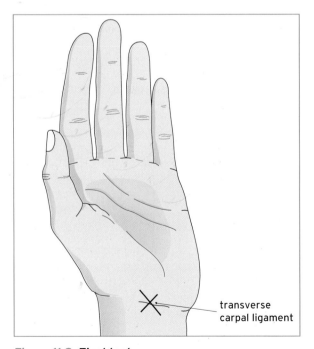

transverse carpal ligament

Figure 11.2 Tinel test.

WORK-RELATED UPPER LIMB DISORDER

Work-related upper limb disorder, sometimes known as 'cumulative trauma disorder' or 'repetitive strain injury' (RSI), is a term often used when describing various disabling upper limb pains caused by repetitive activities. It occurs when forces are repeatedly applied to the same muscle group, joint or tendon over a prolonged period. This can lead to tendon and synovial disorders, degenerative joint disease, nerve compression or muscle and ligament problems. Typically, arm pain in patients with RSI does not follow a specific anatomical or pathological pattern (Barton *et al.*, 1992), but may occur in any area between the neck and digits. It may include conditions such as CTS, epicondylitis and cervical/thoracic spine problems as well as adverse mechanical tension in the brachial plexus.

The prevalence of the condition is high amongst workers in high speed manufacturing industries (Zimmerman *et al.*, 1992) and has reached epidemic proportions in computer keyboard operators. Work related risk factors associated with RSI include repetition, high force, awkward joint posture, direct pressure, vibration, prolonged constrained posture and psychological stress. Perceived stress levels are significantly associated with perceived RSI while in those people who feel that their workstation is ergonomically correct fewer symptoms are reported (Hess, 1997).

TREATMENT AND PREVENTION
The reduction or elimination of repetitive activity usually relieves symptoms, as may rest, splinting and exercises including stretches and strengthening of local muscles. Corticosteroid injections and NSAIDs may be useful, as may surgery such as median nerve release.

Ergonomics has a great deal to offer in designing and organising work for maximum productivity with minimal risk of injury. It includes risk assessment, the introduction of work/rest pauses, assessing occupational stress and redesigning the workplace and equipment. For example, holding straight handled tools requires almost 19^0 of ulnar deviation at the wrist and so handles that are angled to bring the wrist into a neutral position help to decrease stress on vulnerable structures (Zimmerman *et al.*, 1992). Although such modifications may appear expensive, this is offset by the reduced costs in terms of employee sick leave.

Upper limb RSI should always be looked at holistically and all structures from the neck to the digits should be considered as possible contributors to the problem.

COMPLEX REGIONAL PAIN SYNDROME

This is a complex group of disorders which may develop as a consequence of trauma (with or without obvious nerve lesion) or idiopathically.

Conditions sometimes considered under the umbrella of reflex sympathetic dystrophy (RSD) include (Herrick, 1994):

- Algodystrophy.
- Causalgia (major or minor).
- Painful osteoporosis.
- Post-traumatic dystrophy.
- Post-traumatic osteoporosis.
- Shoulder–hand syndrome.
- Sudeck's atrophy.

The term 'sympathetically mediated pain' is sometimes used (Herrick, 1994) but does not completely equate with RSD, although it seems likely that the sympathetic nervous system plays a role in the majority of cases.

CLINICAL FEATURES OF REFLEX SYMPATHETIC DYSTROPHY

Autonomic (sympathetic) motor and sensory symptoms develop in the distal region of affected extremities. The most prominent feature is persistent pain, often described as burning. Tenderness, which is frequently generalised, usually accompanies the pain, often with oedema and vasomotor changes (Blumberg & Janig, 1994).

The evolution of RSD is sometimes divided into the following stages:
- Acute: vasomotor changes are predominately vasodilatory with redness and increased temperature, swelling, shiny skin, decreased range of movement and decreased function.
- Dystrophic: the limb may be dusky in colour, cold and clammy; in addition, autonomic changes occur which alter the pattern of sweating. Early dystrophic changes may occur with the start of contractures.
- Atrophic: pain and vasomotor changes may decrease but irreversible atrophic changes and contracture of skin and soft tissue lead to severe limitations in functional ability.

INVESTIGATIONS

No diagnostic test exists for RSD but X-rays may show patchy osteoporosis of the affected extremity and sometimes erosive changes. Isotope bone scanning shows increased uptake, which is not confined to the periarticular areas, indicating vascular and non-vascular changes in the bone (Atkins et al., 1993).

PATHOLOGY

The precise mechanism is unknown but the pathology is thought to involve both peripheral and central mechanisms and sensitisation of neurones in the dorsal horn (see Chapter 4). This incorporates the concept of sympathetically maintained pain (Roberts, 1986). Whatever the mechanism, it seems probable that alteration of central information processing results (Janig, 1990).

MANAGEMENT

Early active mobilisation of injuries with potential to develop RSD should be encouraged, along with functional use of the limb. Once the condition has progressed to the atrophic stage then treatment is likely to be difficult and lengthy. Continuous passive motion may be helpful, especially in RSD affecting the knee. Some authors have advocated the use of acupuncture (Fialka et al., 1993) and TENS (Kesler et al., 1988). Other measures include sympathetic blockade by intravenous guanethidine at paravertebral or regional level or stellate ganglion blocks.

Many patients with RSD demonstrate marked pain behaviour, with disability and complaints of pain which are out of proportion to symptoms, so the therapist's approach should be multidisciplinary to incorporate pain-management strategies. Overall, however, RSD is a difficult condition to treat as it covers a wide range of disease and disability. The therapist therefore needs to recognise the early signs of the condition to prevent disability.

FIBROMYALGIA

Fibromyalgia is a non-articular rheumatic syndrome in which there is widespread locomotor pain, fatigue and non-refreshing sleep. Other features may include early morning stiffness, low mood, tension headaches, irritable bowel syndrome and Raynaud's phenomenon as well as complaints of joint swelling in the absence of actual swelling. There is an absence of clinical and laboratory evidence of active joint disease, and no clear abnormality in the physiology of the affected tissues (Ledingham et al., 1993).

CLINICAL FEATURES

Features include widespread pain, bilateral pain, both above and below the waist, as well as axial skeletal pain. There must also be pain in 11 of 18 tender point sites on digital palpation (McCain, 1994). The 18 tender spots of fibromyalgia are illustrated in Figure 11.3, and listed in Table 11.1. For a tender point to be 'positive' the patient must state that the palpation with a force of $4\,kg/cm^2$ is painful and not merely tender (McCain, 1994). Muscular aching should also be present for longer than 3 months and, in general, the symptoms are more proximal than distal (Leavitt et al., 1986).

The exact prevalence of the condition is unknown, but about 73 % of patients are women between 35 and 55 years of age (Wolfe, 1989). However, it may present in any age group, including the elderly.

AETIOLOGY

The aetiology is unknown, but theories include muscle abnormalities, immune system alterations, sleep pattern disturbances and psychological factors.

MUSCLE ABNORMALITIES

The fatigability of muscle in fibromyalgia has not been fully explained, but abnormalities in energy handling, histological changes, inability to relax between muscle contractions and reduced muscle blood flow have been postulated as mechanisms in the generation of fibromyalgia (Bennett & Jacobsen, 1994). Physical fitness training including aerobic exercise has been shown to decrease the reported intensity of pain and number of tender spots in patients, although a physiological mechanism has not been clearly identified.

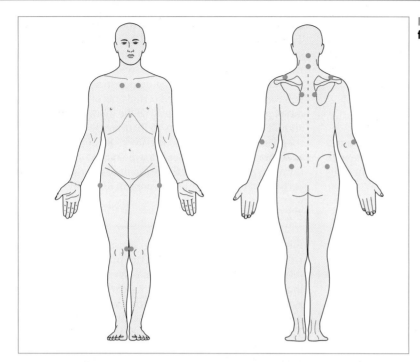

Figure 11.3 **Sites of tender points in fibromyalgia.**

Table 11.1 **List of tender spots of fibromyalgia.**

List of tender spots of fibromyalgia	
Occiput	At site of suboccipital muscle insertion
Low cervical	Anterior aspect of intertransverse spaces at C5–C7
Trapezius	Mid-point of upper border
Supraspinatus	Bilaterally, at origins above the medial border of the scapular spine
Second rib	Just lateral to the costochondral junctions at the upper surfaces
Lateral epicondyle	2cm distal to the epicondyles
Gluteal	In the upper outer quadrants of the buttocks in the anterior fold of muscle
Greater trochanter	Posterior to the trochanteric prominence
Knee	Proximal to the joint line at the medial fat pad

(All the above points are bilateral)
American College of Rheumatology (1990), cited in McCain (1994)

PAIN SENSING CHANGES/SLEEP DISTURBANCE

Fibromyalgia may reflect a generalised change in pain threshold, and certain neurotransmitters have been implicated. One of these, serotonin, has been shown to be at low levels in fibromyalgia patients and has also been linked to sleep disturbances and increases in depression and perceived pain (Russell *et al.*, 1986).

IMMUNE SYSTEM ALTERATION

Fibromyalgia has a possible link with immune system abnormalities, although this has not been conclusively proven. Immune system function may possibly be linked with the sleep/wake cycles (Kruger & Karnovsky, 1987).

PSYCHOLOGICAL FACTORS

A premorbid 'perfectionist personality' has been linked with fibromyalgia (Smythe, 1985). Anxiety and depression appear to be important elements in the problem but it is not clear whether they are reactive or an integral part of fibromyalgia, and stress may contribute to worsening symptoms.

MANAGEMENT

Fibromyalgia patients present a difficult management problem and often multiple treatments are used over a protracted period with limited success. Antidepressants may have a place in the management of fibromyalgia, but NSAIDs and steroids are not beneficial (Simms, 1994). Non-pharmacological treatments include cardiovascular fitness training, cognitive behavioural therapy and physiotherapy.

Physiotherapy

An holistic approach is necessary, involving the patient in joint goal-setting. Graded exercise, including hydrotherapy, is helpful, but it is important that patients work only to their limit and do not exceed it. Most pain-relieving modalities at the physiotherapist's disposal may be used—however, these should not be viewed as 'treatment' but rather as a means to facilitate exercise, stretching and restoration of function (Rosen, 1994). Pacing and energy conservation advice may be useful to manage fatigue. Sleep disturbance must be addressed, and patient education is important (Burckhardt & Bjelle, 1994).

TROCHANTERIC BURSITIS

The onset of pain in trochanteric bursitis is often insidious. Pain increases with active or resisted abduction and external rotation of the hip due to the attachment of these muscle groups in the greater trochanter area. There is often marked tenderness on deep palpation either behind or above the greater trochanter. The patient also complains of aggravation of the problem by lying on the affected side or walking, and pain may radiate to the lateral thigh and the buttock. Immediate relief of pain following injection of local anaesthetic is a major diagnostic criterion.

Trochanteric bursitis often accompanies hip or lumbar spine joint disease and differential diagnosis is necessary. Lateral thigh pain may be caused by:

- Lumbar facet syndrome—facet blocks may confirm the diagnosis if this is suspected on clinical and radiological examination and joint distension during facet joint injection often reproduces the patient's symptoms (Traycoff, 1991).
- Referred pain from the thoracolumbar junction and upper lumbar spine.
- Peripheral nerve entrapment—the pain differs from bursitis in quality rather than location, with complaints of burning or stinging being common.
- Abductor muscle strain, often gluteus medius—the pain occurs on resisted abduction of the hip but passive range of the hip in the neutral position is usually painless.

- Tensor fascia lata pain—often more diffuse and generally involves the more distal area of the lateral thigh.
- In the elderly, stress fracture of the femur is also a possible cause of thigh pain (Morgan & Power, 1986).

PHYSIOTHERAPY

Local electrotherapy such as pulsed electromagnetic energy and ultrasound may be helpful in relieving symptoms, but it is also important to examine the hip and lumbar spine and treat any underlying problem. In some cases a full biomechanical assessment may result in modifications to the footwear, which may improve hip pain by altering the orientation of the lower limb.

PLANTAR FASCIITIS

This term is most often used to describe pain that arises on the anteromedial surface of the calcaneal tuberosity, but may be applied to any painful disorder arising anywhere in the plantar fascia. The cause is not specific and there are many contributory factors including excessive loading, degeneration or abnormal/altered biomechanics. In young patients or those with bilateral symptoms, ankylosing spondylitis, Reiter's syndrome and psoriatic arthritis should be considered as possible causes (Kier, 1994). It is also useful to check for signs of adverse mechanical tension in the lower limb as some foot pain can be attributed to a neural cause. In these cases the pain may be elicited by increasing straight leg raise whilst maintaining ankle and knee positions, i.e. without increasing stretch on the plantar fascia. Heel spurs (bony extensions on the calcaneum) have been described in association with plantar fasciitis (Kwong et al., 1988).

Predisposing factors to the condition include pes planus or cavus foot deformities as well as running, playing basketball, tennis or dancing (Kier, 1994). Obesity and occupations that involve prolonged standing or walking may also be implicated in development of plantar fasciitis (Campbell & O'Lawton, 1994) and pronation deformity is present in 80% of patients with the condition (Gibbon & Cassar-Pullicino, 1994).

Patients describe a gradual onset of pain, which is worse when they take their first step in the morning. Climbing stairs or going up on the toes may also exacerbate the symptoms. On physical examination, sufferers have pain and tenderness in the area of the calcaneal tuberosity where the central and thickest portion of the plantar fascia is attached.

PATHOLOGY

Repetitive trauma produces micro-tears in the plantar fascia close to its attachment, with chronic inflammation developing as healing is attempted amidst recurrent trauma.

TREATMENT

Most patients can be successfully treated conservatively using anti-pronation orthoses and energy absorbing heel cushions (Karr, 1994), as well as rest and anti-inflammatory drugs. Occasionally local steroid injections may be helpful, although multiple injections should be avoided as they may lead to atrophy of the heel fat pad. Physiotherapy for this condition includes local electrotherapy in combination with stretching exercises; reduction of precipitating activities and the introduction of non-weightbearing sports such as swimming or cycling should also be advised.

HYPERMOBILITY SYNDROME

CRITERIA FOR HYPERMOBILITY

Joints are said to be hypermobile when excessive ranges of movement are permitted by ligamentous laxity.

Beighton Criteria for Hypermobility

Score 1 point for each of the following:
- Passive dorsiflexion of the fifth fingers beyond 90° (L and R).
- Passive opposition of thumbs to the forearm (L and R).
- More than 10° of elbow hyperextension (L and R).
- More than 10° of knee hyperextension (L and R).
- Putting palms flat on the floor on forward flexion with straight knees.

These tests give a score of 0–9. A score of 2 or more indicates hypermobility (Jónsson & Valtysdóttir, 1995).

SYMPTOMS

Pain may be experienced around the joints and the patella, shoulder or hip may even sublux. In some cases swelling may be more pronounced than pain.

MANAGEMENT

Physiotherapy

Slow static contractions throughout a range of joint movement just short of end range and active movements throughout this range help to develop extra muscle tone to protect vulnerable joints. Care must be taken during pregnancy or just before menstruation when women are often unable to tell where movement is naturally restricted due to hormonal changes, and the tissues can overstretch.

Drugs

Simple analgesia such as paracetamol and NSAIDs may be useful to relieve symptoms.

CONCLUSION

Soft tissue symptoms often have a complex aetiology, and the therapist needs to be mindful not only of the presenting lesion but also of possible differential diagnoses. Management of these conditions may require a combination of approaches.

REFERENCES

Atkins RM, Tindale W, Bickerstaff D, Kanis JA. Quantitative bone scintigraphy in reflex sympathetic dystrophy. *Br J Rheum* 1993, **32**:41-45.

Barton NJ, Hooper G, Noble J, Steel WM. Occupational causes of disorders in the upper limb. *BMJ* 1992, **304**(6822):309-311.

Bennett RM, Jacobsen S. Muscle function and the origin of pain in fibromyalgia. *Baillières Clin Rheumatol* 1994, **8**:721-746.

Blumberg H, Janig W. Clinical manifestations of reflex sympathetic dystrophy and sympathetically maintained pain. In: Melzack R, Wall P, eds. *Textbook of pain*. Edinburgh: Churchill Livingstone; 1994:685-696.

Bulgen DY, Binder AI, Hazelman BL, Dutton J, Roberts S. Frozen shoulder: Prospective clinical study with an evaluation of three treatment regimens. *Ann Rheum Dis* 1984, **43**:353-360.

Burckhardt CS, Bjelle A. Education programmes for fibromyalgia patients: description and evaluation. *Baillières Clin Rheumatol* 1994, **8**:935-956.

Campbell P, O'Lawton J. Heel pain: diagnosis and management. *Br J Hosp Med* 1994, **52**:8380-8384.

Chard MD, Hazleman BL. Tennis elbow, a reappraisal. *Br J Rheum* 1989: **28**:3,186-190.

Chop WM. Tennis elbow. *Post-Grad Med* 1989, **86**:301-308.

Cyriax J. Diagnosis of soft tissue lesions. In: *Textbook of orthopaedic medicine, 8th edition*, chapter 9, London: Ballière Tindall; 1984:134-135.

Emig EW, Schweitzer ME, Karasick D, Lubowitz J. Adhesive capsulitis of the shoulder. *Am J Roentgenol* 1995, **164**:1457-1459.

Fialka V, Resch KL, Ritter-Dietrich D *et al*. Acupuncture for reflex sympathetic dystrophy. *Arch Int Med* 1993, **153**:661-665.

Gibbon WW, Cassar-Pullicino VN. Heel pain. *Ann Rheum Dis* 1994, **53**:344-348.

Herrick AL. *Topical reviews: reflex sympathetic dystrophy*. Reports Rheum Dis Arthritis and Rheumatism Council; 1994:2.

Hess D. Employee perceived stress. Relationship to the development of repetitive strain injury symptoms, 1997. *AAOHN J* 1997, **45**:115-123.

Janig W. The sympathetic nervous system in pain - physiology and pathophysiology. In Stanton-Hicks M, ed. *Pain and the sympathetic nervous system*. Massachusetts: Kluwer Academic Publishers; 1990:17-89.

Jónsson H, Valtysdóttir S. Hypermobility features in patients with hand osteoarthritis. *Osteoarthritis Cartilage* 1995, **3**:1-5.

Karr SD. Subcalcaneal heel pain. *Orthopaed Clin North Am* 1994, **25**:161-173.

Kesler RW, Salisbury FT, Miller LT, Rowlingson JC. Reflex sympathetic dystrophy in children treatment with transcutaneous electric nerve stimulation. *Pediatrics* 1988, **82**:728-732.

Kier R. Magnetic resonance imaging of plantar fasciitis and other causes of heel pain. *MRI Clin North Am* 1994, **2**:97-107.

Kingsley G, Gibson T. Frozen shoulder - a comparative clinical and radiographic study. *Br J Rheum* 1986, **25**:suppl 2,58.

Kruger JM, Karnovsky ML. Sleep and the immune response. *New York Acad Sci* 1987, **496**:517.

Kruger VL, Kraft GH, Deitz JC, Ameis A, Polisar L. Carpal tunnel syndrome - objective measures and splint use. *Arch Phys Med Rehabil* 1991, **72**:517-520.

Kushner S, Reid DC. Manipulation in the treatment of tennis elbow. *J Orthopaed Sports Phys Ther* 1986, **7**:No 5, 265-272.

Kwong PK, Kay D, Voner RT. Plantar fasciitis - mechanics and pathomechanics of treatment. *Clin Sports Med* 1988, **7**:119-126.

Leavitt F, Katz RS, Golden BE, Glickman PB, Layfer LF. Comparison of pain properties in fibromyalgia patients and rheumatoid arthritis patients. *Arth Rheum* 1986, **29**:6, 775-781.

Ledingham J, Doherty S, Doherty M. Primary fibromyalgia syndrome - an outcome study. *Br J Rheum* 1993, **32**:139-142.

McCain GA. Fibromyalgia and myofascial pain syndromes. In: Melzack R, Wall P, eds. *Textbook of pain*. Edinburgh: Churchill Livingstone; 1994:475-493.

Molsberger A, Hille E. The analgesic effect of acupuncture in chronic tennis elbow pain. *Br J Rheumatol* 1994, **33**:1162-1165.

Morgan CA, Power BM. Unapparent fractures in the elderly. *Med J Austr* 1986, **20**:424-426.

Morris IM, Mattingly PC, Thomson AJ. Radiological erosions in frozen shoulder. *Br J Rheum* 1990, **29**:293-294.

Neviaser TJ. Arthroscopy of the shoulder. *Orthopaed Clin North Am* 1987, **18**:361-372.

Neviaser TJ. Intra-articular inflammatory diseases of the shoulder. *Instructional Course* 1989, Lecture **38**:199-204.

Noteboom T, Cruver R, Keller J, Kellogg B, Nitz AJ. Tennis elbow: a review. *J Orthopaed Sports Physiother* 1994, **19**:357-366.

Rizk TE, Pinals RS. Frozen shoulder. *Sem Arthritis Rheumat* 1982, **11**:440-450.

Roberts WJ. A hypothesis on the physiological basis for causalgia and related pains. *Pain* 1986, **24**:297-311.

Rosen NB. Physical medicine and rehabilitation approaches to the management of myofascial pain and fibromyalgia syndromes. *Baillières Clin Rheumatol* 1994, **8**:881-916.

Russell IJ, Vipraio GA, Morgan WM, Bowden CL. Is there a metabolic basis for fibrositis syndrome? *Am J Med* 1986, **81**:50.

Schneider G. Restricted shoulder movement. Capsular contracture or cervical referral - a clinical study. *Austr J Physiother* 1989, **35**:97-100.

Segmullèr BE, Taylor DE, Hogan CS, Saies AD, Hayes MG. Arthroscopic treatment of adhesive capsulitis. *J Shoulder Elbow Surg* 1995, **4**:403-408.

Shaffer B, Tibone JE, Kerlan RK. Frozen shoulder. *J Bone Joint Surg* 1992, **74A**:738-745.

Simms RW. Controlled trials of therapy in fibromyalgia syndrome. *Baillières Clin Rheumatol* 1994, **8**:917-934.

Simmonds FA. Shoulder pain with particular reference to frozen shoulder. *J Bone/Joint Surg* 1979, **31B**:426-432.

Sipos DA. Carpal tunnel syndrome. *Orth Nurs* 1995, **14**:17-20.

Smythe H. Fibrositis and other diffuse musculoskeletal syndromes. In: Kelly WN, Harris ED Jnr, Ruddy S, Sledge CB, eds. *Textbook of rheumatology*. Philadelphia: WB Saunders; 1985:481-489.

Stratford PW, Levy DR, Gouldie S, Miseferi D, Levy K. The evaluation of phonophoresis and friction massage as treatment for extensor carpi radialis tendinitis: a randomized controlled trial. *Physiother Canada*; 1989:**41**, No 2, 93-98.

Thompson JS, Phelps TH. Repetitive strain injuries. *Postgrad Med* 1990, **88**:143-149.

Totten PA, Hunter JM. Therapeutic techniques to enhance nerve gliding in thoracic outlet syndrome and carpal tunnel syndrome. *Hand Clin* 1991, **7**:505-519.

Traycoff RB. 'Pseudotrochanteric bursitis'. The differential diagnosis of lateral back pain. *J Rheum* 1991, **18**:1810-1812.

Whitley JM, McDonnel DE. Carpal tunnel syndrome. *Postgrad Med* 1995, **97**:89-96.

Wolfe F. Fibromyalgia - the clinical syndrome. *Rheum Dis Clin North Am* 1989, **15**:1-18.

Zimmerman NB, Zimmerman SI, Clark GL. Neuropathy in the workplace. *Hand Clin* 1992, **8**:255-262.

12 C David

SERONEGATIVE ARTHRITIDES

CHAPTER OUTLINE

- Spondyloarthropathies
- Seronegative rheumatoid arthritis
- Viral arthritis
- Infective (septic) arthritis
- Lyme disease (borreliosis)
- Behçet's syndrome
- Physiotherapy management of seronegative arthritides

INTRODUCTION

Seronegative arthritis is inflammatory arthritis in which the blood concentration of rheumatoid factor (RF) is within normal limits. Some of these conditions, for instance the spondyloarthropathies, are a distinct group with many features in common. Behçet's syndrome, on the other hand, has only superficial similarity with other seronegative arthritides and is in fact a vasculitic syndrome. It is included in this chapter due to its previous classification as a spondyloarthropathy, although this classification has been questioned for some time (Moll, 1994). Some seronegative arthritides are associated with infection; those associated with HIV infection are described in Chapter 16.

SPONDYLOARTHROPATHIES

As the name suggests, many of these conditions include spinal as well as peripheral joint involvement. The group includes psoriatic arthritis (PsA), enteropathic spondyloarthropathy, reactive arthritis, Reiter's syndrome and ankylosing spondylitis (AS). Since AS is of major importance to physiotherapists, it is described separately in Chapter 10.

Table 12.1 lists the common features which characterise spondyloarthropathies. They can occur in all ages. There is a strong association with human leukocyte antigen (HLA) B27, ranging from 50% of patients with psoriatic and enteropathic arthritis to 95% of patients with AS (Calin, 1993).

PSORIATIC ARTHRITIS

Psoriatic arthritis is an inflammatory arthritis associated with psoriasis, classified as a distinct entity in 1964 by the American Rheumatism Association (Blumberg et al., 1964). The exact relationship between psoriasis and arthritis is unclear, and severity of joint disease does not always correlate with severity of skin involvement. However, psoriasis is found in 3–7% of patients with arthritis compared with less than 3% in the general population, and arthritis is found in 7–42% of psoriatic patients compared with 2–3% in the general population (Gladman, 1994). PsA justifies inclusion among the seronegative spondyloarthropathies since it may present as a spondyloarthropathy (Gladman, 1993). A severe form of PsA is associated with HIV infection, described in Chapter 16.

There are five distinct subgroups of PsA (Moll & Wright, 1973), which are summarised in Table 12.2.

Diagnostic criteria for spondyloarthropathy	
Clinical symptoms or history of:	**Score**
1. Lumbar or dorsal pain during the night, or early morning stiffness lumbar or dorsal region	1
2. Asymmetrical oligoarthritis	2
3. Alternate buttock pain	1 or 2
4. Dactylitis	2
5. Heel pain enthesitis	2
6. Iritis	2
7. Urethritis or cervicitis, non gonococcal, accompanying or within 1 month of arthritis onset	1
8. Acute diarrhoea accompanying or within 1 month of arthritis onset	1
9. Presence or history of psoriasis, balanitis, ulcerative colitis, Crohn's	2
10. Radiologically Grade ≥2 bilateral or ≥3 unilateral sacroiliitis	3
11. HLA B27 or family history of ankylosing spondylitis, Reiter's, uveitis, psoriasis or chronic enteropathy	2
12. Clear cut response to non steroidal anti-inflammatory drugs	2
If the total score is 6 or more, spondyloarthropathy is present: reactive arthritis if items 7 and 8 present. (Amor *et al.*, 1990)	

Table 12.1 **Diagnostic criteria for spondyloarthropathy.**

Classification of psoriatic arthritis	
% of total cases	**Subgroup of psoriatic arthritis**
1. 10%	Asymmetrical distal interphalangeal joint involvement of hands and feet, with resorption of the distal phalanx and onycholysis
2. Up to 5%	Arthritis mutilans – particularly disabling form involving osteolysis of affected joints, especially in fingers and toes, leading to shortening and telescoping of digits ('opera-glass hands')
3. 5%	Symmetrical polyarthritis, seronegative but otherwise indistinguishable from rheumatoid arthritis
4. 70%	Asymmetrical oligoarthritis of large joint, e.g. knee, plus a few distal interphalangeal joints, proximal interphalangeal joints and metacarpo interphalangeal joints, and possibly dactylitis of fingers or toes
5. Up to 5%	Ankylosing spondylitis, enthesitis, possibly peripheral arthritis. Conjunctivitis in 33%, iritis in 7%

Table 12.2 **Classification of psoriatic arthritis.**

Systemic symptoms such as early morning stiffness (EMS), fatigue and fever are most common in the symmetrical polyarticular pattern. Dactylitis ('sausage digit') is a characteristic swelling of the whole finger or toe indicating tendinitis as well as proximal interphalangeal (PIP) and distal interphalangeal (DIP) inflammation, and is seen in several of the seronegative arthritides (Figure 12.1). Nail involvement takes the form of onycholysis (separation of the nail from the nail bed) and pitting, ridging or erosion of the nail. This may occur independently of DIP involvement. Nail lesions are found in 90% of patients with PsA compared with 46% of psoriatic patients without arthritis.

In this chapter, forms of PsA involving mainly peripheral joints will be termed 'rheumatoid arthritis (RA)-type' and those more closely resembling AS, 'AS-type'.

Incidence

The incidence of PsA is difficult to ascertain but is thought to affect almost 1% of the population (Gladman, 1993). The peak age of onset is between 20 and 40. Sex distribution is equal, and it is most common in North European and North American Caucasians. Spinal involvement is linked with HLA B27 while the polyarthritis is linked with HLA DR4. In 75% of cases the psoriasis precedes the arthritis, 15% have synchronous onset and in 10% the arthritis precedes psoriasis (Helliwell & Wright, 1994). The psoriasis may be a small patch and hard to find.

Diagnosis

Diagnosis is difficult as other forms of arthritis may exist with concurrent psoriasis. Diagnostic criteria have been developed by Vasey & Espinoza (1984).

Diagnostic Criteria for Psoriatic Arthritis

Mandatory skin or nail involvement plus one of the following:
- Pain and soft tissue swelling of DIP joints for more than 4 weeks.

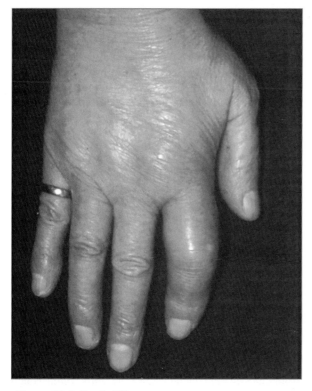

Figure 12.1 Dactylitis.

- Pain and soft tissue swelling of peripheral joints in asymmetrical pattern for more than 4 weeks.
- Symmetrical peripheral arthritis for more than 4 weeks in absence of RF or subcutaneous nodules.
- Peripheral radiological features; 'pencil in cup' deformity, erosion of terminal phalanges, fluffy periostosis and bony ankylosis.
- Spinal pain and stiffness with restriction of movement for more than 4 weeks.
- Spinal radiological features: grade 2 bilateral sacroiliitis or grade 3/4 unilateral sacroiliitis.

Investigations

Inflammatory indices, e.g. erythrocyte sedimentation rate (ESR), correlate with the degree of synovitis but not with the severity of spondylitis symptoms. Radiology may show axial changes which are similar to AS. However, sacroiliitis and syndesmophytes are more usually asymmetrical, and squaring of the vertebral bodies is not as common (Porter, 1994). Cervical involvement may be severe, with erosion of the odontoid peg and atlanto-axial subluxation, facet joint erosions and serial subluxation. Anterior longitudinal ligament ossification and fusion between vertebral bodies may also be seen.

Peripheral changes are most marked in the hands and feet. Asymmetrical destructive lesions are seen, mainly involving the DIP joints of fingers and toes. Erosions progress from the periphery of the joint to the centre (Figure 12.2). Bony proliferation and fusion may also occur, particularly in the interphalangeal joints. New bone may be formed at the sites of enthesitis, for instance the insertion of the plantar fascia leading to heel spurs.

Treatment

Basic principles of medical management are along similar lines to RA. Drugs used are:
- Non steroidal anti-inflammatory drugs (NSAIDs): generally produce a good response but may possibly exacerbate psoriasis.
- Slow acting anti-rheumatic drugs (SAARDs).
- Azathioprine and sulphasalazine are useful.
- Methotrexate is effective in psoriasis and can also help nail lesions.
- Gold is useful in RA-type disease but may cause photosensitivity and exacerbate psoriasis.
- Cyclosporin A suppresses the psoriasis, but effects on the arthritis are not so good. Discontinuation usually exacerbates skin and joint involvement.
- Penicillamine may be as effective as for RA but the evidence is limited.
- Steroids: topical steroid is useful for skin lesions. Oral steroids may be necessary to control severe joint symptoms, but the skin may flare up during reduction in dose. Intra-articular injection is beneficial but careful skin preparation is needed to avoid introduction of infection into the joint. For details of drugs and their side effects, see Chapter 3.

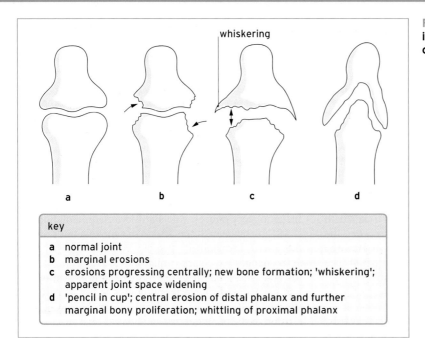

Figure 12.2 **Progression of distal interphalangeal joint radiological changes.**

whiskering

a   b   c   d

key

a normal joint
b marginal erosions
c erosions progressing centrally; new bone formation; 'whiskering'; apparent joint space widening
d 'pencil in cup'; central erosion of distal phalanx and further marginal bony proliferation; whittling of proximal phalanx

- Psoralens plus ultraviolet A (PUVA) has been found to improve joint symptoms in RA-type PsA, but not in the AS-type group (Cuellar *et al.*, 1994).
- Surgical indications are the same as for RA. However, as skin involvement in PsA increases the risk of wound infection systemic prophylactic antibiotics may be necessary.

Prognosis

The course tends to be mild in terms of hospital admission and time off work. Although there is a gradual progression over time, this may not necessarily be associated with major changes in function. Significant functional limitation occurs in about 11%; about 2% have severe arthritis affecting five or more joints (Cuellar *et al.*, 1994).

REACTIVE ARTHRITIS
Pathology

Reactive arthritis is defined as 'Aseptic arthritis triggered by an infectious agent located outside the joint' (Amor & Toubert, 1993). The original infection may be enteric, most commonly caused by shigella, yersinia, salmonella and campylobacter, or genitourinary, chiefly chlamydial. Around 1–2% of patients with these infections go on to develop arthritis. The term 'Reiter's syndrome' describes the classic triad of arthritis, urethritis and ocular involvement, but is interchangeable with reactive arthritis (Toivanen, 1994).

Joint involvement is usually an asymmetrical oligoarthritis affecting knees, ankles and metatarsophalangeal joints, often accompanied by fatigue and low-grade fever. Onset is usually sudden, and within days or weeks of infection. Occasionally the onset is acute with fever, severe weight loss and diffuse polyarticular involvement. Inflammatory dorsal or buttock pain is found in 50% of cases; enthesitis is common, especially plantar fasciitis and tendo-achilles insertion. Dactylitis is a common feature. (For further information on enthesitis, see Chapter 10.)

Urethritis may be present even in the absence of sexually transmitted disease. Conjunctivitis or uveitis is found in up to 30% of cases (Veys & Mielants, 1994). Rarely heart and neurological lesions may be found, such as heart block, pericarditis, myelopathy or cranial nerve lesions. Balanitis and oral mucosal ulceration are found in about 10%; these lesions are often painless. Keratoderma blennorrhagica (pustular psoriasis) may occasionally be found on the palms and soles in disease of genitourinary origin, and is associated with a poor prognosis. It is not found in disease of enteric origin (Veys & Mielants, 1994).

Incidence

The annual incidence is 30–40 per 100,000 (Toivanen, 1994). A total of 75% of cases are young adults under 40, and three times as many men as women are affected. Between 70 and 80% are HLA B27 positive (Inman, 1993).

Investigations

In some cases no causative organism is found. Enteric organisms have usually disappeared from the gut by the time the arthritis appears. Synovial fluid is usually sterile although non-viable organisms may be found (Amor & Toubert, 1993) and white count is raised (Inman, 1993). ESR is raised. Asymmetrical sacroiliitis may be found on X-ray.

Treatment

Antibiotics do not generally affect the course of the condition, with the exception of tetracycline which may shorten the course of post-chlamydia disease. Methotrexate, sulphasalazine, azathioprine and NSAIDs may be helpful, as may intra articular steroids provided synovial fluid cultures are negative. Steroid eye drops are useful in the treatment of uveitis, but systemic steroids are of no proven benefit (Amor & Toubert, 1993).

Prognosis
The prognosis is generally good. Most recover over 3 or 4 months, but 25–40% follow a chronic course having either persistent disease activity or intermittent attacks, often triggered by fresh infection. A minority have long-term functional disability.

ENTEROPATHIC ARTHRITIS
The most common inflammatory bowel diseases associated with arthritis are ulcerative colitis (UC), which affects 50–100 per 100,000 people, and Crohn's disease (CD) which is a little more common (Veys & Mielants, 1994).

Pathology
There are two patterns of joint involvement associated with UC and CD: peripheral and axial. Peripheral arthritis is seen in 2–22% of UC patients and 10–20% of CD patients, while axial involvement is present in about 6% of both groups (Amor & Toubert, 1993). The peripheral arthritis is usually a symmetrical oligoarthritis which starts suddenly and is often migratory. Knees and ankles are most commonly affected. Up to 75% of joint flare-ups coincide with flares of underlying bowel disease. There is equal sex distribution and no link with HLA. Axial involvement is indistinguishable from idiopathic AS and includes enthesitis, particularly heel pain. 75% of patients are HLA B27 positive, with a slight male predominance. Bowel and spinal symptoms flare up independently of each other, and the spondylitis often precedes the enteropathy by many months or years.

Investigations
ESR is raised. Cultures are negative (Veys & Mielants, 1994).

Treatment
NSAIDs may be contra-indicated during acute bowel episodes. Bowel resection may help to prevent recurrence of the peripheral arthritis but has little effect on the spondylitis (Gibofsky, 1993).

Prognosis
Prognosis for peripheral disease is usually good, with 50% of attacks normally lasting for less than 6 months although 20% may last for more than a year (Amor & Toubert, 1993). The arthritis is non-erosive and does not lead to permanent joint damage or deformity, even when recurrent (Haslock & Wright, 1973). Some 25% have minor limitation or contracture. Amyloidosis may be a feature, especially in CD, and is usually fatal (Veys & Mielants, 1994). Progress and prognosis for axial disease are similar to AS (see Chapter 10.)

SERONEGATIVE RHEUMATOID ARTHRITIS

The concentration of RF in the blood of a patient with RA varies with the level of disease activity, and may at times be within the normal range. However, up to 25% of patients with RA never have clinically significant levels of RF (Williams, 1994). For this group of patients non-articular features are less prominent and the prognosis may be better than in seropositive disease, but otherwise there is no difference in clinical presentation and management. Seronegative RA may prove to be a subgroup of RA with a different aetiological basis (Maini & Feldmann, 1993).

VIRAL ARTHRITIS

Viruses may either infect the synovium directly or trigger an immune response. Most viral arthritides are short lived and require symptomatic therapy only. The most common viral causes of arthritis are:

RUBELLA
The reported frequency of arthritis varies from 15–65% of rubella cases. Up to 90% of those affected are adult women. Symmetrical pain and stiffness develop within a week of rubella rash, and may also follow immunisation with live vaccine. Knees, wrists and small joints of hands are most commonly affected, but shoulders, elbows, ankles and hips may also be involved. Symptoms usually improve in a few weeks but may persist for up to 2 years (Woolf, 1993).

PARVOVIRUS
Although parvovirus B19 does not play a significant part in the aetiology of RA, the arthritis it triggers may be indistinguishable from RA (Nikkari *et al.*, 1995). About 40% of parvovirus infections occur between the ages of 6 and 16, but all ages may be affected. Children have a characteristic 'slapped cheeks' facial rash. About 5% of children with parvovirus go on to develop an acute symmetrical arthritis mainly affecting knees, feet and small joints of hands. Occasionally the onset is similar to systemic juvenile chronic arthritis with fever, intermittent rash, high ESR and low haemoglobin. 60% of adults with parvovirus arthritis are women (Kalden, 1994). The arthritis usually lasts for about 10 days but may persist for up to 5 years in some cases. Despite the long duration of symptoms no disability or erosions result and prognosis is good.

HEPATITIS B
Transient symmetrical arthritis and morning stiffness may affect knees and small joints of hands, and sometimes wrists, ankles, shoulders and elbows, after an incubation period of 40–180 days following infection. Only symptomatic treatment is required.

INFECTIVE (SEPTIC) ARTHRITIS

PATHOLOGY

Joint sepsis may result directly from puncture into the joint, from adjacent bony or soft tissue infection or, more commonly, through bacteraemia. A wide variety of organisms is involved, most commonly staphylococcus and streptococcus in adults, *Haemophilus influenzae* in children (Kavanagh *et al.*, 1995). In young adults, gonococcus is an important cause of arthritis and may be difficult to distinguish from reactive arthritis. Predisposing factors to septic arthritis include:

- Age—10% are under 5; 55% are 60 or over (Kavanagh *et al.*, 1995).
- Extra-articular infection.
- Previous damage to the joint—RA, OA, crystal arthropathy, neuropathic, trauma, surgery.
- Underlying chronic conditions—malignancy, diabetes, cirrhosis, intravenous drug abuse, systemic lupus erythematosus.
- Immunosuppressive or steroid therapy.

The onset is acute, with joint pain, swelling, warmth, erythema and tenderness, occasionally accompanied by rash. Usually only one joint is affected, but 10–20% have polyarthritis. Knees and hips are most commonly affected, but when bacteraemia results from intravenous drug abuse sepsis may involve sternoclavicular, sacroiliac or shoulder joints. Joint pain is often referred, and increased on extremes of movement and weightbearing. Fever is found in 90% and septic shock may occur in vulnerable patients. Occasionally the arthritis may follow a subacute or even chronic pauci-articular course with less virulent organisms.

INVESTIGATIONS

ESR and C-reactive protein (CRP) will be high; blood cultures will be positive in a third of cases. Purulent synovial fluid is not always indicative of infection as it can occur in long-standing RA, gout, pseudogout or subchondral fractures. A negative culture may not always indicate absence of infection. The polymerase chain reaction (PCR) is a sensitive genetic engineering technique used to detect small quantities of bacterial genetic material, and may be needed to detect bacteria such as *Borrelia* which are difficult to culture. Infection may still be present within joints despite negative PCR results (Highton & Poole, 1993). X-rays may show peri-articular soft tissue swelling, periarticular osteopaenia, uniform joint space narrowing, erosions, and eventually fibrous or bony ankylosis if chronic.

TREATMENT

Antibiotics and immobilisation of the joint until the pain begins to resolve, then non-weightbearing range of movement exercises which may aid cartilage nutrition (Brause, 1993). Surgical drainage may be needed in cases of hip infection, loculation or lack of response to antibiotics. Infected prostheses often need removal, but any invasive procedure carries the risk of introducing new pathogens (Hughes, 1996).

LYME DISEASE (BORRELIOSIS)

First recognised in 1975, Lyme disease is caused by a spirochaete, *Borrelia burgdorferi*, carried by the tiny *Ixodes* tick. Although not common in the UK (200 cases per year) it is the most common vector-borne disease in the US, where incidence has risen from 497 in 1982 to 9344 in 1991 (Rees & Axford, 1994). The mechanism is unknown but is possibly a delayed hypersensitivity reaction.

PATHOLOGY

In 75% of patients, a characteristic 'bulls-eye' rash develops within a few weeks of a tick bite, often accompanied by flu-like symptoms. In some cases the presentation may be similar to polymyalgia rheumatica (Schwartzenberg *et al.*, 1995). Lyme arthritis shows significant geographical variation. In North America about 50% of infected patients will develop recurrent flitting arthritis. This most commonly affects the knee, lasting a few days to a few months. Between 10 and 20% will go on to develop chronic arthritis, a third of whom will have erosive changes (Rees & Axford, 1994). Arthritis is less common in Europe, affecting about 33% of infected patients, and only rarely reported in UK (about 14%).

Neurological symptoms may develop within several weeks, months, or even years following an untreated infection, and include meningitis, Bell's palsy, numbness or weakness in the limbs, poor co-ordination, loss of memory or concentration and changes in sleeping habits. Symptoms often last for weeks or months and may recur. About 10% develop transient heart arrhythmias.

INVESTIGATIONS

Lyme disease is difficult to diagnose because symptoms mimic those of other disorders and many patients will not recall being bitten by a tick. *B. burgdorferi* is difficult to culture but antibodies may be detected in blood or cerebrospinal fluid, or PCR may be used (National Institutes of Health (NIH), 1992).

PROGNOSIS

Most cases recover fully with antibiotics. In 70% of patients with chronic arthritis resistant to treatment, the organism is eradicated but reactive arthritis persists. HLA DR4 is linked with resistant disease (Rees & Axford, 1994). Patients with severe arthritis may need intravenous antibiotics, anti-inflammatory drugs, joint aspiration or synovectomy (NIH, 1992). Fatigue and general malaise can take months to subside but do so spontaneously without additional antibiotic therapy.

PREVENTION

Development of an effective vaccine for Lyme disease has been difficult since acquired immunity to *B. burgdorferi* is not consistent, and re-infection is common. Tick-infested areas should be avoided during the summer, skin should be covered and insect repellent applied.

BEHÇET'S SYNDROME

This syndrome, first described in 1937, seems to share some features with spondyloarthropathies – eye involvement, diarrhoea, mucocutaneous ulceration and peripheral arthritis are common. However, there is no link with psoriasis or inflammatory bowel disease, and little familial clustering. In addition, sacroilitis and spondylitis are not a feature (Chamberlain & Robertson, 1993) and HLA B51 is associated rather than B27. The underlying pathology is a vasculitis of unknown cause, although it is possibly triggered by streptococci or herpes simplex.

The vast majority of patients with Behçet's Syndrome (BS) have oral ulceration, 80% have genital ulceration and 50–80% have skin lesions similar to erythema nodosum (see Chapter 16). Gastrointestinal symptoms are secondary to mucosal ulceration. Up to 50% have arthritis, mainly mono- or oligoarthritis of knees, ankles, wrists and elbows. The arthritis usually lasts for a few weeks but may become chronic. Avascular necrosis may occur as a result of vasculitis (Yazıcı, 1994). Vasculitis affects all sizes and types of vessels, especially veins, including the vena cava. Up to 25% of patients have thrombophlebitis, which may lead to vena cava obstruction. Arterial aneurysms may also develop; these are particularly dangerous in the pulmonary artery (Hamuryudan et al., 1997).

Eye involvement is the most serious manifestation of BS, affecting 50% of patients overall. In 90% of cases both eyes are affected. Eye disease usually starts about 2 or 3 years after the onset of BS. Uveitis and retinal vasculitis lead to scarring and secondary glaucoma. Conjunctivitis is rare. Hypopyon, the deposition of white cells and debris in the anterior chamber of the eye, is typical of BS and indicates severe eye involvement (Hamuryudan et al., 1997).

Other features include pulmonary infarcts, aneurysms, and thromboses, and occasional myositis or amyloidosis. 5% have neurological involvement, mainly pyramidal and cerebellar signs and meningeal irritation. Pathergy, a condition unique to BS, is an extreme tissue response to minor trauma which may lead to recurrence of aneurysms after reconstructive surgery and synovitis after joint aspiration (Yazıcı, 1994).

INCIDENCE

Behçet's Syndrome has a clearly defined geographical distribution, being most common in Turkey (80–300 per 100,000) and Japan (10–15 per 100,000). It is less common in Europe (1 per 300,000). The exact prevalence is unknown due to lack of data (Yazıcı, 1993). Onset is usually between the ages of 20 and 35 years. Sex distribution is equal, but males have more severe disease.

INVESTIGATIONS

There are no specific diagnostic tests for BS. There may be a slight rise in CRP and ESR but this does not correlate with disease severity.

TREATMENT

Azathioprine and cyclosporin prevent recurrence and worsening of eye disease but cannot reverse damage. Steroids may be needed for neurological symptoms, sulphasalazine or bowel resection for gastrointestinal involvement. Skin lesions and arthralgia respond to colchicine, while cyclophosphamide may be required for severe skin and systemic vasculitis. Treatment can usually be stopped 2 years after remission.

PROGNOSIS

The disease generally runs a palindromic course with a good prognosis. However, the outlook is worse for males and younger patients, and amyloidosis carries a grave prognosis. Eye involvement leads to severe visual loss and blindness in 10–20%. The mortality rate from BS is 0.8%.

PHYSIOTHERAPY MANAGEMENT OF SERONEGATIVE ARTHRITIDES

Assessment of the patient with seronegative arthritis will be similar to that for RA (see Chapter 8). However, the therapist needs to bear in mind the possibility of spondyloarthropathy, and if the spine is involved assessment following the guidelines for AS is indicated (see Chapter 10). Psoriatic patients may be embarrassed about their skin condition and must be assessed with sensitivity.

Depending on the presenting problems, treatment follows the same principles as for AS and/or RA; treatment is detailed in the relevant chapters. Exercise may need to be modified to take into consideration peripheral arthritis in a patient with AS-type PsA. Psoriasis is not a contraindication to hydrotherapy provided the skin is not broken, although the chlorine may cause irritation. Wearing leotards or tee-shirts in the pool will help to overcome self-consciousness. Plastic gloves will protect psoriatic or onycholytic hands when using wax.

The acute stage of reactive arthritis may be difficult to control and can be extremely painful. Although it is vital to regain joint mobility as soon as possible, especially in the hands, adequate pain relief should accompany physiotherapy.

Ultrasound is inadvisable in septic arthritis due to the theoretical risk of spread of infection (Low & Reed, 1990).

REFERENCES

Amor B, Dougados M, Mijiyawa M. Critères de classification des spondylathropathies. *Revue du Rheumatisme et des Maladies Ostéoarticulaires* 1990, **57**:85-89.

Amor B, Toubert AA. Reactive arthropathy, Reiter's and enteric arthropathy in adults. In: Maddison PJ, Isenberg DA, Woo P, Glass DN, eds. *Oxford textbook of rheumatology*. Oxford: Oxford Medical Publications; 1993:699-709.

Brause BD. Infectious arthritis. In: Paget S, Pellici P, Beary JF, eds. *Manual of rheumatology and outpatient orthopaedic disorders*. Boston: Little, Brown; 1993:294-302.

Blumberg BS, Bunim JJ, Calkins E, Pirani CL, Zvaifler NJ. American Rheumatism Association nomenclature and classification of arthritis and rheumatism (tentative). *Arthritis Rheum* 1964, **1**:491-523.

Calin A. Spondylarthropathy, undifferentiated spondarthropathies and overlap. In: Maddison PJ, Isenberg DA, Woo P, Glass DN, eds. *Oxford textbook of rheumatology*. Oxford: Oxford Medical Publications; 1993:666-674.

Chamberlain MA, Robertson RJH. A controlled study of sacroiliitis in Behçet's disease. *Br J Rheum* 1993, **32**:693-698.

Cuellar ML, Citera G, Espinoza LR. Treatment of psoriatic arthritis. In: Wright V, Helliwell P, eds. *Baillières Clin Rheumatol*: Psoriatic arthritis 1994, **8**:2483-2498.

Gibofsky A. Enteropathic arthritis. In: Paget S, Pellici P, Beary JF, eds. *Manual of rheumatology and outpatient orthopaedic disorders*. Boston: Little, Brown; 1993:260-263.

Gladman DD. Psoriatic arthritis. In: Maddison PJ, Isenberg DA, Woo P, Glass DN, eds. *Oxford textbook of rheumatology*. Oxford: Oxford Medical Publications; 1993:691-698.

Gladman DD. Natural history of psoriatic arthritis. In: Wright V, Helliwell P, eds. *Baillières Clin Rheumatol*: Psoriatic Arthritis 1994, **8**:2379-2394.

Hamuryudan V, Ödzogan H, Yazıcı H. Other forms of vasculitis and pseudovasculitis. In: Yazıcı H, Husby G, eds. *Baillières Clin Rheumatol*: Vasculitis 1997, **11**:2335-2355.

Haslock I, Wright V. The musculoskeletal complications of Crohn's disease. *Medicine* 1973, **52**:217-225.

Helliwell PS, Wright V. Psoriatic arthritis: clinical features. In: Klippel JH, Dieppe P, eds. *Rheumatology*. London: Mosby Year Book Europe; 1994, 3:31.1-8.

Highton JE, Poole E. Sexually acquired reactive arthritis - inflammation or sepsis? *Br J Rheum* 1993, **32**:649-652.

Hughes RA. Septic arthritis. *Arthritis and Rheumatism Council reports on rheumatic diseases* 1996, practical problems. Series 3, No. 7.

Inman R. Reiter syndrome. In: Paget S, Pellici P, Beary JF, eds. *Manual of rheumatology and outpatient orthopaedic disorders*. Boston: Little, Brown; 1993:267-269.

Kalden JR. Viral arthritis. In: Klippel JH, Dieppe P, eds. *Rheumatology*. London: Mosby Year Book Europe; 1994, 4:6.1-8.

Kavanagh R, Ryan MJ, Wall P, *et al*. Bacterial joint infections in England and Wales 1990-93. *Br J Rheum* 1995, **34**:No. 55 (abstract).

Low J, Reed A. *Electrotherapy explained: principles and practice*. Oxford: Butterworth-Heinemann; 1990.

Maini RN, Feldmann M. Immunopathogenesis of RA. In: Maddison PJ, Isenberg DA, Woo P, Glass DN, eds. *Oxford textbook of rheumatology*. Oxford: Oxford Medical Publications; 1993:621-638.

Moll JMH. The place of psoriatic arthritis in the spondarthritides. In: Wright V, Helliwell P, eds. *Baillières Clin Rheumatol*: Psoriatic Arthritis. 1994, **8**:2395-2417.

Moll JM, Wright V. Psoriatic arthritis. *Sem Arthritis Rheum* 1973, **3**:55-78.

National Institute of Health. *Lyme disease: the facts, the challenge*. United States Department of Health and Human Services Publications National Institute of Health 1992; April. NIH 92-3193 (20).

Nikkari S, Roivainen A, Hannonen P, *et al*. Persistence of parvovirus B19 in synovial fluid and bone marrow. *Ann Rheum Dis* 1995, **54**:597-600.

Porter GG. Plain radiology and other imaging techniques. In: Wright V, Helliwell P, eds. *Baillières Clin Rheumatol*: Psoriatic Arthritis. 1994, **8**:2465-2481.

Rees DHE, Axford JS. Lyme arthritis. *Ann Rheum Dis* 1994, **53**:553-556.

Schwartzenberg M, Weber CA, Musico J. Lyme borreliosis presenting as a polymyalgia-like syndrome. *Br J Rheum* 1995, **34**:392-393.

Toivanen A. Reactive arthritis. In: Klippel JH, Dieppe P, eds. *Rheumatology*. London: Mosby Year Book Europe; 1994, 4:9.1-8..

Vasey FB, Espinoza LR. Psoriatic arthropathy. In Calin A, ed. *Spondylarthropathies*. Orlando: Grune and Stratton; 1984:151-185.

Veys EM, Mielants H. Enteropathic arthropathies. In: Klippel JH, Dieppe P, eds. *Rheumatology*. London: Mosby Year Book Europe; 1994, 3:35.1-8.

Williams DG. Autoimmunity in rheumatoid arthritis. In: Klippel JH, Dieppe P, eds. *Rheumatology*. London: Mosby Year Book Europe; 1994, 3:9.1-14.

Woolf AD. Viral arthritis. In: Maddison PJ, Isenberg DA, Woo P, Glass DN, eds. *Oxford textbook of rheumatology*. Oxford: Oxford Medical Publications; 1993:521-560.

Yazıcı H. Behçet's syndrome. In: Maddison PJ, Isenberg DA, Woo P, Glass DN, eds. *Oxford textbook of rheumatology*. Oxford: Oxford Medical Publications; 1993:884-889.

Yazıcı H. Behçet's Syndrome. In: Klippel JH, Dieppe P, eds. *Rheumatology*. London: Mosby Year Book Europe; 1994, 6:20.1-6.

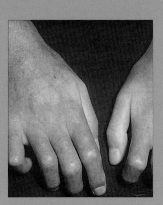

13

C David & J Lloyd

CONNECTIVE TISSUE DISORDERS

CHAPTER OUTLINE

- Systemic sclerosis
- Systemic lupus erythematosus
- Dermatomyositis and polymyositis
- Mixed connective tissue disorder

IXNTRODUCTION

Connective tissue disorders, also known as collagenoses, comprise a varied group of conditions, all of which have systemic complications and which can affect virtually any organ system. The ways in which these conditions may present are extremely variable, posing problems in classification and diagnosis. The conditions may present singly or in combination with other connective tissue disorders, rheumatoid arthritis (RA) or Sjögren's syndrome. They are not common, but knowledge of the varied nature of their features is useful since the physiotherapist may encounter patients with these conditions in wards and specialities other than rheumatology.

SYSTEMIC SCLEROSIS

Systemic sclerosis (SSc) is one of a closely related group of conditions with the title of scleroderma, from the Greek sklera, meaning hard, and derma, skin. Four subsets are recognised:
- 'Pre-scleroderma'—Raynaud's syndrome nailfold changes and digital ischaemic changes, presence of disease-specific antibodies.
- Diffuse cutaneous—skin thickening on the trunk, face, proximal and distal extremities. Early interstitial lung disease, renal failure, myocardial and gastrointestinal involvement.
- Limited cutaneous—skin changes restricted to hands, face, feet and forearms. Possibly late pulmonary and gastrointestinal involvement.
- Sine scleroderma—internal organ, vascular and serological changes without skin thickening; Raynaud's may possibly be present (Black, 1996).

Limited cutaneous SSc is sometimes known as CREST (LeRoy et al., 1988):
- **C**alcinosis.
- **R**aynaud's.
- **E**sophageal dysfunction.
- **S**clerodactyly.
- **T**elangiectasia (dilatation of groups of superficial capillaries).

PREVALENCE

SSc is an uncommon connective tissue disorder affecting a population estimated at between 28 and 130 per million and an annual incidence of 2–10 per million adults worldwide (Black & Stevens,1989). In a study in the West Midlands region Silman et al. (1988) reported prevalence rates of 13 and 48 per million in males and females respectively, and annual incidence rates of 1 and 6 per million. The condition is strongly linked with gender; in all ages the estimated female:male ratio is 3:1, rising to 8–10:1 between the ages of 15 and 44 years (Black & Stevens, 1989). Studies are being conducted into familial aggregation. There does also appear to be some clustering with other autoimmune diseases (Valenta & Elias, 1987). 93% of patients are reported to carry the human leukocyte antigen (HLA)-DR5 or C4AQO markers and 6% carry both (Briggs *et al.*, 1986).

AETIOLOGY

SSc-like illness has been linked with exposure to epoxy resins, organic substances such as trichloroethane, vinyl chloride, silica dust, silicone implants, denatured rapeseed oil ('toxic oil syndrome') and drugs such as bleomycin (Bennett 1993). However, it is likely that SSc is caused by a combination of factors rather than individual substances. Occasionally local scleroderma in children may follow local trauma, such as thorn puncture or tetanus vaccination (Wallace, 1994).

PATHOGENESIS

SSc is a multi-system condition with a broad spectrum; the milder forms of the disease may be unrecognised, while the more severe forms are life threatening. Fibrosis is the hallmark of the disease. Several events occur either simultaneously or as a cascade and contribute to the disease process.

The normal turnover of connective tissue increases, possibly as the result of an inflammatory event, and becomes disrupted with an increase in collagen metabolism (McWhirter *et al.*, 1987). This causes increased deposition of extra cellular matrix in the skin and certain internal organs. There are also marked changes in the microcirculation and immune cell activation, and damage to the intima resulting in increased vascular permeability (Black, 1996). Lymphocytes, macrophages and monocytes collect around the vessels, provoked perhaps by tissue damage or by genetic or environmental factors. T cells then release mediators which facilitate the development of fibroblasts, leading to fibrosis after the inflammatory response has subsided.

Over 97% of cases are associated with Raynaud's phenomenon, which may predate the development of scleroderma by many years (Black, 1996). There are also abnormalities in the microcirculation, with proliferation of intimal arterial lesions and obliteration of the vessels leading to ischaemia. Affected vessels may be in the skin, muscle, subcutaneous tissue or internal organs.

CLINICAL FEATURES

Changes appear first in the hands, face and feet. Initially the hands may be swollen, with an appearance similar to inflammatory arthritis. Fibrosis, leading to thickening of the skin, contractures, tethering and tendon friction rubs, may at first appear as a subcutaneous swelling which the patient may report as feeling warm, itchy or tight.

Skin

The skin may appear dry, shiny and hairless due to obliteration of sebaceous glands and hair follicles; ultimately the skin can become dry and coarse with a possible 'peau d'orange' texture.

Alteration in the appearance due to facial involvement is a striking feature of the disease and is often noticed first by patient and family. Figure 13.1 shows a patient with SSc. The mouth becomes smaller and tight (microstomia) which compromises dental hygiene and eating habits, with a possible resultant effect on nutrition. The nose becomes more pointed and beak-like and the eyes seem larger and more staring due to loss of fatty tissues surrounding them. The patient may look younger, since the normal lines of ageing become obliterated with excess collagen deposition. Facial expressions may be more static due to tightness of the skin and possible alterations in the latent power of the muscle. It is quite often the facial changes that worry the patient the most.

The hand deformity in SSc is characteristic. Fingers become semiflexed with fixed extension at the metacarpophalangeal (MCP) joints and the wrist fixed in a midposition. The fat pads of the fingers may be lost leading to hard, pointed fingers (sclerodactyly, see Figure 13.2). The mechanism causing these deformities is fibrosis and contracture of soft tissues such as joint capsules, tendons and ligaments.

Musculoskeletal

Joint range of movement may be limited by fibrosis and tethering of the skin and structures overlying the muscle, compromising expansion during muscle contraction. Weakness may be due to disuse atrophy; in addition, muscle power may be further compromised by a myositis, leading to proximal weakness. Synovitis has been found in SSc, and it appears that a subset of patients may exist who exhibit features overlapping with RA (Misra *et al.*, 1995).

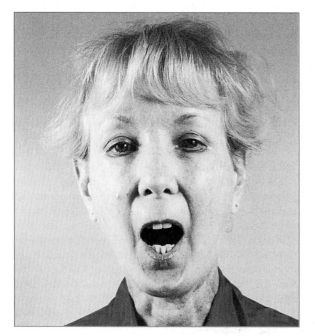

Figure 13.1 Patient with systemic sclerosis.

Vascular

Capillaries show dilated loops, which may disappear leaving avascular areas. Most of the scleroderma patients with vasculitis have CREST syndrome. Only very rarely are large vessels involved (Breedveld, 1997). Diffuse fibrosis and vasculitis may involve internal organs and cause interstitial lung disease. This will affect medical interventions and prognosis.

MANAGEMENT
Physiotherapy

Assessment of the patient will usually reveal limited range of movement and contractures in the hands and the face. In the early stages careful examination will be required to detect minor contractures. The degree of deformity will vary with the extent of the condition and the patient's response to the drug therapy and possibly with his or her compliance to exercise therapy, although this has yet to be evaluated. Exercise tolerance is likely to be limited, hampering both assessment and management. Additionally severe internal sclerosis and life threatening disease may present the patient with more urgent needs that must be attended to before physiotherapy can be instigated.

There has been no formal evaluation of physiotherapy techniques in the management of SSc at the time of writing; consequently the following will be largely anecdotal. but it is an area that would benefit from research.

Attention should be given to those areas identified by the patient as the ones causing most problems and intervention should be directed towards function rather than attempting to regain full joint range and muscle power. Following thorough measurement of all joint ranges and muscle power, problem areas can be highlighted. Accurate baseline data are useful for a number of reasons: they can be used to identify actual and potential problems, and can be employed as retrospective research data or for audit purposes. They may also be used to evaluate the efficacy of drug therapies and physiotherapeutic interventions, and act as an incentive to the patient's efforts.

Techniques used to treat the effects of SSc will clearly vary with the presentation and the patient's identification of the main problems. However, education, either from the physiotherapist, occupational therapist or the nurse specialist, is essential and a regular review and monitoring session would be recommended.

Exercise programmes for stretching the tightened structures and maintaining the length of all tissues must be accurately taught and steadfastly adhered to. Minor contractures should be pointed out to the patient, who may be unaware that the joint is limited. Mouth closure can be maintained by closing the lips with the neck in extension. Application of heat prior to exercise may facilitate stretching of soft tissues. Exercise may include endurance training, for example walking or low-impact aerobics. Muscle strengthening, possibly with weights, may help to prevent deformity. Isotonic exercises should be avoided in the presence of active myositis or severe restrictive lung damage. Range of movement programmes for functional preservation should also be incorporated into the programme. Likewise, breathing exercises, including active cycle of breathing techniques, which are essential to maintain excursion of the ribs and also to optimise lung function in early pulmonary fibrosis.

Skin care is a potential problem for the patient with SSc, and massage techniques to protect and mobilise structures should be taught with emphasis on safe and accurate application. Products designed for the infant skin and inert oils such as olive oil may be the most suitable.

Splinting for prevention of deformities ought theoretically to be beneficial; however, in practice it is not

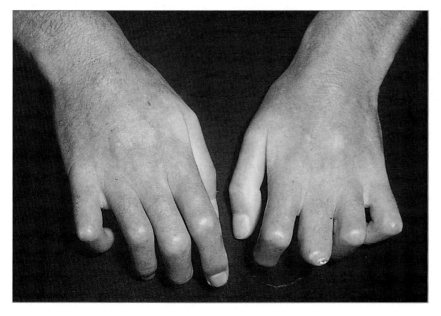

Figure 13.2 **Typical finger deformities and sclerodactyly associated with scleroderma.**

effective in preventing loss of range of movement, and night splinting has resulted in negative consequences including ischaemia over pressure points such as the tips of the fingers.

Many patients are helped by relaxation and this could be incorporated into holistic patient care.

Drug Therapy

Drug treatment is directed at modulating the immune response, controlling the fibrosis and treating the effects of Raynaud's syndrome. Many of the drugs used are still experimental—there is currently no cure for this condition. Immunosuppressive agents may include:
- Cyclosporin A—helps skin and renal manifestations.
- Methotrexate—being evaluated.
- Cyclophosphamide—of anecdotal benefit ± steroids.
- Anti-thymocyte or anti-lymphocyte globulin.
- Photophoresis or plasmaphoresis—trial needed.

Anti-fibrotic therapy may include:
- D-penicillamine—widely used. Benefits lung, skin and kidney disease.
- Interferon alpha or gamma—trials currently in progress.

Raynaud's therapy may include:
- Calcium channel blockers, e.g. nifedipine.
- 5-hydroxytryptamine (HT) antagonist, e.g. ketanserin.
- Angiotensin-converting enzyme (ACE) inhibitors, e.g. captopril
- Topical vasodilators, e.g. glyceryl trinitrate (GTN) patches.
- Parenteral vasodilators, e.g. prostaglandin (iloprost).
- Antibiotics for secondary infection.
- Surgical procedures, e.g. sympathectomy for Raynaud's, debridement or amputation for necrosis.

(Adapted with permission from Arthritis Research Campaign (ARC) Topical Reviews Series 3 (Black, 1996).)

PROGNOSIS

This varies with the severity of internal organ involvement. Recent studies show a four-fold increased mortality rate, higher in females (Bryan et al., 1996). A total of 79% of these excess deaths were related to scleroderma, probably due to lung disease and renal disease.

SYSTEMIC LUPUS ERYTHEMATOSUS

Systemic lupus erythematosus (SLE) is a chronic auto-immune disease that can affect any organ with episodes of remission and relapse. It can be difficult to diagnose due to the great variability in symptoms, which range from mild to life threatening. The term 'lupus' is from the Latin 'wolf', because it was thought that healed skin lesions resembled wolf bites, and was used in the 18th century to describe a variety of skin conditions. Lupus erythematosus was first described in 1833; originally it was thought to be a skin disorder, until its systemic nature was recognised in 1872 (Gladman & Urowitz 1994).

PREVALENCE

SLE affects 4–280 cases per 100,000, with wide geographical variation. In the UK it affects 12 per 100,000 of the population (Gladman & Urowitz, 1994). It is most common in Afro-Caribbeans, followed by Asians, and affects 13 times as many women as men. SLE may affect any age but the peak onset is between 16–55 years, being milder and more rare in the elderly. There is a strong familial tendency, and it is linked with HLA A1, B8, DR2 and DR3 (Emery, 1994). Different genes may be associated with different patterns of disease presentation.

INVESTIGATION

SLE is difficult to classify as it is variable both between patients and within a single patient over time (Hay, 1995).

Diagnostic Criteria for SLE

SLE is diagnosed if four or more of the following are present during the course of the illness:
- Malar (cheek) rash.
- Discoid rash.
- Photosensitivity.
- Oral ulcers.
- Arthritis.
- Serositis (pleuritis or pericarditis).
- Renal disorder.
- Neurologic disorder.
- Haematological disorder.
- Immunological disorder.
- Raised titre of antinuclear antibody (Tan et al., 1982).

CLINICAL FEATURES

Features are extremely variable but may include any of the following:

Skin

The classical 'butterfly' malar rash is found in 50% of patients (Figure 13.3). Discoid lesions, annular plaques which leave scarring, telangiectasia and depigmentation may occur without systemic symptoms, although 10% of patients with discoid lesions will go on to develop systemic lupus. Ultraviolet (UV) exposure causes a photosensitivity rash in about 60% of patients, and can also cause generalised disease exacerbation. About 70% of patients suffer from alopecia.

Musculoskeletal

A migratory non-erosive arthritis, usually symmetrical, commonly affects the knees, wrists and proximal interphalangeal (PIP) joints. The arthritis mainly consists of soft tissue swelling with little effusion. It is possible that differences in the cytokines produced may account for the non-destructive nature of the arthritis compared with other inflammatory arthropathies. However, deformities may occur due to soft tissue contractures and joint subluxation (Gladman & Urowitz, 1994). Tenosynovitis may lead to tendon rupture. Avascular necrosis of bone may occur, especially the femoral head—this may be due to disease itself or to high dose steroids used to treat the disease. Osteoporosis or muscle weakness may develop secondary to steroids. Myalgia is frequently found, but myositis is not common.

Pulmonary

Pleuritic chest pain affects 45% of patients but is rarely severe. Interstitial fibrosis and pulmonary hypertension carry a poor prognosis.

Cardiovascular

Systolic murmurs and mild pericarditis may be present. Hypertension can be a serious problem, causing renal deterioration. Raynaud's disease affects 25%, and vasculitis may lead to micro infarcts at fingertips and toes, best treated non-surgically (Emery, 1994).

Renal

Virtually all patients have a histological abnormality and about 50% develop clinical abnormalities, commonly proteinuria and glomerulonephritis.

Haematological

A normochromic/normocytic anaemia is common, and reflects the inflammatory process. Haemolytic anaemia is found in 25%. Leucopenia and thrombocytopenia are common, the latter usually due to antiplatelet antibodies. The risk of a bleed increases significantly when platelet count falls below 20,000. Acute phase response (see Chapter 2): erythrocyte sedimentation rate (ESR) is elevated in virtually all patients, particularly during active disease. C-reactive protein (CRP) is usually normal or only slightly raised.

Neuropsychiatric

Patients may present with depression, anxiety or psychosis. Headaches are frequent and may be associated with double vision, personality change or minor seizure. No specific abnormality has been found—it is assumed that seizures are secondary to the disease process. Peripheral neuropathy is present in about 10%, and can involve cranial nerves and multiple individual nerves. Cerebro-vascular accident (CVA) and transverse myelitis may be secondary to vasculitis or thrombus or embolus. The central nervous system (CNS) lupus is hard to diagnose as there may be little correlation with disease activity elsewhere. An electroencephalogram may help, or magnetic resonance imaging in the case of vasculitis.

Systemic

Virtually all patients suffer from lethargy, fatigue and low exercise tolerance to some degree. Increased fatigue may herald a lupus flare; if constant, with additional symptoms, it is usually due to active SLE. If the patient has good and bad days this may be due to either active SLE or inadequate drug control. Fatigue with sleep disturbance may be due to depression, fibromyalgia or sleep apnoea; if it occurs together with weakness, it may be drug induced or due to myopathy (Liang, 1994).

AETIOLOGY

It is thought that much of the tissue damage, especially in the blood vessels and kidneys, is due to deposition of antibody/antigen complexes in the tissues (Woods, 1993). Starting oestrogen oral contraceptives may flare the disease, as may pregnancy. Although this poses little risk to the patient about 30% miscarry, often recurrently. Retardation in foetal growth has been reported but most babies are normal, although often premature (Schur, 1993).

SLE may also be drug induced—most frequent causes are hydralazine, procainamide, isoniazid, chlorpromazine, D-penicillamine and methyldopa. The lupus is mild and reverses when the drug is discontinued. The mechanism of drug-induced lupus is not clear.

Lupus may also be triggered by emotional stress. Rarely, discoid lupus develops in an area of skin trauma through an unknown mechanism that relates to chronic inflammation and activation of pro-inflammatory factors (Wallace, 1994).

PROGNOSIS

Overall the outlook is good. Prognosis has improved from less than 50% survival at 5 years in 1955, to over 90% at 5 years and greater than 80% survival at 10 years presently. This improvement is due to earlier diagnosis, better treatment and better antibiotics (Gladman & Urowitz, 1994). Mortality is usually due to cerebral vasculitis, intractable bleeding, intestinal perforation, or renal, cardiac or pulmonary failure. Nephropathy and central nervous system

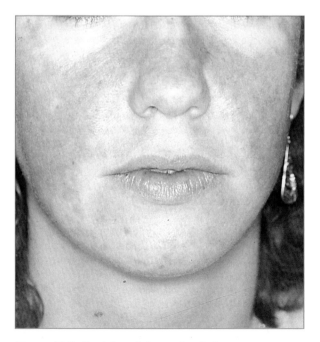

Figure 13.3 Facial rash in systemic lupus erythematosus.

(CNS) involvement carry a poorer prognosis (Gladman & Urowitz, 1994). Lupus flares require urgent referral and screening for infection, especially if immunosuppressed, as unusual infections (for instance, fungal) may be present. A normal CRP is helpful in excluding infection. Blood pressure should be monitored regularly as poor control leads to renal deterioration.

MANAGEMENT
Drugs
Non-steroidal anti-inflammatory drugs (NSAIDs) may be used for arthritis, arthralgia and myalgia. Antimalarials and steroid joint injections are useful if the symptoms are not controlled by NSAIDs. Low dose oral steroids or methotrexate may also be necessary.

Flare up of systemic and skin problems due to UV may be prevented by use of protective clothing and sunscreens, factor 15 or higher. Topical steroids may be useful for dermatitis but discoid lupus usually needs management by a dermatologist. Lupus rash responds to antimalarials although the exact mechanism is not clear.

Weight loss and fatigue may be managed by steroids; often only a small dose is required. Fatigue is frequently underestimated by physicians. Much is written about the side effects of steroids, but little about side effects of active disease and effects on quality of life (Emery, 1994). Azathioprine is used for maintenance once steroids have induced a remission.

Cyclophosphamide is indicated for life-threatening conditions such as vasculitis, renal disease and severe thrombocytopaenia, while CNS disease is treated with anticoagulants for thrombi or emboli, and steroids or cytotoxics for vasculitis.

Physiotherapy Management
Exercise programmes for SLE should emphasise strengthening and low-impact aerobic endurance workouts. Programmes should include isometric and isotonic strengthening of the muscles surrounding the large joints, and maintenance of joint range of movement. If avascular necrosis is present, only isometric exercise is indicated (Hicks, 1990). Aerobic training during active SLE flare can increase symptoms (Liang, 1994); aerobics should also be avoided if the haemoglobin is less than 11 (Hicks, 1990).

Neurological complications will require appropriate programmes depending on the presentation.

DERMATOMYOSITIS AND POLYMYOSITIS

As the names would suggest, dermatomyositis (DM) and polymyositis (PM) are inflammatory myopathies of striated muscles. DM has a characteristic skin rash in addition. There is no known cause, although there may be a weak association with neoplasia in the elderly. It can also develop as a rare reaction to infection or to some medications, particularly in children. There may additionally be immunological abnormalities or a viral component; it may be associated with a family history of autoimmune disease. Juvenile DM is covered in Chapter 19.

The ratio of women to men affected is 2–3:1, and onset peaks in childhood and adulthood; adolescent onset is rare. Incidence is around 5–10 new cases per million of the population each year and so it is a rare condition but one in which physiotherapists are keenly involved, both in ongoing assessment and consequent adjustment of drug therapy, and in its management. The condition is more common in adults than the muscular dystrophies but much less common in children (Dieppe et al., 1985).

PATHOLOGY
Skeletal muscle becomes inflamed, with degeneration and atrophy of muscle fibres, although some attempted regeneration also occurs. Infiltration of lymphocytes, plasma cells and polymorphs is present around vessels and also between muscle fibres. In DM with skin involvement there is epidermal atrophy, liquefaction and degeneration of the epidermis, and infiltration of the dermis with mononuclear cells (Dieppe et al., 1985).

CLASSIFICATION
There are various ways of classifying PM and DM:
- Adult PM.
- Adult DM.
- Myositis associated with malignancy.
- Childhood poly or DM.
- Myositis accompanying other connective tissue diseases (Dieppe et al., 1985).

CLINICAL FEATURES
Onset is usually insidious and fairly rapid, progressing over weeks or months. Occasionally, however, muscle weakness can develop very slowly over 5–10 years.

Muscle Involvement
Initially the limb girdle muscles are involved, particularly lower limb. The weakness is generally symmetrical and may be painless, although in 50% it may be accompanied by pain and tenderness. The patient will complain of functional problems including inability to get out of a chair or roll over in bed, difficulty climbing stairs and problems with personal hygiene. The gait may be waddling as proximal stability is lost. The neck flexors are also involved, leading to problems in raising the head from the pillow. Distal strength is usually well maintained, although Medsger & Oddis (1994) report distal involvement in 10–20%. Ocular and facial involvement is uncommon.

In severe and untreated cases (around 4%) there may be involvement of the respiratory and bulbar muscles affecting swallowing, speech and exercise tolerance (Dieppe et al., 1985).

The pattern of muscle involvement in DM and PM is summarised in Table 13.1. Later muscle atrophy will be seen. Shoulder joint contractures are most common, but knees, hips and elbows may also be affected. Children with type IV disease and calcinosis are particularly prone to elbow, knee and ankle/foot complex contractures. Children can develop contractures over a short time interval, and develop new contractures up to 7–8 years after disease onset.

Skin

The classic skin rash of DM is variously described as violet, heliotrope or dusky bluish. The rash can occur on the upper eyelids, bridge of nose and malar area, over the MCP joints, knees, elbows, medial malleoli, neck, upper chest and back. Periorbital oedema, telangiectasia and nail fold capillary dilatation may be present. Calcinosis is a late complication of chronic juvenile DM, but rare in adult-onset disease (Medsger & Oddis, 1994). Gottron's papules, elevated plaques of rash, may be present on the knuckles and dorsum of the hand. Raynaud's is present in 30% of patients with DM (Bohan & Peter, 1975). Vasculitic lesions occur more frequently in children than adults; vessels of various diameters are affected, including ischaemic gastro-intestinal or pulmonary involvement, which indicates a poor prognosis (Breedveld, 1997).

Other Sites Involved

The joints may be affected by a mild, transient rheumatoid-like arthritis. Deformity is unusual, but may be found in some cases with serum anti-Jo-1 antibody (Medsger & Oddis, 1994). The arthritis is non-erosive but joint subluxation is common.

The lungs may be affected by alveolitis, pulmonary fibrosis, aspiration pneumonia or methotrexate toxicity. Heart involvement is common but seldom symptomatic.

There is still doubt over the association between DM and neoplasia. The incidence varies with age but can be as high as 75% in males above the age of 50. Tumour sites may include the lungs, ovary and breast and discovery can occur years after the onset of muscle disease. Treatment of the underlying malignancy often resolves the myopathy (Medsger & Oddis, 1994).

DIAGNOSIS

Diagnosis is based on the presenting clinical signs in addition to a raised ESR, creatinine phosphokinase (CPK), aldolase and transaminase. Auto-antibodies, particularly Jo-1, have been reported in around half the patients with DM/PM. Electromyographic studies can be a helpful aid to diagnosis and show a typical picture:
- Polyphasic short small motor-unit potentials.
- Spontaneous fibrillation.
- Bizarre high frequency repetitive discharges.

Muscle biopsy may be required to confirm the diagnosis and can demonstrate:
- Degeneration, necrosis, phagocytosis, fibrosis and some regeneration of muscle fibres.
- Mononuclear cell infiltrate.
- Variation in cross sectional diameter.

MANAGEMENT

Steroids may be required initially to prevent the condition from progressing to involve the respiratory muscles. The patient will generally be on a fairly high dose (e.g. 60 mg) to gain control before reduction is attempted. Immuno-suppressive agents can be used in patients who fail to respond and in those where the dose of steroid should be reduced. Azathioprine, cyclophosphamide, chlorambucil and methotrexate have all been reported as inducing remission.

Whilst DM may be brief and remit completely, most PM cases exacerbate and remit. Mortality rate for PM is up to 50% without treatment; with treatment the prognosis is good—over 95% survival rate after 5 years in the absence of malignancy.

Physiotherapy

Management should be tailored to the stage of inflammation (Wortmann, 1993). It may be necessary to assess and grade the patients' muscle power prior to commencement of drug therapy, and vital before commencement of a physiotherapy programme. It is clearly important to maintain contact with the same therapist at each assessment to avoid inter-observer error and to assess muscle power using the most accurate method possible. Simple reproducible functional tests, such as sitting to standing, step-ups and walking times, are also useful, although checks need to be made for trick movements.

For the physiotherapist, there are four main stages of the condition: acute, early recovery, late recovery and chronic (Hicks, 1994). During the acute phase, whilst the inflammatory markers remain high and muscle weakness is at its most apparent, the role of the physiotherapist is to maintain muscle length and prevent contractures. The

Pattern of muscle involvement in dermatomyositis and polymyositis		
Upper limbs:	proximal proximal & distal	86% 39%
Lower limbs:	proximal proximal & distal	92% 32%
Neck:	flexors extensors	47% 14%
Respiratory muscles:		4%
Bulbar muscles:		6%
Facial muscles:		4%

Table 13.1 **Pattern of muscle involvement in dermatomyositis and polymyositis (Dieppe et al., 1985).**

patient will be nursed on strict bed rest with minimal active movement. Joints should be moved through their full range at least once daily, passively if necessary, and care must be taken to maintain muscle length whilst respecting pain.

Respiratory impairment should be assessed and treated appropriately. Some patients may need assisted ventilation.

During the early recovery phase the patient will be able to begin a supervised graduated exercise and rehabilitation programme designed to regain muscle power and maximise function; care should be taken that progress is designed to fit around ESR and CPK values (Schroeder, 1988). Once muscle power has improved to about 3/5, active assisted range of movement and isometric exercises may be added (Hicks, 1994). During the late stage of recovery, isotonic and low weight exercise may be added. During the chronic stage aerobic exercise should be added, working at 60% VO2max (Hicks, 1994). Muscle power and inflammatory markers should be reviewed regularly, and the programme modified if muscles become sore, strength deteriorates or muscle enzyme levels increase. The myalgia of myositis is often difficult to distinguish from post-exercise soreness; however, the latter is generally of shorter duration (Hicks, 1994). Communication with the other members of the multidisciplinary team is essential throughout the course of the therapy.

MIXED CONNECTIVE TISSUE DISORDER

The connective tissue disorders overlap in about 25% of cases (Bennett, 1993). Sjögren's syndrome may be a feature of any of the conditions. About 5% of patients with SSc also have PM/DM, but overlap with SLE is uncommon. Mixed connective tissue disorder, an overlap syndrome consisting of features of SLE, SSc and PM, was described in 1972 by Sharp *et al.*, although there is debate over its status as a distinct syndrome rather than a subgroup of SLE (Bennett, 1993). The prevalence is unknown, but estimated at 10 per 100,000; female:male ratio is about 9:1 (Venables, 1994). There is a possible link with HLA DR4. Diagnosis is usually made on serological grounds; diagnosis on the basis of clinical features is difficult as it may take several years for sufficient features of each overlapping syndrome to appear. Patients present most commonly with fatigue, swollen hands, arthralgia, myalgia, Raynaud's and, occasionally, fever.

The features of connective tissue disorders overlapping in MCTD are different to the features found in those conditions presenting in isolation. For example, the arthralgia in MCTD is more severe than in classic SLE; about 60% develop obvious arthritis and deformities similar to those seen in RA, although erosions are infrequent. MCTD has also not been found to be precipitated by UV or drugs. Up to 50% have renal involvement (Venables, 1994) but this is usually not as severe as in SLE. Unlike SLE, CNS involvement is not common, although headaches are frequent. In comparison with SSc, which has been linked with a number of causative chemicals, only vinyl chloride has been implicated in the aetiology of MCTD (Farhey & Hess, 1997).

There are often no objective signs to accompany the myalgia, which is thought to be due to low-grade myositis, physical deconditioning, vasculitis or associated fibromyalgia. Systemic involvement may include tachycardia or galloping heart rhythm and dyspnoea disproportionate to pulmonary involvement. The prognosis is variable; mortality, which is most commonly caused by pulmonary hypertension, is around 13% over 17 years (Farhey & Hess, 1997). Management will depend on presentation.

REFERENCES

Bennett RM. Mixed connective tissue disease and other overlap syndromes. In: Kelley WN, Harris ED, Ruddy S, Sledge CB, eds. *Textbook of rheumatology, 4th edition*. Philadelphia: WB Saunders; 1993:1057-1076.

Black CM. Systemic sclerosis. *ARC Topical Reviews*, ARC Series **3**;1996:7.

Black CM, Stevens WM. Scleroderma. *Rheum Dis Clinics North Am* 1989, **15**:89.

Bohan A, Peter JB. Polymyositis and dermatomyositis. *N Engl J Med* 1975, **292**:344-347.

Breedveld FC. Vasculitis associated with connective tissue disease. In: Yazici H, Husby G, eds. *Baillières Clin Rheumatol:* Vasculitis 1997, **11**:315-334.

Briggs DC, Welsh KI, Pereira RS *et al*. A strong association between null alleles at the C4A locus in the major histocompatability complex and systemic sclerosis. *Arthritis Rheum* 1986, **29**:1274-1277.

Bryan C, Howard Y, Brennan P, *et al*. Survival following the onset of scleroderma: results from a retrospective inception cohort study of the UK population. *Br J Rheum* 1996, **35**:1122-1126.

Dieppe PA, Doherty M, Macfarlane DG *et al. Rheumatological medicine*. London: Churchill Livingstone; 1985.

Emery P. Systemic lupus. *Reports on Rheumatic Diseases*, ARC 1994:2.

Farhey Y, Hess EV. Mixed connective tissue disease. *Arthritis Care Res* 1997, **10**:333-341.

Gladman DD, Urowitz MB. Systemic lupus erythematosus: clinical features. In: Klippel JH, Dieppe P, eds. *Rheumatology*. London: Mosby Year Book Europe; 1994:2.1-2.20.

Hay EM. Systemic lupus erythematosus. *Baillières Clin Rheumatol* 1995, **9**:437-470.

Hicks J. Exercise in inflammatory arthritis and connective tissue disease. *Rheum Dis Clinics North Am* 1990, **16**:845-870.

Hicks JE. Rehabilitation of patients with myositis. In: Klippel JH, Dieppe P, eds. *Rheumatology*. London: Mosby Year Book Europe; 1994:15.4-15.6.

LeRoy EC, Black C, Fleischmajer R *et al*. Scleroderma (systemic sclerosis): classification, subsets and pathogenesis. *J Rheumatol* 1988, **15**:202-205.

Liang MH. Fatigue in systemic lupus erythematosus. In: Klippel JH, Dieppe P, eds. *Rheumatology*. London: Mosby Year Book Europe; 1994:7.3-7.4.

McWhirter A, Kirk JME, Laurent GJ, *et al*. Changes in serum type 111 procollagen peptide concentrations in patients with systemic sclerosis and Raynaud's phenomenon. *Conference Proceedings for Control Mechanisms in Scleroderma*. ARC; 1987 (abstract no 14).

Medsger TA, Oddis CV. Inflammatory muscle disease: clinical features. In: Klippel JH, Dieppe P, eds. *Rheumatology*. London: Mosby Year Book Europe; 1994:12.1-12.14.

Misra R, Darton K, Jewkes RF, *et al*. Arthritis in scleroderma. *Br J Rheum* 1995, **34**:831-837.

Schroeder LK. Physical therapy protocol for polymyositis/dermatomyositis. In: Branwell B, Gall V, eds. *Physical therapy management of arthritis*. London: Churchill Livingstone; 1988.

Schur PH. Clinical features of SLE. In: Kelley WN, Harris ED, Ruddy S, Sledge CB, eds. *Textbook of rheumatology, 4th edition*. Philadelphia: WB Saunders; 1993:1017-1042.

Sharp GC, Irvin WS, Tan EM *et al*. Mixed connective tissue disease: an apparently distinct rheumatic disease syndrome associated with a specific antibody to an extractable nuclear antigen (ENA). *Am J Med* 1972, **52**:148.

Silman A, Jannini S, Symmons D, Bacon P. An epidemiological study of scleroderma in the West Midlands. *Br J Rheum* 1988, **27**:286-290.

Tan EM, Cohen AS, Fries JF *et al*. The 1982 revised criteria for the classification of systemic lupus erythematosus. *Arthritis Rheum* 1982, **25**:1271-1277.

Valenta LJ, Elias AN. Familial scleroderma in a kindred with high incidence of auto-immune disease: a correlation with HLA-A1/B8 haplotype. *Arch Dermatol* 1987, **123**:1438-1440.

Venables PW. Overlap syndromes. In: Klippel JH, Dieppe P, eds. *Rheumatology*. London: Mosby Year Book Europe; 1994:28.1-28.8.

Wallace DJ. Does stress or trauma cause or aggravate rheumatic disease? *Baillières Clin Rheumatol* 1994, **8**:1,149-159.

Woods VL. Pathogenesis of systemic lupus erythematosus. In: Kelley WN, Harris ED, Ruddy S, Sledge CB, eds. *Textbook of rheumatology, 4th edition*. Philadelphia: WB Saunders; 1993:999-1016.

Wortmann RL. Inflammatory diseases of muscles. In: Kelley WN, Harris ED, Ruddy S, Sledge CB, eds. *Textbook of rheumatology, 4th edition*. Philadelphia: WB Saunders; 1993:1159-1188.

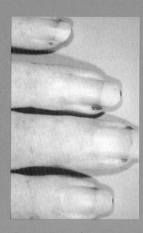

14

A Chadwick

VASCULITIDES

CHAPTER OUTLINE

- Pathology of vasculitides
- Management of vasculitides
- Physiotherapy

- Case history—Wegener's granulomatosis

INTRODUCTION

Vasculitis is characterised by inflammation within or through a blood vessel wall, which hampers blood flow and may damage the vessel's integrity. One or many vessels may be involved and this may affect many organ systems. There are several different vasculitic syndromes which all result in ischaemia to the tissues supplied by the damaged vessels. Patients may present with systemic features of fever, weight loss and anorexia accompanied by widespread vascular inflammation (Lightfoot, 1994). There are no specific laboratory tests for individual syndromes. Multisystem investigations are often necessary. The patient with vasculitis may feel unwell. This is due not only to active disease but also to damage to organs caused by chronic disease or the drugs used (Luqmani et al., 1997). The incidence and epidemiology of vasculitis is summarised in Table 14.1.

PATHOLOGY OF VASCULITIDES

Inflammation occurs in the intimal layers of the blood vessel, followed by a dramatic infiltration of neutrophils and eosinophils responsible for phagocytosis and histamine production. The vascular lumen is consequently decreased by oedema. The intimal lining fragments and in the latter stages fibrinoid necrosis occurs. Granulation tissue may form, further weakening the blood vessel wall.

The mechanism triggering this response is unknown. The extent of arteritis may be variable within the one vessel, and different phases of inflammation, healing and granulation tissue formation may be seen in the same region concurrently.

Figure 14.1 is a summary of the vasculitic syndromes which will be discussed in this chapter.

POLYMYALGIA RHEUMATICA, GIANT CELL ARTERITIS, TAKAYASU'S ARTERITIS
Pathology and Clinical Presentation

In each of these conditions large arteries are affected by the cellular immune response. In Takayasu's arteritis, stenosis of the aorta results from the inflammatory process. Extensive intimal irregularity occurs with narrowing in some areas and aneurysmal dilatation in others. This can be life-threatening.

In giant cell arthritis (GCA), also known as temporal arteritis, the cranial arteries are especially affected, including the occipital, external carotid, the temporal, lingual and external maxillary arteries. Vasculitis may also be present in other regions including intestinal vessels, causing abdominal complaints, intermittent claudication of the lower limb and even angina.

A patient with polymyalgia rheumatica (PMR) may complain of diffuse shoulder girdle and pelvic girdle pain, which is muscular in origin, but will not demonstrate any true muscle weakness. Patients may complain of stiffness, especially after a period of inactivity. Some studies suggest patients may additionally present with swelling and pitting oedema of distal extremities (Salvarani *et al.*, 1996). These may also cause symptoms similar to carpal tunnel, described by 10–20% of patients who may have had a mono-neuropathy of the median nerve with PMR. 20% of patients with PMR go on to develop GCA, often in the first few weeks. Classical symptoms are headaches, tenderness near the temples, jaw pain, difficulty in swallowing, a sore throat and visual disturbances. They may also complain of ear pain or sudden deafness.

Aetiology

The aetiology of PMR, GCA and Takayasu's arteritis is largely unknown. However, a sudden onset of symptoms in GCA may be caused as a result of exposure to infection. It has also been suggested that solar radiation may damage the internal elastic lamina of the temporal artery, which may initiate the infiltration of giant cells (phagocytes). Human leukocyte antigen (HLA) B8 is more common in PMR and GCA (59 and 50% respectively) compared with an incidence of 27% in a generalised arthritis population.

Prognosis

Both PMR and GCA have good prognoses with treatment, but if the erythrocyte sedimentation rate (ESR) is greater than 90 mm/h at diagnosis there is often increased risk of complications. Only 6–10% of GCA patients experience visual loss. Relapses are most likely within 18 months of starting treatment and are often linked with the withdrawal of steroids (Berlit, 1992). Some will need medication for 4 years or more (Ayoub, 1985). GCA is considered to be self-limiting and has no influence on life expectancy.

Takayasu's arteritis has an unpredictable prognosis and may progress rapidly or spontaneously remit. In one study at 10 years there was a 58% survival of patients with severe disease.

Diagnostic Tests

Blood tests are the best indicator of disease activity in PMR and GCA. The ESR will often be raised. Patients may be anaemic with a haemoglobin (Hb) of less than 8 g/dl. Examination of synovial fluid may reveal mild inflammatory changes, while a urine specimen usually shows normal glucose and protein levels. A total of 5% of PMR patients may be hypothyroid (Hellman, 1993). Creatinine phosphokinase (CPK) is usually normal, as are muscle biopsy findings. Electromyography is also usually normal and no abnormalities are seen on X-ray. C3 and C4 complement levels are often decreased, but immunoglobulin levels are increased with evidence of circulating immune complexes. Liver function tests (LFTs) too are frequently abnormal—serum alkaline phosphatase is increased in a third of patients but a liver biopsy often reveals nothing. The reasons for this are unclear.

Incidence and epidemiology of vasculitis				
Syndrome	Incidence/100,000	Male:Female	Average age onset (years)	Population
Polymyalgia rheumatica	70-133 over age 50	1:3	60s often following an upper respiratoy tract infection (URTI) or severe emotional upset	15% black
Giant cell arteritis	17	1:3		Almost exclusively Caucasian population
Takayasu's arteritis	0.2	1:9	15-25	Worldwide
Polyarteritis nodosa	4.6 in England	2:1	40-60 but any age	All racial groups
Churg-Strauss syndrome	Unknown	2:1	Middle age	2% black
Wegener's granulomatosis	Unknown	1:1	40s	97% Caucasian
Henoch-Schönlein purpura	1	1.5:1	<18 or 30-70	Japan and developed countries
Kawasaki disease	70-80 in Japan	1.5:1	<5	Mainly in Japan

Table 14.1 **Incidence and epidemiology of vasculitis.**

Diagnosis of PMR and GCA is frequently confirmed by a dramatic and prompt reduction in symptoms within 48 hours of corticosteroid therapy. If GCA is suspected, a temporal artery biopsy may be performed in which a 1–2 cm segment of artery may be serially sectioned.

Takayasu's arteritis is characterised by arterial bruits. The patient complains of headaches, malaise, night sweats and general fatigue and may have visual disturbance and dizziness. The patient may also have absent pulses and describe symptoms of upper limb claudication (Hughes, 1987).

POLYARTERITIS NODOSA
Pathology
In polyarteritis nodosa (PAN) the large and medium-sized vessels are primarily affected. The 'nodosa' in PAN are multiple aneurysms occurring in the vascular tissue which forms scar tissue. In some areas blood flow may be totally occluded. Blood vessels associated with nerves are also frequently involved, accounting for other widespread symptoms.

Aetiology
Polyarteritis nodosa is thought to be associated with the circulating hepatitis B antigen (Hughes, 1987).

Prognosis
The prognosis of PAN depends on the presence and extent of visceral and central nervous system (CNS) involvement. Most deaths occur within a year of diagnosis and are due to uncontrolled vasculitis. The prognosis of untreated polyarteritis is poor and 5-year survival less than 15%, but with treatment this rises to between 50 and 60%.

Diagnostic Tests
Patients with PAN need a thorough multi-system assessment to include musculoskeletal assessment of arthralgias and arthritis. Neurological, renal and gastrointestinal systems should be reviewed. The cardiovascular system is assessed. Arteriography assesses aneurysmal formation or occlusions of visceral arteries. Arteries may be biopsied to provide evidence of polymorphonuclear neutrophils, indicative of a vasculitis.

Approximately 50% of patients may have visible skin lesions, including digital infarcts (Figure 14.2). A characteristic mottled skin pattern on the extremities or torso is commonly linked with PAN (Lightfoot, 1994). Fever and anorexia, often with weight loss, may be present and abnormal LFTs may be found.

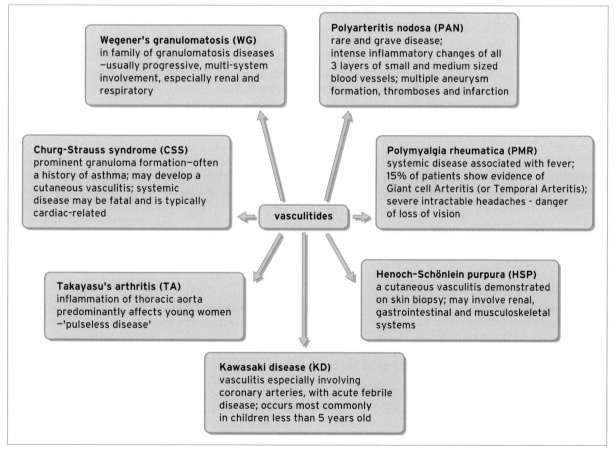

Figure 14.1 Vasculitic syndromes.

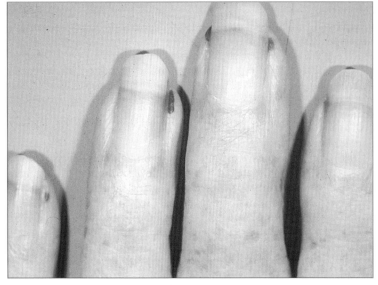

Figure 14.2 **Digital infarcts.**

CHURG-STRAUSS SYNDROME
Pathology
As in PAN, inflammation occurs in the smooth muscle fibres of large- and medium-sized vessels. Granuloma may also form around the vessels. The patient will present with systemic illness, nodular skin lesions and possible peripheral neuropathies. A history of asthma is common. The systemic vasculitis occurring in Churg–Strauss syndrome (CSS) only occurs in its final phase, when fever and weight loss are common. The patient may present with congestive cardiac failure, as the vasculitis affects the cardiac system, while the bowel and stomach may also be affected with a resulting bloody diarrhoea. Palpable abdominal masses may indicate granulomas of the bowel.

Aetiology
The aetiology of CSS is unclear but it is thought that it may be initiated by an allergy.

Prognosis
At 5 years the survival rate is approximately 60% if the condition is treated.

Diagnostic Tests
Anti-nuclear cytoplasmic antibodies (ANCA) will be positive in 50% of patients with CSS and an elevated serum immunoglobulin (Ig)E will be found. Diagnosis will be confirmed on skin or lung biopsy. Serial monitoring of respiratory, cardiac and dermatological features is important.

WEGENER'S GRANULOMATOSIS
Pathology
In Wegner's granulomatosis (WG) the muscle fibres of small- and medium-sized vessels are primarily affected. An antigen–antibody response primes the neutrophils to release enzymes, creating tissue damage. The subsequent granuloma (granular tissue) then triggers the production of further antibodies. Different phases of inflammation occur through the vessels. Table 14.2 summarises the clinical presentation in WG.

Aetiology
Humoral immune mechanisms are thought to be associated with the initiation of WG and possibly Henoch–Schönlein purpura (HSP), but their aetiologies are largely unknown.

Prognosis
Wegner's granulomatosis is usually progressive but the prognosis is much improved with early treatment. Age and gender are not relevant to outcome. If leukocytosis is present the patient is more likely to have active aggressive disease. Renal and pulmonary involvement is probably the most useful prognostic indicator of a poor outcome (Briedigkeit et al., 1993). The 10-year survival rate is less than 50% with lung involvement and less than 60% with renal involvement (De Remee, 1994).

Diagnostic Tests
The diagnosis of WG is often made following a history of sinusitis and/or epistaxis, recurrent ear or chest infections. A nasal scrape for cytology may demonstrate numerous neutrophils and occasional giant cells (Granados, 1994). Pulmonary function tests (PFTs) will often be inconclusive. A chest X-ray may identify masses or nodules and a renal biopsy may help confirm the diagnosis. Creatinine levels may be raised. Blood tests will often show a raised ESR and the Hb will frequently be less than 10 gm/dl. In 80% of patients with WG, the ANCA is positive. These antibody titres may parallel the disease activity and can be used to monitor the response to treatment if measured serially.

Table 14.2 **Clinical presentation in Wegener's granulomatosis.**

% involved	System	Symptom
85	Respiratory	Pulmonary masses/nodules Paranasal sinus–crusting, epistaxis
60-75	Renal	Necrotising glomerulonephritis
30-40	Neurological	Peripheral neuropathy/mononeuritis multiplex
20-35	Musculoskeletal	Non-erosive, transient arthritis
20	Ocular	Episcleritis
10-20	Dermatological	Palpable purpura
10	Cardiac	Coronary arteritis, angina, pericardial effusions

Clinical presentation in Wegener's granulomatosis

(De Remee, 1994)

HENOCH-SCHÖNLEIN PURPURA

Pathology

In HSP immune complexes are deposited within the blood vessels and the kidney. Symmetrical involvement of ankles, knees, metacarpophalangeal and metatarsophalangeal joints is found in 60–90% of patients.

Aetiology

The aetiology of HSP is largely unknown but may be linked to an infectious agent affecting the upper respiratory tract.

Prognosis

Henoch–Schönlein purpura has a very good outlook, often with complete resolution. Gastrointestinal and renal involvement are uncommon but complications may lead to gastrointestinal bleeds, perforation and renal failure.

Diagnostic Tests

There are no specific tests but any relevant systems are reviewed.

Clinical Presentation

A patient may present with an acute rash affecting the lower extremities and buttocks. There may be a history of arthritis or abdominal symptoms.

KAWASAKI DISEASE

Little is known about the aetiology or prognosis of Kawasaki disease. A vasculitis affecting the coronary arteries may be diagnosed by echocardiography. Children may present with a fever, lymphadenopathy and erythematous rash, which may later cause extensive peeling of the hands and feet. Conjunctivitis and oral soreness and bleeding are other diagnostic features.

FULMINANT VASCULITIS

A patient may have very sudden onset of widespread severe symptoms (fulminant vasculitis). Pulmonary and renal failure may necessitate admission to an Intensive Therapy Unit for close monitoring of all body systems and ventilation if required. The risk of infection must be minimised in order to avoid a relapse of the underlying vasculitis in the already immunosuppressed patient.

MANAGEMENT OF VASCULITIDES

MEDICAL MANAGEMENT

Prompt diagnosis is vital. Where multi-organ failure is present, early and aggressive management is needed. Oral or intravenous corticosteroids are used for most forms of vasculitis (Table 14.3). Cytotoxic medication, for example cyclophosphamide or azathioprine may also be required. Methotrexate can be used as an effective corticosteroid-sparing agent. There are significant risks associated with using cytotoxic agents. Side effects to monitor initially are leukopaenia (white cell count less than four), haemorrhagic cystitis and an increased risk of opportunistic infections. Long-term studies indicate that the risk of all malignancies increases by a factor of 2.4, risk of lymphoma increases 11-fold and there is a 33-fold increase in risk of bladder cancer (Hellman, 1993). The activity of the disease process may however necessitate such intervention. Constant monitoring over many months is then needed to minimise the risk of iatrogenic complications and ensure optimum prognosis. The ESR and C-reactive protein (CRP) will be regularly reviewed. The CRP will reflect disease activity most accurately over the first 2 months of treatment (Kyle, 1989).

Rarely, plasmaphoresis is used to remove circulating antibodies.

PHYSIOTHERAPY

PHYSIOTHERAPY ASSESSMENT

No literature has been found regarding physiotherapy or occupational therapy management of vasculitis patients. Treatment is therefore based on other documented research-based practice.

History

The patient's current functional difficulties and perception of the main problems should be elicited. A psychosocial history is necessary to identify the extent of family support and the effect that the patient's condition is having on work, leisure and personal relationships. Current and past medication should be included. Blood results, biochemistry and abnormal findings should be documented, with attention to ESR and CRP.

Specific Considerations in Polymyalgia Rheumatica and Giant Cell Arthritis Assessment

Medical staff should be alerted if the therapist identifies:
- Hearing loss.
- Headaches.
- Scalp or temple tenderness, e.g. discomfort on combing hair or wearing a hat.
- Visual disturbances require emergency medical consultation to avoid permanent loss of vision (Berlitt, 1992).
- Swallowing problems, speech difficulties, or complaints of tongue pain also require a prompt medical opinion.

- Muscle pain—on palpation, proximal muscle groups may feel hot and tender; CPK levels will be raised with a myositis.
- The patient's pain should be documented on a body chart with a visual analogue score.
- The duration of early morning stiffness (EMS) should be noted.
- Paraesthesia should be differentiated from a nerve root irritation, symptoms of carpal tunnel syndrome or claudication.

Physical Examination

Physical examination should include:
- Posture.
- Skin condition.
- Joint range and quality of movement, active and passive.
- Joint palpation—effusions, synovitis.
- Muscle power and bulk.
- Muscle functional analysis.
- Transfers, gait analysis, activities of daily living.

The cardiovascular system may need particular assessment. Labile blood pressure or heart rate should be noted along with history of hypertension, angina, claudication or absent pulses. Peripheral oedema should also be noted. Dyspnoeic patients (often in WG or PAN) may require a respiratory assessment and may need peak flows and other spirometry. Findings on auscultation effectiveness and productivity of cough should be noted. Cytology may be

Management of vasculitis	
Syndrome	**Management**
Polymyalgia rheumatica	10-20 mg oral steroid (Lestico et al., 1993)
Giant cell arteritis	Initial dose 40-60 mg oral or IV corticosteroids 120 mg if ocular symptoms present 20-50% suffer side effects of steroid, especially vertebral collapse (Hellman, 1993)
Polyarteritis nodosa	Corticosteroids +/- cytotoxic agents
Churg-Strauss syndrome	Corticosteroids
Wegener's granulomatosis	IV methylprednisolone may achieve a faster initial remission and suppress the progression of renal involvement In active disease IV cyclophosphamide, especially if respiratory tract involved
Takayasu's arteritis	Corticosteroids. Angioplasty for renal artery stenosis
Henoch-Schönlein purpura	Corticosteroids and immunosuppressive agents. Renal failure treated as necessary
Kawasaki disease	IV gammaglobulin with anticoagulants. Occasionally coronary artery by-pass surgery is needed

Table 14.3 **Management of vasculitis.**

requested. An assessment of exercise tolerance, involving a timed walk or activity (with or without pulse oxymetry), may also be valuable. A more detailed neurological assessment may be indicated with WG and PAN patients. Psychological factors are also important. Any loss of independence and/or function will cause stress and anxiety.

TREATMENT
Pain Relief
Local treatment can be given for painful active joints. Hydrotherapy may maximise joint range and muscle function and relieve pain. Patients may find great benefit from local heat treatment, e.g. hot packs. Transcutaneous electrical nerve stimulation has also been found to be of value for patients with myalgic pain.

Exercise
Mobilising exercises of all upper limb and lower limb joints are often important to relieve EMS and improve muscle function. These are progressed to include specific strengthening exercises for shoulder and pelvic girdle muscle groups in PMR/GCA patients. The muscle imbalance approach maximises stability in these regions and helps regain normal movement patterns (McConnell, 1993). If myositis is present, a minimal daily programme to maintain muscle length and minimise muscle wasting should be followed and progressed to add eccentric and resisted exercises as symptoms diminish and ESR and CPK levels return towards normal limits.

All exercises should be linked to a function relevant to the individual patient. The patient's exercise tolerance should be improved. Physiotherapists have a vital role in progressing patients gradually and helping them regain their confidence. A progressive exercise plan will be necessary, possibly including increased walking distance and speed on a treadmill, static bike, etc. Patients can be taught to monitor their own heart rate (HR) and respiratory rate (RR). Compliance and motivation will be further increased if they complete their own record sheets of achievement. The patient should aim to have no higher than 60% of their maximum HR during the exercise period. The length of time or number of repetitions of an exercise can be increased initially and then worked up to 70–80% of maximum HR (Kavanagh, 1995).

A guide to increasing exercise tolerance is:
(220 – patient's age) = 100% maximum HR desirable

Precautions
Patients on cytotoxic therapy, e.g. cyclophosphamide, will have a lowered immunity and precautions should be taken to avoid infection. Hydrotherapy is probably ill-advised for immuno-suppressed patients.

OTHER TEAM MEMBERS
All team members have an educational and supporting role. The patient and family should understand the disease process, the medication he or she is taking and the possible side effects. A clinical nurse specialist may be valuable in this role. A dietician may offer advice to patients taking cytotoxic medication who may feel nauseous and have poor nutritional intake. Dietary supplements may be included or dry diets with minimal odour. Occupational therapists can assess for activities of daily living, the need for assistive devices or the provision of splints to maximise independence.

Outcome Measures used with Vasculitis Patients
- VAS—pain (Waterfield & Sim, 1996).
- EMS—timed.
- Functional 10 m walk test—or other set distance activity timed.
- Exercise tolerance—monitoring heart rate/respiratory rate/O_2 saturation:
    Set activity in a given distance.
    Set activity in a measured time.
    Set number of repetitions in a measured time.
- Joint range of movement—use of goniometry or eye (Williams & Callaghan, 1990).
- Spirometry.
    Peak flow.
    Vital capacity.
    Auscultation.
- Short form health survey (SF 36)—36 Questionnaire assesses functional ability incorporating mobility, pain, emotional health, work, social life and perception of own health (Ware & Sherbourne, 1992).
- Health assessment questionnaire (Kirwan & Reeback, 1986).

CASE HISTORY – WEGENERS GRANULOMATOSIS

A 29-year-old female, previously in good health, initially complained of ear infections and multiple skin abscesses, and was investigated by the ear, nose and throat physicians. Four months subsequently the patient complained of iritis, cellulitis of her ankle and presented with subcutaneous nodules and nephritis.

A chest X-ray revealed a large opacity in the right lung. Bronchoscopy and renal ultrasound were inconclusive. The patient's ESR was raised, 48 mm/h; Hb was 7.8 and 4 units of blood were transfused. The patient was started on prednisolone and cyclophosphamide. A renal biopsy confirmed the diagnosis of WG.

Over the following year the patient suffered mouth ulcers, recurrent chest infections and deteriorating renal function. She required four admissions to hospital in the ensuing months for treatment including chest physiotherapy for alveolitis. The opacity on chest X-ray measured 5 × 3.5 cm.

The patient soon required home oxygen therapy and was re-admitted in sputum retention. She had severely reduced mobility, was chairbound and complained of general weakness reporting a 5-stone gradual loss in weight over the previous year.

The patient was taught the active cycle of breathing techniques, advised on positioning and encouraged to use saline nebulisers. The patient started to expectorate, but her respiratory function remained poor and it was decided that a lung transplant was necessary.

Post-operatively the patient's mobility improved and she was able to walk 50 metres, limited by shortness of breath and severe weakness in her legs. The patient no longer required oxygen therapy, but continued to expectorate. She was taught self-management techniques, including the use of an incentive spirometer. Increasing mobility and exercise tolerance were encouraged throughout the patient's admission and exercises to maintain full joint range of movement were taught.

Following discharge the patient was seen as an out-patient in the physiotherapy department.

PHYSIOTHERAPY PROBLEMS

- Decreased muscle power of all lower limb muscle groups—Quads lag of 10^0. The patient was unable to get on/off floor to play with her children.
- Decreased distance mobilising—timed walk was 34 seconds, limited by shortness of breath.
- Decreased exercise tolerance, HR at rest 112/min.
- Potential recurrence of chest infection.

TREATMENT PLAN

- Teach specific free active strengthening exercises through range:
  Auto resisted exercises.
  Resisted exercises with weights.
  Practise getting on and off the floor.

- Teach:
  Controlled sitting—standing.
  Step ups—increase repetitions as shortness of breath allows.
  Static bike—increase time as able.
  Tread mill—increase time, increase speed.
- The patient's fitness was calculated and monitored at each treatment session:
  100% maximum HR = 220 – the patient's age
  100% = 220 – 33 = 187 and the patient was advised to work between 60 and 70% of maximum HR
  = 112–131/min
- Monitor chest.
  Check incentive spirometry technique.

The patient was able to get on/off floor independently after a fortnight. After a month of physiotherapy the patient's HR at rest was 108 per minute, and timed walk was 28 seconds. After 2 months the patient's HR at rest was 90/minute and timed walk 21 seconds, while after 3 months her HR at rest was 76/minute and timed walk 18 seconds. Exercise programme and timed daily walks were charted on the patient's record card.

After 3 months the patient was cycling up to 20 minutes per day and able to walk for up to 1 hour. The patient continued to manage her chest independently. Throughout, the patient had no specific joint problems. Six months after her lung transplant the patient was discharged from physiotherapy and given a contact number to use if she needed further advice.

(Case History is courtesy of G Dainty.)

REFERENCES

Ayoub WT. Polymyalgia rheumatica–duration of therapy and long-term outcome. *Am J Med* 1985, **79**:309-315.

Berlit P. Clinical and laboratory findings with giant cell arteritis. *J Neurol Sci* 1992, **111**:1-12.

Briedigkeit L, Kettritz R, Gobel U, *et al*. Prognostic factors in Wegener's granulomatosis. *Postgrad Med J* 1993, **69**:856-861.

De Remee RA. Sarcoidosis and Wegener's granulomatosis–a comparative analysis. *Sarcoidosis* 1994, **11**:7-18.

Granados R. Nasal scrape cytology in diagnosis of Wegener's granulomatosis–a case report. *Acta Cytologica* 1994, **38**:463-466.

Hellman D. Immunopathogenesis, diagnosis and treatment of giant cell arteritis, temporal arteritis, polymyalgia rheumatica and Takayasu's arteritis. *Curr Opinion Rheumatol* 1993, **5**:25-32.

Hughes GRV. Polyarthritis, Wegener's granulomatosis, Takayasu's arteritis, other vasculitides, polymyalgia rheumatica and giant cell arteritis. In: Hughes GRV, ed. *Connective tissue diseases, 3rd edition.* Oxford: Blackwell Scientific Publications;1987:200-252.

Kavanagh T. The role of exercise training in cardiac rehabilitation. In: Jones D, West R, eds. *Cardiac rehabilitation.* London: BMJ Publishing Group; 1995:75.

Kirwan JR, Reeback JS. Stanford health questionnaire–modified to assess disability in British patients with rheumatoid arthritis. *Br J Rheumatol* 1986, **25**:206-209.

Kyle V. Laboratory Investigations including liver in polymyalgia rheumatica/giant cell arteritis. *Baillières Clin Rheumatol*, 1989, **8**:475-484.

Lightfoot RW. Vasculitides. In: Klippel JH, Dieppe P, eds. *Rheumatology.* London: Mosby; 1994:16.1-26.9.

Luqmani RA, Exley AR, Kitas GD *et al*. Disease assessment and management of the vasculitides. In: Yazici H, Husby G, eds. *Baillières Clin Rheumatol: Vasculitis* 1997, **11(2):**423-440.

McConnell J. *Promoting effective segmental alignment. Key issues in musculo-skeletal physiotherapy.* In: Crosbie J, McConnell J, eds. Oxford: Butterworth-Heinemann; 1993:172-194.

Salvarani C, Gabriel S, Hunder G. Distal extremity swelling with pitting oedema–a manifestation of polymyalgia rheumatica. *Arthritis Rheum* 1996, **39**:73-80.

Ware JE, Sherbourne CD. The MOS 36-item short form health survey (SF36). *Med Care* 1992, **30**:473-483.

Waterfield J, Sim J. Clinical assessment of pain by the visual analogue scale. *Brit J of Ther and Rehab* 1996, **3**:94-97.

Williams JG, Callaghan M. Comparison of visual estimation and goniometry in determination of a shoulder joint angle. *Physiotherapy* 1990, **76**:655-657.

GENERAL READING

Jones J, Hazleman BL. Prognosis and management of polymyalgia rheumatica. *Ann Rheum Dis* 1981, **40**:1-5.

Lestico MR, Boh LE, Schuna AA. Therapy review–polymyalgia rheumatica. *Clin Pharm* 1993, **12**:571-578.

Soding P, Locoweed C, Park G. The intensive care of patients with fulminant vasculitis. *Anaesth Intensive Care* 1994; **22**:81-89.

Wilson AK. *Arthritis: an equipment guide.* Oxford: The Disability Information Trust; 1991.

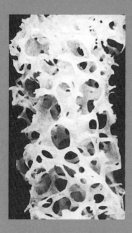

15

C David &
K West

METABOLIC DISORDERS

CHAPTER OUTLINE

- Osteoporosis
- Paget's disease

- Diabetes mellitus
- Crystal arthropathies

INTRODUCTION

Metabolic conditions may play a part in rheumatological problems in a variety of ways. The structure of bone may be affected, as in Paget's disease and osteoporosis; joints may be damaged secondary to neuropathy, as in diabetic Charcot's joints; or crystals may be deposited in the joints and tissues, as in gout.

This chapter aims to cover these conditions. Some, such as osteoporosis, are extremely common and becoming increasingly important to the therapist due to an ageing population and better diagnosis. Other conditions are less common, and an overview is presented.

OSTEOPOROSIS

Osteoporosis is a common metabolic bone disease affecting both sexes, predominantly women. It is characterised by a lower than average bone mineral density with disorganised bone micro-architecture and an increased risk of fractures, which often occur with trivial trauma.

Osteoporosis differs from osteomalacia in that the mineral/matrix ration is equal, whereas in osteomalacia there is a disproportionately low ratio of mineral to matrix (Dequeker 1994).

Figure 15.1 shows osteoporotic bone.

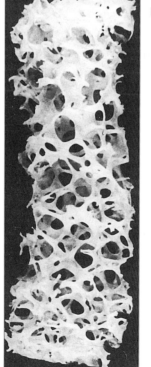

Figure 15.1 **Osteoporotic bone.**

INCIDENCE

This is difficult to establish because only about a third of patients with vertebral fractures seek medical attention as a consequence of the fracture; therefore it is likely to remain undiagnosed (Cooper & Melton, 1992).

Most patients with osteoporosis are over the age of 60, and the female:male ratio is 5:1 (Mundy, 1995). The recognised incidence of osteoporosis is rising in men, due partly to the ageing population but also to greater awareness and better diagnosis. Additional evidence that the disease is on the increase is that there are now 60,000 hip fractures per year in the UK, as opposed to only 10,000 in the 1960s. Elderly patients with fractured femoral necks occupy 20% of all orthopaedic beds. Mortality is high, at 5–25% around the time of the fracture, and only 20–50% of older patients regain their former mobility.

The National Osteoporosis Society estimates that osteoporosis costs over £500 million per year. There is also the human cost in terms of reduction in quality of life due to pain, immobility, loss of confidence and restriction of social life.

AETIOLOGY

The density of bone varies in response to mechanical stress, hormones, genetic factors, disease, toxins and drugs in an adaptive process called remodelling.

Bone remodelling occurs by the action of osteocytes: osteoclasts and osteoblasts. Osteoclasts are involved with resorption of bone, while osteoblasts produce the bone matrix and initiate bone mineralisation. The bone remodelling balance results in up to 30% of the adult skeleton being replaced each year. Cortical bone, which comprises 80% of the skeleton, is densely packed and surrounds trabecular (cancellous) bone. Cancellous bone, with its intermeshing structures of trabeculae, is most responsive to remodelling signals within the body (Aloia, 1993). In long bones, osteoporotic fractures tend to occur where there is the greatest proportion of cancellous bone (proximal femur and distal radius).

The response of bone to mechanical stresses is especially evident in the higher bone mass of athletes, for example the higher density in the dominant arm of tennis players (Rutherford, 1990). Conversely, individuals who have been immobilised due to injury or who are physically inactive are predisposed to bone loss. This has been demonstrated through the rapid loss of bone mass in astronauts due to the effect of weightlessness. Obesity, however, is a protective factor against the development of osteoporosis, partly due to the weightbearing stress on the bones and partly because fat acts as a reservoir for oestrogens. Bone mass, then is directly related to lean muscle mass (Cohn et al., 1997). Muscle strength declines with age and therefore bone mass will decrease at a similar rate. Figure 15.2 illustrates the relationship between age and bone density.

Osteoporosis is categorised into primary or secondary types, described below.

Primary Osteoporosis

Primary osteoporosis accounts for approximately 95% of osteoporotic patients. There are three main types:

- Type I: mainly affecting women, this is hormone-related and due to overactive osteoclasts. Bone loss is most rapid in the 10 years after the menopause, especially in the first 2–3 years (Lindsay et al., 1976). This is particularly apparent in the vertebrae but shows individual variation in the rate of loss (Woolf & Dixon, 1988).
- Type II: affecting both sexes, this is age related and due to underactive osteoblasts. Osteoblasts have a decreased capacity to form new bone in the elderly, and fractures heal more slowly than in the young (Mundy, 1995).
- Idiopathic: less common, affecting younger people.

Secondary Osteoporosis

This is associated with factors which predispose individuals to reduced bone density. These factors are listed below.

Nutrition

There is convincing evidence linking dietary calcium deficiency and osteoporosis. A high calcium intake is recommended for children and adolescents in order to establish a good peak bone mass, and in the elderly since calcium absorption from the gut decreases with age. Other crucial times include pregnancy, lactation and the menopausal years. Recommended daily intakes for postmenopausal women are 1,000 mg/day with hormonal replacement or 1.500 mg/day without, together with an adequate supply of vitamin D (NIH Consensus Development Panel, 1994).

Other dietary causes include protein malnutrition, excessive caffeine and excess alcohol consumption. Vitamin C deficiency leads to reduced collagen formation, therefore less osteoid tissue formation.

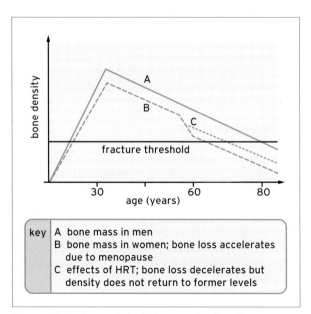

Figure 15.2 Age-related changes in density.

Hormonal

Transient osteoporosis may occur in the third trimester of pregnancy, a major period of calcium input to the skeleton of the growing foetus. This osteoporosis affects the vertebrae and the head of femur; bone density recovers soon after birth, and bed rest for symptomatic relief is all that is required.

Amenorrhoea caused by extreme physical exercise can predispose female athletes to an increased risk of fractures, particularly stress fractures of the tibia or metatarsals.

Osteoporosis is associated with poorly controlled Type I diabetes. Type II diabetics tend to have higher than average bone mineral density as insulin promotes calcification (Forgács, 1994). Hyperthyroidism speeds up bone turnover; women treated with thyroid hormones may have reduced bone density at the femoral neck, spine and radius.

Drugs

Corticosteroids contribute to spinal bone loss (Chevalier & Larget-Piet, 1994). Oral steroid doses of more than 10 mg/day short-term or 7.5 mg long-term have a detrimental effect on bone mass. Heparin and methotrexate may also contribute to osteoporosis.

Disease

Chronic liver disease may lead to osteoporosis due to impaired vitamin D metabolism. Organ transplant patients are at risk of osteoporosis due to the large doses of steroids used (Johnell & Obrant, 1997). Other conditions predisposing patients to osteoporosis include inflammatory bowel disease, coeliac disease and anorexia nervosa (Johnell & Obrant, 1997).

Rheumatological conditions

Inflammatory mediators affect bone resorption (Jones & Bhalla, 1993). In addition, patients with rheumatoid arthritis (RA) are generally less mobile than the normal population and are therefore not weightbearing through their skeleton.

Ankylosing spondylitis may lead to spinal fractures in areas of most inflammation. Rigid spines do not absorb stress forces well and recover less successfully from vertebral fractures, particularly if spinal movement was restricted previously.

FACTORS INFLUENCING PEAK BONE MASS

Following cessation of growth, the skeleton increases in density for about 15 years. Peak bone mass is attained at about the age of 35 years, after which it starts to decline. It will gradually drop to half its maximum value by the age of 80 or 90 years. Peak bone mass is determined by genetic factors, dietary intake of calcium and physical activity in childhood and adolescence (Johnston et al., 1992). It varies between different ethnic groups; for example, African races have greater bone density than Caucasians, who in turn have greater peak bone mass than Oriental races (Mundy, 1995). The vitamin D receptor gene may be responsible for changes in calcium resorption or bone remodelling, and thus the attainment of peak bone mass (Kelly et al., 1991). Women generally have a lower peak bone mass than men.

INVESTIGATIONS

Dual Energy X-ray Absorptiometry

Bone density dual energy x-ray absorptiometry (DEXA) scanning provides a safe, rapid, non-invasive and accurate measurement of bone mineral density and thereby a prediction of risk of future fracture. Measurements are standardised, usually the body of L4 and the right femoral neck (Fordham et al., 1994).

Radiology

Conventional X-rays are of limited value in showing the degree of bone loss in generalised osteoporosis because changes will only show when around 30% of bone mass has already been lost. However they will show:
- Thinning and accentuation of the bone cortex.
- Accentuation of the primary trabeculae and loss of secondary trabeculae.
- Changes in vertebral shape (biconcave, wedge shape compression).
- Fractures of bones predisposed to osteoporosis: spine, femur, wrist and ribs.

Ultrasound Measurements

There is potential for the widespread use of this method, but it requires further research (Hans et al., 1997).

Laboratory Measurements

Investigations may be required to exclude causes of secondary osteoporosis.

CLINICAL FEATURES OF OSTEOPOROSIS

Many patients with osteoporosis do not realise that they have the disease because they do not experience any symptoms. When there is a problem it will be in terms of pain, fracture or deformity.

Pain

Back pain is a characteristic feature in osteoporotic patients through either microfractures of the vertebral bodies or wedge compression fractures. The pain may be severe initially, becoming worse on movement. Wedge fractures also lead to deformities, which in turn give rise to more chronic persistent pain due to abnormal stresses on the soft tissues.

Fractures

The most common osteoporotic fractures are found in the mid-thoracic vertebral bodies, later the lower thoracic and upper lumbar levels. Fractured femoral necks are the second most common but carry the greatest mortality. Fractures of the distal forearm are less common and occur more frequently in the younger age group, who tend to fall forwards. The elderly are more likely to fall sideways on to the femoral trochanter thereby sustaining femoral fractures.

Deformity

Osteoporotic patients have usually lost height and appear to have disproportionately long legs. This is because loss of height occurs in the trunk. Walking aid height needs to be adjusted as the patient's height changes, and should be measured to the wrist as opposed to the greater trochanter.

The patient will frequently develop kyphotic posture with increasing angulation of the spine. This is often referred to as a dowager's or bison's hump. Patients consequently will complain that their clothes will no longer fit because of a protruding abdomen. Skin creases will appear around the abdomen because of the loss of vertebral height and in advanced disease the thoracic cage will rest uncomfortably on the iliac crests. Deformities of the chest wall may lead to respiratory difficulties, and stress incontinence may result from compression of the abdominal contents. Figures 15.3A & B highlight these changes due to osteoporosis.

MEDICAL MANAGEMENT

Drug management aims to increase bone mass. However, increase in bone mass in established osteoporosis may not necessarily lead to increase in bone strength since the trabecular architecture is lost. Drugs most commonly used are bisphosphonates, for example etidronate and alendronate; hormone replacement therapy (HRT); calcium and vitamin D. Fluoride has an anabolic effect on the osteoblasts, but its use is controversial. It is now generally recognised that HRT has a protective role against the development of cardiovascular disease as well as its ability to prevent bone loss in women, but it may be associated with the development of certain cancers and deep vein thrombosis. For further discussion on the drugs used for osteoporosis, see Chapter 3.

PHYSIOTHERAPY MANAGEMENT
Acute Vertebral Fractures

Until the acute pain subsides bedrest is recommended in a comfortable position, possibly supported by beanbag cushions to accommodate existing deformity. Analgesic drugs are usually required and the various pain-relieving modalities of physiotherapy including transcutaneous electrical nerve stimulation (TENS), interferential or acupuncture may be useful. Patients should be mobilised as soon as possible. Gentle exercise in the hydrotherapy pool may promote relaxation and give the patient confidence to start moving. Extension exercises should be started as soon as patients can tolerate them.

Later Stage Vertebral Fractures

Patients with established osteoporosis will need full assessment of pain, deformity, posture, joint range of movement, balance, gait and confidence level. Physiotherapists will be involved in re-educating posture and teaching exercises to strengthen the areas affected by osteoporosis, for example the trunk and femur. Specific exercises will also help to maintain ranges of movement, improve co-ordination and balance and increase confidence. Patients will be encouraged to practise

their own exercises at home on a regular basis. Other forms of treatment may be useful at this stage, for example relaxation techniques and electrotherapy.

Management of Other Types of Fractures

Femoral fractures occur at either the femoral neck or the intertrochanteric region. Femoral neck fractures have the risk of non-union or avascular necrosis. They are usually stabilised with internal fixation methods using screws, plates or rods. Arthroplasty may be necessary.

Colles fractures are usually immobilised in plaster of Paris for 4–6 weeks unless they are severely comminuted or displaced and require surgical fixation. Physiotherapy

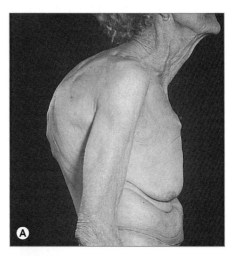

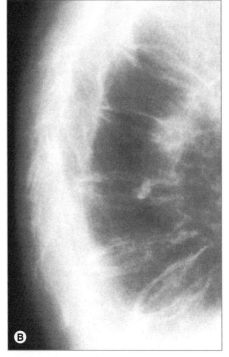

Figures 15.3A & B **Postural changes due to osteoporosis.**

may be required to improve range of movement after plaster removal.

Pelvic fractures usually affect the ischium or pubis unilaterally, but sometimes they can occur bilaterally. Osteoporotic pelvic fractures are stable but bedrest is recommended until the patient can tolerate mobilising within the limits of pain.

Fractured ribs may require pain relief, such as TENS or Entonox. The physiotherapist should encourage the patient to keep the chest clear of secretions, teaching relaxed deep breathing exercises and forced expiratory techniques rather than coughing.

Orthotics

Lumbosacral supports or a more rigid type of brace provide localised support, decrease pain, limit motion and attempt to realign the vertebrae, but their effect is of limited value (Aloia, 1993). Collars may be useful for support in lifting the head upwards from the chest, and a soft collar may make sleeping more comfortable.

Exercise in Established Osteoporosis

While some mechanical stress is needed to maintain optimal bone mineral density (BMD), it is not clear which exercises are most valuable. It is likely that a combined programme of weightbearing, mobilising and aerobic exercises is necessary (Gutin & Kasper, 1992). A physical exercise programme for osteoporotic patients should aim to:
• Restore confidence.
• Improve or maintain joint mobility.
• Reduce pain.
• Improve posture.
• Reduce stress.
• Increase muscle strength and bulk.
• Maintain bone density.

Exercises which may help include:
• Postural exercise including spinal stretches.
• Deep breathing exercises.
• Abdominal muscle strengthening.
• Spinal extension and strengthening.
• Hip and gluteal strengthening.
• Co-ordination and balance exercises.
• Pelvic floor exercises.

Walking will provide weightbearing stresses. Swimming, although non-weightbearing, can improve posture, mobility and confidence.

Postural Considerations

Patients should be instructed in good static and dynamic posture and safe lifting practice. Loads should be carried symmetrically. Spinal flexion should be discouraged, since flexion increases vertebral fractures even if counterbalanced by extension exercises (Sinaki & Mikkelson, 1984). In addition, sustained static postures, such as sitting for long periods to knit or sew, tighten the spinal flexors, stretch the extensors and reinforce poor posture. If sneezing or coughing, patients should straighten up and support their lumbar spine with their hands to minimise flexion forces.

Environmental Considerations

Foam blocks may be required in chairs and car seats to compensate for the loss of trunk height.

Safety in the home environment is paramount to prevent falls. The patient should beware of tripping over trailing leads, loose rugs, pets or children's toys, and slipping on greasy or wet floors. Poor lighting and the distorting effect of bifocal spectacle lenses may present a hazard, especially on stairways.

Footwear should be practical, avoiding loose shoes and high heels. Outdoor footwear should have good treads, especially for the ice and snow. Ferrules on walking aids should be checked regularly for wear. Hip protector pads have been successful in preventing femoral fractures, although compliance may be a problem (Lauritzen *et al.*, 1993).

PAGET'S DISEASE

This common bone disease of elderly people was first described in 1877 by Sir James Paget who named it 'osteitis deformans'. Its main features are enlargement and thickening of bone, resulting in spongy bone with a tendency to bend and which will become brittle in later stages with an increased likelihood of fracture (Figure 15.4).

INCIDENCE

Great Britain and continental Europe have the highest incidence, affecting as many as 4% of the population over the age of 40 and 10% of over 85 year olds. It is rare under the age of 40. It is common in Eastern Australia and in the

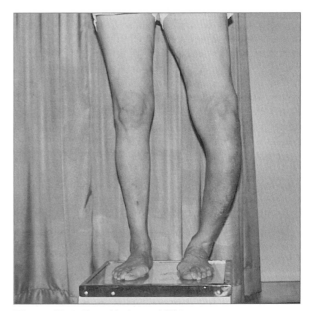

Figure 15.4 **Paget's bowed tibia.**

Eastern states of the USA where there are many British descendants, but rare in Scandinavia, Africa, Asia and the Middle East (Duckworth, 1995). There is a 16% incidence with a family history of Paget's disease and it affects men and women at a ratio of 4:3 (Dieppe *et al.*, 1985).

AETIOLOGY

The cause of the disease is unknown although a slow virus of the paramyxovirus (measles) family is thought to be responsible because of the characteristic inclusion bodies found consistently in the osteoclasts of the affected bones. Paget's disease in Manchester has been linked with dog ownership (O'Driscoll & Anderson, 1985).

PATHOLOGY

Any bone can be affected by Paget's disease. The frequency of involvement in different bones is:

- Pelvis 71%.
- Lumbar spine 50%.
- Femur 49%.
- Humerus 40%.
- Skull 28%.
- Tibia 8%.

Defective osteoclast functioning leads to alternating phases of rapid bone resorption and formation. Rates of bone remodelling may be increased 20-fold. During the resorption phase bone is soft, vascular and bleeds freely, whilst during the formation phase, it is hard and sclerotic.

Marrow spaces are filled with fibrous tissue. Haversian systems are disrupted with coarse, disorganised trabeculae. Weightbearing bones such as the tibia and femur become bowed anteriorly and laterally.

INVESTIGATIONS

Radiology

X-rays may reveal reduced density of the bone cortex in the early stages, followed by increased bone density and characteristic coarsening of the bone trabeculae in the later stages of the disease. Bony deformity may be apparent; for example, compression of the vertebral bodies, deformity of the pelvis and skull and bowing of the long bones. The skull often has a cotton wool appearance on X-ray. Radio-isotope scanning with technetium-labelled diphosphonate will show increased uptake in the affected bones.

Other Investigations

Blood alkaline phosphatase levels may be raised. Raised levels of hydroxyproline in the urine indicate increased bone matrix resorption (Mundy, 1995). Occasionally bone biopsy may be required to rule out osteosarcoma.

CLINICAL FEATURES

Most patients with Paget's disease are asymptomatic, although dull bone pain (especially nocturnal) is a common feature. Deformities of the long bones may result in awkward gait or restriction of functional range of movement. Degenerative joint disease is a common feature, especially in the hips. Spinal kyphosis follows vertebral involvement and root pain may occur due to thickened vertebrae. Headaches may be attributed to enlargement of the skull.

COMPLICATIONS

Many patients with Paget's disease present with complications associated with increased bone turnover. Pathological fractures are especially common in the weightbearing bones, and often occur with minimal trauma especially in the tibia and femur. There is a high incidence of non-union in femoral fractures due to Paget's disease. Stress fractures are common, especially on the convex borders of weight-bearing bones, and protrusio acetabuli is frequently occurs due to softening of the pelvic bones. Paraplegia is an uncommon complication, caused by change of shape or collapse of a vertebra. It may also be due to vascular changes affecting the spinal cord.

Compression of the auditory or optic nerves due to bone thickening around the foramina of the skull may cause deafness or visual disturbances.

Sarcoma affects 1% of elderly patient with Paget's disease. Usually the long bones are affected and sometimes the skull or vertebrae. It is highly malignant and rapidly fatal. Sudden pain, swelling, deformity or tenderness may be an indication of osteosarcoma.

MEDICAL MANAGEMENT

Drugs including calcitonin and bisphosphonates are used to inhibit osteoclastic bone resorption (Mundy, 1995). Femoral neck fractures are usually treated with prosthetic replacements. Fractured bone shafts are more successfully stabilised with internal fixation methods because of the high rate of non-union. Tibial osteotomy may be required for painful knee malalignment.

PHYSIOTHERAPY MANAGEMENT

The goals of management are to reduce pain and increase mobility. Patients with Paget's disease will usually complain of pain, deformity and reduced functional activity. Physiotherapy should be tailored to the individual's presenting problems and should include exercises to mobilise affected joints and strengthen muscles.

Many patients will present with back pain, sometimes because of localised disease activity in the lumbar spine or possibly due to leg-length discrepancy. Back-care education and gentle mobilising exercises may be of help, and a shoe raise may be required to correct gait biomechanics.

The physiotherapist will be involved before and after orthopaedic surgery. Some patients may require extended hospital stays because of the associated complications. Many members of the multidisciplinary team will be involved with the assessment and rehabilitation of these patients.

DIABETES MELLITUS

Diabetes affects about 2% of the population. It may be Type I (juvenile onset, insulin dependent) or Type II (adult onset, non-insulin dependent) (Forgács, 1994). Diabetic patients have an increased tendency to develop septic arthritis, bone infections and diffuse idiopathic skeletal hyperostosis (see Chapter 16). They are also more predisposed to soft tissue problems such as Dupuytren's contracture, carpal tunnel syndrome (Swedler *et al.*, 1995), trigger finger, adhesive capsulitis and trophic ulceration. Arthropathies particularly associated with diabetes are diabetic cheiroarthropathy and neuropathic joints.

DIABETIC CHEIROARTHROPATHY

This is characterised by symmetrical flexion contractures of the fingers, starting with the ring and little fingers (Figure 15.5). Wrists, elbows and ankles are occasionally involved. Joint stiffness is related to the duration of the disease and occurs in up to 50% of Type I diabetics, with equal male to female ratio. It is rare in Type II diabetes (Forgács, 1994). The condition runs a slowly progressive course over a few years; it tends not to be painful and leads to minimal functional impairment except in severe cases. Patients have normal X-rays and erythrocyte sedimentation rate (ESR).

Therapy includes improved diabetic control, vasodilators, anti-inflammatory medication and gentle exercise. (Forgács, 1994, Swedler *et al.*, 1995). Wax, passive stretches and a home programme of hand exercises may be appropriate. Tenolysis may be considered for patients with disabling deformities.

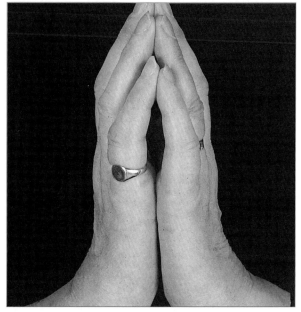

Figure 15.5 **Diabetic cheiroarthropathy.**

NEUROPATHIC JOINTS (CHARCOT'S JOINTS)

A total of 0.1% of all diabetics, and 5% of those with diabetic neuropathy, develop neuropathic joints. 80% of cases involve the foot, most commonly the tarsal and metatarsal joints. The condition is monoarticular in 70% of patients. (For further information on Charcot's joints, see Chapter 16.)

CRYSTAL ARTHROPATHIES

Arthritis may be caused by the deposition of crystals in the tissues and within the joints, most commonly:
• Monosodium urate monohydrate (gout).
• Calcium pyrophosphate dihydrate (CPPD).
• Calcium phosphate (hydroxyapatite) (Poór, 1995).

GOUT

Gout is an umbrella term for several different metabolic disorders involving deposition of monosodium urate monohydrate (MSUM). The incidence is world-wide, affecting men aged between 40 and 50 years and women over 60 years of age. The prevalence is 1–3 per 1000 men, 0.2 per 1000 women (Cohen & Emerson, 1994). Gout is caused by excess uric acid in the blood (hyperuricaemia), although 95% of hyperuricaemic patients remain asymptomatic (Nuki, 1993). The reasons for this are unclear (Terkeltaub, 1995).

Causes of Hyperuricaemia

Hyperuricaemia may be caused either by overproduction or undersecretion of uric acid:
Overproduction:
• Purine, alcohol, fructose intake.
• Polycythaemia, leukaemia, infectious mononucleosis.
• Psoriasis.
• Drugs – cytotoxics, nicotinic acid.

Undersecretion:
• Idiopathic.
• Alcohol.
• Renal disease, low urine output, hypertension, low plasma volume.
• Metabolic/hormonal: vasopressin, lactic acidosis, ketosis, angiotensin.
• Miscellaneous: myxoedema, respiratory acidosis, toxaemia of pregnancy, acute myocardial infarction, hyperparathyroidism (Cohen & Emerson, 1994).

Renal urate excretion is increased by high dose aspirin, high dose phenylbutazone, diflunisal, radiographic contrast medium and oral anticoagulants. It is decreased by low dose aspirin and phenylbutazone, and thiazide diuretics. Gout may be also be a complication of cyclosporine to prevent organ rejection in transplant recipients (Howe & Edwards, 1995).

Clinical Features

There are four stages of gout (Nuki, 1993):
• Asymptomatic hyperuricaemia.
• Acute arthritis of the wrist, elbow, small joints hands and feet.
• Intercritical (remission).
• Chronic tophaceous (Figures 15.6A&B).

The American College of Rheumatology Criteria (Wallace *et al.*, 1977) are listed in Table 15.1 Back pain is an occasional feature (Leventhal *et al.*, 1990).

Investigations

Polarised light microscopy of synovial fluid may reveal urate crystals; these are needle shaped, around 5–25 mm in length and negatively birefringent. This means that crystals lying parallel to the line of slow vibration will be yellow, and at 90° will be blue. Crystals may also be seen in neutrophils.

Common features of X-rays are punched out erosions due to tophi, with sclerotic margins and overhanging edges due to new bone formation. Although cartilage is not eroded, late stage disease may be difficult to tell apart from RA. Secondary osteoarthritis (OA) is common, leading to spurs, osteophytes and sclerosis (Cohen & Emerson, 1994).

Medical Management

Medication is the mainstay of arthritis management, and varies according to the stage. During acute arthritis the joint should be rested and non-steroidal anti-inflammatory drugs (NSAIDs) and intra-articular steroid used to relieve inflammation and pain. Repeated attacks of acute gout may require hypouricaemic agents such as probenecid, sulfinpyrazone or allopurinol (Star & Hochberg, 1994).

Management of chronic gout is determined by the patient's renal status, concomitant drug use, and the cause of the hyperuricaemia (Table 15.2). Allopurinol is used in patients with tophaceous gout (Calin, 1995).

CALCIUM PYROPHOSPHATE DEPOSITION DISEASE

This is a common idiopathic condition in the elderly, affecting more than 50% of people over the age of 85 (Terkeltaub, 1994). It may be acute, subacute, chronic or asymptomatic, and may be familial or associated with certain metabolic disorders or pre-existing joint damage. Calcium pyrophosphate deposition disease (CPDD) is diagnosed by radiological changes (commonly calcification of articular cartilage, see Figure 15.7) and identification of calcium pyrophosphate dihydrate crystals in synovial fluid. Management consists of NSAIDs, joint aspiration and intra-articular corticosteroid. Physiotherapy management is similar to that for OA (see Chapter 9).

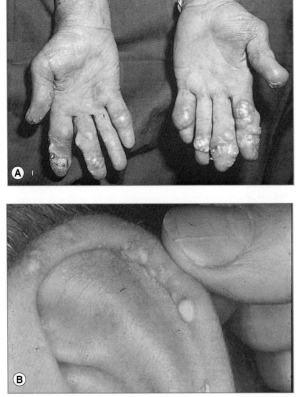

Figures 15.6A & B **Gouty tophi.**

American College of Rheumatology Criteria
1 More than 1 attack of acute arthritis
2 Max inflammation developed within 1 day
3 Mono/oligoarthritis
4 Redness over joints
5 1st MTP joint attack
6 Unilateral 1st MTP joint attack
7 Unilateral tarsal attack
8 Tophus: a proved   b suspected
9 Hyperuricaemia
10 Asymmetrical swelling within joint on radiograph
11 Subcortical cysts without erosion on radiograph
12 Monosodium urate monohydrate crystals in joint fluid during attack
13 Joint fluid culture negative for organisms during attack
12 or 8a are diagnostic, or 6 out of 12 features (excluding 12 and 8a)

Table 15.1 **The American College of Rheumatology Criteria (Wallace *et al.*, 1977).**

CALCIUM PHOSPHATE DEPOSITION DISEASE

This may be primary, familial or associated with chronic renal failure, progressive systemic sclerosis or dermatomyositis. Acute, subacute and chronic musculoskeletal symptoms, e.g. bursitis, tendinitis, periarthritis and arthritis, may be related to calcium phosphate deposition, commonly in the shoulder, greater trochanter, lateral epicondyle of elbow and tendons around wrist and knee. 'Milwaukee shoulder' is a rapidly destructive progressive arthritis of shoulder accompanied by large cool effusions. Calcium phosphate crystals are difficult to isolate as they are very small (Poór, 1995).

PHYSIOTHERAPY MANAGEMENT

Little has been found in the literature on physiotherapy for crystal deposition diseases although ice is effective in decreasing pain, resolving swelling and helping to resolve inflammation in the acute phase of gout (Schlesinger *et al.*, 1996). Occasionally the patient may need assistance to remobilise joints after an acute attack, or may need maintenance management in chronic arthritis.

Table 15.2 Difference between gout and pseudogout (Cohen & Emerson).

Difference between gout and pseudogout (Cohen & Emerson, 1994)	Gout	Calcium pyrophosphate
Sex (male:female)	2–7:1	4:1
Peak age	40–50 years	>60
Common joints	1st metatarsophalangeal joints	Knee
Serum urate	Raised	Normal
Radiology: calcification erosion	No Characteristic – punched out erosions	Chondrocalcinosis Often degenerative
Crystals: type shape birefringence	Monosodium urate monohydrate Needle Strong negative	Calcium pyrophosphate dihydrate Small rod Weakly positive

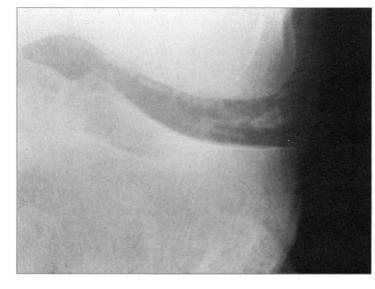

Figure 15.7 Calcification of cartilage.

REFERENCES

Aloia JF. A colour atlas of osteoporosis. London: Wolfe (Mosby-Year); 1993.

Calin A. Managing hyperuricemia and gout: challenges and pitfalls. *J Musculoskeletal Med* 1995, **12**:42-46.

Chevalier X, Larget-Piet B. General disease of the spine in rheumatoid arthritis. *Curr Opin Rheum* 1994, **6**:311-318.

Cohen MG, Emerson BT. Gout. In: Klippel JH, Dieppe P, eds. *Rheumatology*. London: Mosby Year Book Europe; 1994, 7:12.1-12.6.

Cohn SH, Abesamis C, Yasumura S *et al*. Comparative skeletal mass and radial bone mineral content in black and white women. *Metabolism* 1997, **26**:171-178.

Cooper C, Melton LJ. Epidemiology of osteoporosis trends. *Endocrinol Metab* 1992, **3**:224-229.

Dequeker J. Bone structure and function. In: Klippel JH, Dieppe P, eds. *Rheumatology*. London: Mosby Year Book Europe; 1994, 7:30.1-30.12.

Dieppe PA, Doherty M, MacFarlane DG, Maddison PJ. *Rheumatological Medicine*. London: Churchill Livingstone; 1985.

Duckworth T. *Lecture notes on orthopaedics and fractures, 3rd edition*. Oxford: Blackwell; 1995.

Forgács SS. Diabetes mellitus. In: Klippel JH, Dieppe P, eds. *Rheumatology*. London: Mosby Year Book Europe; 1994, 7:20.1-20.6.

Fordham JN, Simpson DS, Pitcher O *et al*. An open access bone densitometry service: report of first year's operation. *Br J Rheum* 1994, **33**:668-673.

Gutin B, Kasper MJ. Can vigorous exercise play a role in osteoporosis prevention? A review. *Osteoporosis Intl* 1992, **2**:55-69.

Hans D, Fuerst T, Lang T *et al*. How can we measure bone quality? In: Delmas PD, Woolf AD, eds. *Baillières Clin Rheumatol*: Osteoporosis 1997, **11**:495-516.

Howe S, Edwards NL. Controlling hyperuricemia and gout in cardiac transplant recipients. *J Musculoskeletal Med* 1995, **12**:15-7, 21-2, 24.

Johnell O, Obrant KJ. What is the impact of osteoporosis? In: Delmas PD, Woolf AD, eds. *Baillières Clin Rheumatol*: Osteoporosis 1997, **11**:459-478.

Johnston CC, Miller JZ, Slemenda CW *et al*. Calcium supplementation and increases in bone mineral density in children. *New Engl J Med* 1992, **327**:82-87.

Jones SM, Bhalla AK. Osteoporosis in rheumatoid arthritis. *Clin Expl Rheumatol* 1993, **11**:557-562.

Kelly PJ, Hopper JL, Macaskill GT *et al*. Genetic factors in bone turnover. *J Clin Endocrinol Metab* 1991, **72**:808-813.

Lauritzen JB, Petersen MM, Lund B. The effect of external hip protectors on hip fractures. *Lancet* 1993, **341**:11-13.

Leventhal LJ, Levin RW, Bomalaski JS. Peripheral arthrocentesis in the work up of acute low back pain. *Arch Phys Med Rehabil* 1990, **71**:253-254.

Lindsay R, Hart DM, Aitken JM *et al*. Long-term prevention of osteoporosis by oestrogen: evidence of increased bone mass after delayed onset oestrogen treatment. *Lancet* 1976, **i**:1038-1041.

Mundy GR. *Bone remodelling and its disorders*. Texas: Martin Dunitz, 1995:161-173.

NIH Consensus Statement Online. *Optimal calcium intake*; 1994, June 6-8, 12:1-31.

Nuki G. Crystal arthropathy. In: Maddison PJ, Isenberg DA, Woo P, Glass DN, eds. *Oxford textbook of rheumatology*. Oxford: Oxford Medical Publications; 1993:983-1005.

O'Driscoll JB, Anderson DC. Past pets and Paget's disease. *Lancet* 1985, **ii**:919-921

Poór G. Crystal arthritis. In: Silman AJ, Symmons DPM, eds. *Baillières Clin Rheumatol Classification Assessment Rheum Dis*, Part I; 1995, **9**:397-406.

Rutherford OM. The role of exercise in the prevention of osteoporosis. *Physiotherapy* 1990, **76**:522-526.

Schlesinger N, Baker DG, Bentler AM *et al*. Local ice therapy during bouts of acute gouty arthritis. *Arthritis Rheum* 1996, **39**:347.

Sinaki M, Mikkelson BA. Postmenopausal spinal osteoporosis - flexion versus extension exercises. *Arch Phys Med Rehabil* 1984, **65**:593-596.

Star VL, Hochberg MC. Gout: steps to relieve acute symptoms, prevent further attacks. *Consultant* 1994, **34**:1697-1699, 1703-1706.

Swedler WI, Baak S, Lazarevic MB *et al*. Rheumatic changes in diabetes: shoulder, arm, and hand. *J Musculoskeletal Med* 1995, **12**:45-48, 50, 52.

Terkeltaub RA. Gout: questions that still need to be answered. *Ann Rheum Dis* 1995, **54**:79-81.

Terkeltaub RA. Identifying and managing calcium pyrophosphate deposition disease: symptoms range from subtle to goutlike. *J Musculoskeletal Med* 1994, **11**:29-32, 34, 36-37.

Wallace SC, Robinson H, Masi AT. Preliminary criteria for the classification of the acute arthritis of primary gout. *Arthritis Rheum* 1977, **20**:895-900.

Woolf AD, Dixon A St J. *Osteoporosis: a clinical guide*. Martin Dunitz; 1988.

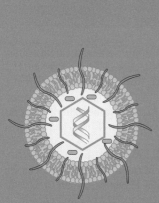

16 N Chettle
MISCELLANEOUS RHEUMATOLOGICAL CONDITIONS

CHAPTER OUTLINE

HAEMOPHILIA

Haemophilia is a rare disorder of the blood clotting mechanism caused by a deficiency of a specific plasma coagulation factor. It is inherited as an X-linked recessive character and produces its greatest morbidity in the musculoskeletal system.

In classic haemophilia (haemophilia A) the individual lacks factor VIII and in Christmas disease (haemophilia B) lacks factor IX. Individuals are classified mild, moderate or severe depending on the levels of circulating coagulation factor.

It is estimated that there are 5000 males in the United Kingdom, with 2000 severely affected, and it is rare in females. There is a family history of haemophilia in 70% and it usually presents in the first years of life. Joint involvement occurs in 90% of patients By 1988, 60% of severely affected haemophiliacs were positive for HIV as a result of contaminated blood products (Buzzard & Jones, 1988). The risk has now been greatly reduced by the screening of donated blood and the use of heat treated blood products.

AETIOLOGY AND CLINICAL FEATURES

In the absence of factor VIII or IX insufficient fibrin is produced to control bleeding. Bleeding into a joint (haemarthrosis) causes a synovitis and the membrane hypertrophies due to resorption of blood and absorption of iron pigment. The synovium forms itself into a pannus (similar to rheumatoid arthritis) and invades the articular cartilage. This then begins to degenerate and fibrillation similar to osteoarthritis occurs. If bleeding is repeated and untreated the subchondral bone becomes osteoporotic and bone cysts develop, leading eventually to collapse of the joint.

The larger joints and muscles are commonly affected with the knee (70%), ankle (20%), elbow, hip and shoulder most often involved. Haemarthrosis may be acute, subacute or chronic.

Acute Haemarthrosis

The sudden onset of a swollen, hot, painful joint is the first manifestation of haemophilia in 25–35% of patients. There is pain at rest which is exacerbated on movement and marked muscle spasm and joint range is limited. Mild systemic features such as fever can occur due to extravasated blood.

Subacute Haemarthrosis

This is determined by the severity, frequency and management of the bleeds and the progression of arthropathy depends on the frequency of bleeds. Clinically the joint is warm and less painful, and a boggy synovium may be palpated. The hypertrophied synovium is very vascular and minimal trauma will produce further bleeding.

Chronic Haemarthrosis

There is synovial thickening with joint degeneration including intra-articular fibrosis and generalised destruction leading to joint stiffness. Marked muscle atrophy is apparent. Loss of extension in the knee leads to a flexion contracture which is then followed by posterior subluxation of the tibia with external rotation and valgus deformity. Bleeding into the muscles around the joint limits range of movement. Initially the muscle will recover but with persistent bleeds it loses its elasticity. The muscle may atrophy and be unable to elongate with normal growth leading to contractures, and there is a danger of compartmental syndrome with possible nerve damage.

INVESTIGATIONS

In the early stages X-rays are normal. With recurrent bleeds there may be evidence of increased soft tissue density and small, irregular superficial erosions or bone cysts. Epiphyseal disturbances may be seen in children. In later stages there is loss of joint space, sclerosis, flattening of the joint surfaces and eventual disorganisation of the joint.

TREATMENT

Treatment involves replacement of the missing factor as soon as possible. There is a trend towards self-administration and these self-therapy programmes have reduced the number and severity of bleeds (Markova *et al.,* 1983). Only major bleeds require hospitalisation. Soft tissue releases may be necessary for contracted structures. If there has been severe joint damage, arthrodesis or arthroplasty may be performed.

PHYSIOTHERAPY

In the acute stage the joint is immobilised in a splint and the patient instructed in isometric exercises. Ice is useful at this stage. Once the risk of re-bleeding has passed, the patient is shown strengthening and mobilising exercises to regain full function and range of movement. Muscle weakness leading to joint instability increases the tendency to re-bleed.

RHEUMATIC MANIFESTATIONS OF HIV INFECTION

AIDS was first recognised in 1981 (Gottlieb *et al.,* 1981). It was 2 years later that HIV, a previously unknown virus, was identified. HIV can directly attack cells of many body systems and damages the immune system allowing opportunistic infections to affect almost any organ. Whilst HIV infection has not in itself been shown to produce rheumatic diseases, it is now recognised that rheumatological problems can affect patients with HIV and in some patients may be the first manifestation of the infection (Rowe *et al.,* 1988).

AETIOLOGY AND CLINICAL FEATURES

It is unclear whether HIV infection is a genuine risk factor for the development of arthritis. However, certain rheumatic lesions occur more than expected in HIV positive individuals (Rowe & Keat, 1989). These include Reiter's syndrome, psoriatic arthropathy and Sjögren's syndrome (SS).

Rheumatic syndromes associated with HIV tend to be oligoarticular with a predisposition for lower limb involvement (Calabrese, 1989). They include several syndromes (Berman *et al.,* 1988).

Rheumatological manifestations of HIV infection are listed in Table 16.1. Reactive arthritis and Reiter's syndrome are the most frequently seen forms of arthritis occurring in 2% of HIV patients. The prevalence of psoriasis in AIDS patients is about three times that observed in the general population (Espinoza *et al.,* 1988). It is associated with the same type of arthritic manifestations as psoriatic arthritis (see Chapter 12). However, patients often exhibit severe and extensive psoriasis which can flare up suddenly.

There are a number of HIV patients whose joint manifestations cannot be classified into any defined arthritic condition and which are described as undifferentiated forms of seronegative arthritis (Table 16.2).

Sjögren's syndrome in HIV-infected patients includes a lower prevalence of xerophthalmia and less severe xerostomia than in patients without HIV. Extraglandular abnormalities include lymphocytic interstitial pneumonia, hepatitis, gastritis, nephritis and aseptic meningitis.

Rheumatological Manifestations of HIV Infection	
Group 1	Opportunistic joint infection
Group 2	Reactive arthritis Psoriatic arthritis Reiter's syndrome
Group 3	Sjögren's syndrome Necrotising vasculitis Systemic lupus erythematosus (SLE)-like syndromes Polymyositis
Group 4	Arthralgia Polyarthritis

Table 16.1 **Rheumatological manifestations of HIV infection.**

INVESTIGATIONS

There are many ways that patients can present and as yet there are no clinical examinations or laboratory tests that are absolutely diagnostic of HIV. However, there are some findings, such as leukoplakia of the tongue, that are suggestive of underlying HIV infection. Patients should be questioned regarding high risk behaviours.

TREATMENT

The rheumatological manifestations tend to respond poorly to treatment (Foster *et al.*, 1988). Non-steroidal anti-inflammatory drugs (NSAIDs) may reduce inflammation and pain in some patients but others respond poorly to these measures. Immunosuppressive drugs may be contra-indicated in HIV patients because of the underlying immunological abnormalities. Glucocorticosteroids possibly increase the likelihood of Kaposi's sarcoma (Schulhafer *et al.*, 1987). Azidothymidine (AZT) has been used early in the treatment of HIV infection but it can interact with NSAIDs and paracetamol.

Physiotherapy management will depend on the presenting signs and symptoms.

SJÖGREN'S SYNDROME

Sjögren's syndrome is a chronic, autoimmune disease characterised by inflammation and destruction of the exocrine glands. The salivary and lachrymal glands are primarily affected leading to a dry mouth (xerostomia) and dry eyes (xerophthalmia) but other exocrine glands can be affected.

SS may be a primary condition, or secondary to almost any systemic autoimmune rheumatic disease.

It is the second most frequently occurring auto-immune disease, affecting nine times as many women as men, mainly in the fourth to fifth decade. A total of 3% of women over 55 years have SS (Price & Venables, 1995).

AETIOLOGY AND CLINICAL FEATURES

The aetiology of SS is poorly understood. It is possibly triggered by environmental factors in genetically predisposed individuals. There is focal lymphocytic infiltration of the exocrine glands which starts around the ducts and results in loss of secretory epithelium.

Exocrine gland manifestations of SS:
• Ocular—Dry gritty, red eyes.
• Oral—Dry mouth with dysphagia.

Other sicca symptoms:
• Hoarseness of voice.
• Parotid gland enlargement.
• Skin dryness.
• Vaginal dryness.
• Epistaxis.
• Dryness of mucous membrane of respiratory tract.

Musculo-skeletal:
• Myositis 3%.
• Myalgias.
• Arthralgias 54%.
• Intermittent, non-erosive synovitis.

Reiter's syndrome and undifferentiated seronegative arthritis	
HIV-associated Reiters syndrome (Winchester *et al.*, 1988)	**Undifferentiated seronegative arthritis (Calabrese, 1989)**
Additive pattern of joint involvement: asymmetric oligoarthropathy of lower extremities	Acute onset of oligoarthropathy: lower limb involvement (knees and ankles). No clinical evidence of antecedent infection
Joint inflammation with some joint destruction and radiological evidence of significant marginal erosions	Chronic mild synovitis, normal radiographs
Severe articular and extra-articular manifestations. Severe, sustained enthesopathy	Severe pain and disability. Possibly dactylitis, tendinitis, enthesopathies, painful heels
Type II (inflammatory) synovial fluid	Type I (non-inflammatory) synovial fluid
No sustained remission. Progressive disease course	Duration of symptoms: 1 week to several months
Negative serology for rheumatoid factor and anti-nuclear antibodies. Most patients HLA-B27 positive	

Table 16.2 **Reiter's syndrome and undifferentiated seronegative arthritis.**

TREATMENT

Sjögren's syndrome has many clinical manifestations and there is no single therapeutic approach that can change the natural course of the condition. Treatment of xerophthalmia includes replacement of the missing secretions with artificial tears and local stimulation of tear secretions. Treatment of xerostomia should include prevention of dental caries by strict oral hygiene, saliva substitutes and systemic therapy to stimulate extraglandular secretions . Systemic corticosteroids and immunosuppressive drugs are used to treat severe disease. NSAIDs are beneficial in arthralgias and myalgias.

PHYSIOTHERAPY

Patients with SS will generally be referred for physiotherapy for their musculo-skeletal complaints and treatment will depend on the presenting problem.

CHARCOT'S JOINTS

Charcot's joints and neuropathic joints are terms used interchangeably when referring to an arthritis associated with a sensory deficit (Sequeira, 1994).

There is a male predominance of 3:2 and although it can occur at any age, there is a peak between 35 and 65 years. The joints affected depends on the underlying pathology and the location of sensory loss. Charcot's joints are monoarticular in 70% of cases.

AETIOLOGY AND CLINICAL FEATURES

The exact pathogenesis is not clear. The initiating factors include mechanical trauma, chronic infection or a metabolic disease (Sequeira, 1994) leading eventually to joint destruction. In unstable joints, lack of sensation accelerates joint destruction (Hurley & Newham, 1993). Charcot's joints may occur secondary to neuropathy associated with diabetes, tabes dorsalis, syringomyelia or occasionally spinal cord and peripheral nerve lesions.

About 50% of patients have an acute onset of pain and swelling, lasting for up to 6 months. The remaining 50% have an insidious swelling and instability, with no history of trauma. There may be further inflammatory episodes during the course of the disease. Subsequent progression leads to chronic instability of the joint with crepitus and marked deformity. However, the joint is often pain free and the resultant disability minimal.

INVESTIGATIONS

The erythrocyte sedimentation rate (ESR) is normal and synovial fluid is non-inflammatory. On plain X-ray loss of joint space can be seen with sclerosis of the bone ends, realignment, remodelling and massive osteophytes with resultant deformity, peri-articular calcification and frequently loose bodies in the joint.

TREATMENT

Rest and splinting to protect the joint is indicated in the acute stage. Analgesics for pain relief and NSAIDs are used to control the synovitis. Joints involved may require stabilisation with the use of orthotics. Arthroplasty is not always successful as the lack of proprioception may lead to loosening of the prosthesis. Arthrodesis may fail for the same reason.

Physiotherapy management should include strengthening exercises to improve stability of the affected joint together with balance and proprioceptive work. Splinting may be needed if gross instability is present.

PIGMENTED VILLONODULAR SYNOVITIS

Pigmented villonodular synovitis (PVNS) is a proliferative disorder of unknown aetiology. It results in villous and/or nodular changes in synovial lined joints, tendon sheaths and bursae (Rao & Vigorita, 1984). PVNS may affect the entire synovial membrane, most commonly seen in joints, or a portion of the membrane, usually seen in tendon sheaths. The synovium shows villous and/or nodular proliferation and can invade subchondral bone and produce cysts.

Pigmented villonodular synovitis is most common in the third and fourth decades and affects both sexes equally. It can affect any joint but tends to be unilateral and involve one joint only, the knee being involved in 80% of cases. Digital tendons are the most frequently affected.

CLINICAL PICTURE

Pigmented villonodular synovitis usually presents as a mild intermittent swelling in one joint over a long period of time, eventually becoming chronic and painful. Occasionally there is an acute episode with severe pain and locking of the joint which may be due to torsion and infarction of a nodule.

INVESTIGATIONS

Diagnosis of PVNS depends on synovial biopsy. Plain X-ray may show soft tissue swelling, increased density of synovium and multiple subchondral cysts. Cartilage narrowing is gradual and occurs late in the disease process. Synovial fluid is often dark brown or frankly bloody. Fluid tends to accumulate rapidly after aspiration.

TREATMENT

Total synovectomy is the recommended treatment. Intra-articular radiotherapy has been used following surgery but its use remains controversial (Gumpel & Shawe, 1991).

DIFFUSE IDIOPATHIC SKELETAL HYPEROSTOSIS

Diffuse idiopathic skeletal hyperostosis (DISH) is a generalised spinal and extraspinal disorder characterised by calcification and ossification of attachments of ligaments, tendons and joint capsules (Hoffman *et al.*, 1995).

AETIOLOGY AND CLINICAL FEATURES

The pathogenesis and aetiology are unknown. The hyperostosis results from proliferative enthesopathy, especially of the anterior longitudinal ligament of the spine, periosteal proliferation and ligamentous ossification.

All regions of the spine can be affected, though it is more commonly seen in the lower thoracic spine where ankylosis can occur. There may be bony proliferation or 'whiskering' at tendon and ligament attachments, especially at the iliac crest, ischial tuberosities, attachments of the tendoachilles and plantar fascia on the calcaneus.

Symptoms tend to be minimal compared to the X-ray changes. They include low grade pain and stiffness in the thoraco-lumbar region. Spinal range of movement is generally only mildly diminished in most patients.

INVESTIGATIONS

X-ray findings form the basis for the diagnosis of DISH. Resnick & Niwayama (1988) have delineated three X-ray criteria:

- The presence of flowing calcification and ossification along the anterolateral aspect of at least four contiguous vertebral bodies, with or without associated localised pointed excrescences at the intervening vertebral bodies at the intervertebral disc junction.
- The presence of relative preservation of the intervertebral disc height in the involved vertebral segment and the absence of extensive X-ray changes of 'degenerative' disc disease, including vacuum phenomenon and vertebral body marginal sclerosis.
- The absence of apophyseal joint bony ankylosis and sacroiliac joint erosion, sclerosis or inter-articular osseous fusion.

TREATMENT

Analgesics and NSAIDs are helpful and physiotherapy depends on the presenting symptoms.

ERYTHEMA NODOSUM

Erythema nodosum is an acute, self-limiting condition characterised by the development of tender nodules in the skin. It usually occurs on the anterior tibial surface but may be present on the thighs, forearms, hands and face.

Erythema nodosum can affect any age group and is five times more common in women than in men. It can be associated with sarcoidosis, Behçet's syndrome, malignant disease and drug sensitivities.

AETIOLOGYAND CLINICAL FEATURES

Erythema nodosum is a panniculitis— i.e. an inflammation within the subcutaneous fat. It is considered to be a vasculitis or a hypersensitivity to a number of possible agents. The cutaneous eruptions are rarely more than 5 cm in diameter and resolve in 1–3 months, though recurrences may occur. They rarely ulcerate and resolve leaving a bruised discoloration.

The patient may present with a non-specific systemic illness with a low grade fever, malaise and loss of appetite, or, apart from the skin eruptions, be well. Arthritis which can affect any joint occurs in 50–75% of patients and is usually synchronous with the skin lesions but may precede them by up to 4 weeks. It generally starts in one joint, the knee being affected in 85% of cases, and is usually symmetrical.

INVESTIGATIONS

In the acute stage the ESR may be raised and the latex test is occasionally positive. Routine diagnostic tests are required for possible causative conditions.

TREATMENT

Treatment is symptomatic and detection of the underlying cause is the main consideration. Acute erythema nodosum is self-limiting; therefore conservative treatment is preferable, but NSAIDs may be helpful (Lehman, 1980). Occasionally corticosteroids are used in persistent cases.

PHYSIOTHERAPY

Patients will be referred because of their arthralgia and management will include home pain relieving techniques and joint care. Resting with the lower legs elevated can relieve the pain and swelling of the cutaneous eruptions and surgical stockings are beneficial.

SARCOIDOSIS

Sarcoidosis is a multi-system inflammatory disorder that is characterised by the presence of granulomas in certain organs and particularly involving the lymph nodes, spleen, liver, lungs and joints. It may be acute or chronic.

The true prevalence of sarcoidosis is unknown as many cases are asymptomatic. It is estimated that in the UK there are 20 per 100,000 cases diagnosed a year. It affects three times as many women as men from the age of 15–50 years with a peak at 20–30 years. It is more common in Afro-Caribbeans than Caucasians and may be familial.

AETIOLOGYAND CLINICAL FEATURES

The cause is unknown but there is an inflammatory response which results in the formation of granulomas which may be triggered by an antigen, possibly mycobacterial in origin (O'Connor & Fitzgerald, 1992). Granulomas may resolve spontaneously or slowly undergo fibrosis.

Acute Sarcoidosis

This may present as an explosive illness with fever, erythema nodosum (70%) and hilar lymphadenopathy. Prognosis is good with an 80% remission rate (Neville *et al.*, 1983). A mild, non-erosive arthritis precedes other symptoms in 65% of patients.

Chronic Sarcoidosis

This is less common and is insidious, progressive and runs a variable course. Chest X-rays show extensive parenchymal infiltration which may affect pulmonary function. The arthritis is characterised by synovial thickening and effusions and may progress to joint deformities and joint destruction. Generally it is monoarticular with one knee or ankle being affected.

INVESTIGATIONS

Radiologically, joints are usually normal although cystic changes are occasionally seen in the hands and feet. Chest

X-ray may show hilar lymphadenopathy in 75% and pulmonary infiltration in 50%, while serology shows raised ESR in the acute phase in 60–80%. Pulmonary function tests usually demonstrate restrictive deficits.

TREATMENT

The prognosis is difficult as sarcoidosis has an unpredictable course which depends on the persistence of disease activity and the organ involved. In most cases symptoms are relatively mild and the condition is self-limiting. Treatment is directed toward suppression of the inflammatory response.

Analgesic drugs and NSAIDs are useful for mild arthritis. Glucocorticosteroids are the drugs of choice in persistent cases but immunosuppressive drugs such as methotrexate have also been used successfully (Lower & Baughman, 1995) and there have been trials into the effectiveness of thalidomide (Carlesimo et al., 1995).

Physiotherapy is aimed at relieving the joint manifestations.

REFERENCES

Berman A, Espinoza LR, Diaz JD et al. Rheumatic manifestations of human immunodeficiency virus infection. Am J Med 1988, **85**:59-64.

Buzzard BM, Jones PM. Physiotherapy management of haemophiliacs: an update. Phsiotherapy 1988, **75(5)**:221-226.

Calabrese LH. The rheumatic manifestations of infection with the human immunodeficiency virus. Semin Arthritis Rheum 1989, **18**:225-239.

Carlesimo M, Guistinis S, Ross A et al. Treatment of cutaneous and pulmonary sarcoidosis with thalidomide. J Am Acad Derm 1995, **32**:866-869.

Espinoza LR, Berman A, Vasey FB et al. Psoriatic arthritis and acquired immunodeficiency syndrome. Arthritis Rheum 1988, **31**:1034-1040.

Forster SM, Seifert MH, Keat AC et al. Inflammatory joint disease and human immunodeficiency virus infection. BMJ 1988, 296:1625-1627.

Gottlieb MS, Schroff R, Schanker HM et al. Pneumocystis Carinii: pneumonia and mucosal candidiasis in previously healthy homosexual men: evidence of a new acquired cellular immunodeficiency. N Engl J Med 1981, **305**:1425-1431.

Gumpel JM, Shawe DJ. Diffuse pigmented villonodular synovitis: non-surgical management. Ann Rheum Dis 1991, **50**:531-533.

Hoffman LE, Taylor JAM, Price D et al. Diffuse idiopathic skeletal hyperostosis (DISH), a review of radiographic features and report of four cases. JMPT 1995, **18**:No. 8.

Hurley MV, Newham DJ. The influence of arthrogenous muscle inhibition on quadriceps rehabilitation of patients with early, unilateral osteoarthritic knees. Br J Rheum 1993, **32**:127-131.

Lehman DW. Control of chronic erythema nodosum with Naproxyn. Cutis 1980, **26**:66-67.

Lower EE , Baughman RP. Prolonged use of methotrexate for sarcoidosis. Arch Int Med 1995, **155**:846-851.

Markova I, Forbes CD et al. The haemophilia patient self-perception of changes in health and lifestyle arising from self-treatment. International Journal of Rehabilitation Reasearch 1983, **6(11)**:11-18.

Neville E, Walker AN, James DG. Diagnostic factors predicting the outcome of sarcoidosis: an analysis of 818 patients. Quart J Med 1983, **208**:525-533.

O'Connor CM, Fitzgerald MX. Speculations on sarcoidosis. Resp Med 1992, **86**:277-282.

Price EJ, Venables PJ. The aetiopathogenesis of Sjögren's syndrome (SS). Sem Arthritis Rheum 1995, **25**:117-133.

Rao AS, Vigorita VJ. Pigmented villonodular synovits (giant cell tumour of the tendon sheath and synovial membrane) A review of 81 cases. J Bone Joint Surg 1984, **66A**:76-94.

Resnick D, Niwayama G. Diagnosis of bone and joint disorders, 2nd edition. Philadelphia: WB Saunders;1988:1563-1600.

Rowe IF, Forster SM et al. Rheumatic lesions in individuals with human immunodeficiency virus (HIV) infection. Br J Rheumatol 1988, **27**:1.

Rowe IF, Keat ACS. Human immunodeficiency virus infection and the rheumatologist. Ann Rheum Dis 1989, **48**:89-91.

Schulhafer EP, Gossamn ME, Fagin G etal. Steroid induced Kaposi's sarcoma in patient with pre-AIDS. Am J Med 1987, **82**:313-331.

Sequeira W. The neuropathic joint. Clin Exp Rheum 1994, **12**:325-337.

Winchester R, Bernstein DH, Fischer HD et al. The co-occurrence of Reiter's syndrome in acquired immunodeficiency. Ann Int Med 1988, **106**:19-26.

SECTION 4

THE HAND AND FOOT IN SPECIFIC RHEUMATIC CONDITIONS

rheumatology (roo′mat·ol·o·je). Branch of medicine which is concerned with the diagnosis and treatment of rheumatic disorders.

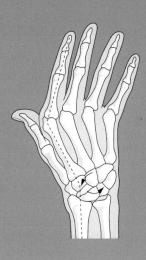

17

D Lloyd

THE HAND IN RHEUMATOLOGY

CHAPTER OUTLINE

- Hand assessment
- Hand involvement in RA
- Common deformities in RA

- Hand involvement in other rheumatological conditions
- Pre-operative assessment
- Surgical outcomes

INTRODUCTION

The hand is the most specialised set of joints in the body. It can perform an infinite number of activities, all of which are group movements learnt gradually. Imagine the number of complex movements required by the hand in a daily routine of washing, dressing, using cutlery, writing, sorting coins etc.

The hand's greatest attribute is, however, its exquisite sensitivity. The fingertip pulp is capable of discriminating between two points no more than 2–3 mm apart and the whole hand has the ability to differentiate between an amazing number of textures and identify objects the eye cannot see.

This chapter covers hand involvement in various rheumatological conditions, causes of typical deformities, hand assessment and common surgical procedures.

HAND ASSESSMENT

Hand function may be virtually normal despite severe deformities (Souter, 1979, Towheed & Anastassiades, 1994). Functional assessment is the only way of judging the significance of deformities.

Hand assessment aims to identify the extent and detail of limitations, and to provide a baseline for treatment (exercise, splintage, surgery). It is also used to set, evaluate and modify treatment goals and provide a tool for research and audit.

ASSESSMENT PRINCIPLES

A systematic and thorough hand assessment requires a good knowledge of anatomy and skill in functional analysis of the problem. Assessing hand function requires examination of the entire upper limb, including the elbow and shoulder but particularly the cervical spine. Both upper limbs need to be assessed too, as disability in one limb may be compensated for by the other side.

Compensatory movements may have developed to make activities of daily living (ADL) easier. If they enable independence to be maintained they should not be discouraged unless they are causing excessive joint strain, wasting important muscles or could result in irretrievable loss of range of movement (ROM) though misuse.

Patients are primarily interested in their ability to perform daily functions. A hand assessment should therefore look at pure movement and grip patterns, comparing these to the patient's own adaptive methods, in order to analyse the degree of any difficulty experienced.

Patients should be reassured that the assessment is not a test which they could fail by clearly explaining the aims of the assessment and what will happen.

The understanding of functional problems is directly influenced by the quality of the information gathered. Therefore, standardised assessment methods, instruments and forms are to be recommended. The use of instruments which have been shown to measure precisely, accurately and consistently allows the therapist to interpret facts gathered objectively rather than making assumptions about the patient's condition. Assessment should include:

Observation:
• Posture of the hand and upper limb.
• Oedema.
• Scars from previous surgery.
• Muscle wasting.
• Deformity.
• Condition of the skin and nails.

Palpation:
• Skin temperature.
• Tissue elasticity.
• Synovitis.
• Pain.
• Tenderness.
• Soft tissue/joint stiffness.

OBJECTIVE TESTS
Pain Scales
For total hand pain, a 100 mm visual analogue scale (VAS) can be used (Scott & Huskisson, 1979). The line is marked to indicate the severity of pain ranging from no pain to the worst pain imaginable. The patient's opinion of joint stiffness can be recorded in the same way.

Range of Movement
There are two methods which can be used to measure ROM.

Measurement in Millimetres (Dellhag *et al.*, 1992)
• Flexion—the distance between the distal palmar crease and each fingertip is measured.
• Extension—with the hand resting supinated on a table, the distance between the table and the nail bed is recorded.
• Abduction—measuring from the thumb tip to the little fingertip with the hand flat, palm down, on a table.

This method has a greater margin for error and is not joint specific, but it is useful for patients to learn to monitor their own ROM.

Goniometer Recordings
• May be taken on either in the dorsal or lateral aspect of a joint, the latter being preferred in the presence of swelling. Consistency of instrument placing is vital.
• Neutral is 0°. It is recommended that hyperextension be recorded as a negative value, making an extension lag a plus value (Fess & Moran, 1980).
• Active and passive motion at each joint should be recorded.

• As proximal joint posture influences distal motion, the position of the elbow, forearm and wrist should be standardised.

Total motion of a digit may also be recorded, along with individual measurements, giving a single number which represents the summation of joint flexion minus the summation of extension deficits. This method facilitates easier comparison of digital movement.

Grip Strength
A sensitive indicator of hand involvement in rheumatoid arthritis (RA) as muscular contraction causes ligamentous tightening around joints, compressing the inflamed synovium, resulting in weakness, with or without pain (Helliwell *et al.*, 1987).

Standardisation, Reliability and Validity of Grip Strength Measurement
The American Society of Hand Therapists has suggested standardising the position of the arm for testing (Fess & Moran, 1980). The patient should be seated with the shoulder adducted and neutrally rotated, elbow flexed to 90° and the forearm and wrist in neutral. No significant difference in grip strength has been noted in wrists positioned between 0° and 15° ulnar deviation and between 0° and 30° extension; however, 15° of flexion significantly reduces strength (Kraft & Detels, 1972).

To improve reliability and validity of testing, the following methods are recommended (Fess & Moran, 1980):
• Standardised positioning and instruction.
• The average of three trials should be used.
• The instrument should measure precisely, accurately and consistently.
• The calibration of the instrument should be checked regularly.
• Scores obtained should be compared to the appropriate age and sex category of normative values for the same instrument.
• The same test instrument should be used for follow-up testing.

Various testing devices are available. The following is a summary of some in current use.

Sphygmomanometer/Pneumodynamometer
These devices involve compression of an air or fluid filled bag. Reproducibility of measurements is limited due to difficulties in exactly replicating the grip position and calibrating the device (Nordenskiold & Grimby, 1993).

Martin Vigorometer
This is an aneroid manometer connected to three different sized rubber bulbs to fit small, medium and large hands. Reliability has been questioned as it has been found that it is difficult for patients with RA to grip the bulb in the same way on different occasions (Jones *et al.*, 1991).

Jamar Dynamometer

Grip is measured by squeezing the handle of the instrument which does not move. As the Jamar is a heavy instrument, rheumatoid patients may require support under the base of the instrument while they grip. These instruments only record maximum grip at a certain moment in time. It is of far more interest, when assessing the rheumatoid hand, to know the rate of development of the grip and what happens to that grip over time.

Grippit Instrument

An electronic instrument which has an arm support and guide to ensure standardisation of positioning (Nordenskiold & Grimby, 1993). It has adjustable handles and is attached to a computer giving three readings:
• The maximum value for a 10-second sustained grip.
• The mean value.
• The value for the final 0.5-second period.

Torsion Dynamometer/Digital Analyser

This device is linked to a microprocessor. Two cushioned handles are squeezed together or pinched at their ends. It provides a more detailed analysis of a timed grip, showing:
• Maximum grip.
• Time to maximum grip.
• Rate of loss of grip from maximum value to the point of release—called the fatigue rate.

The results of grip strength tests in rheumatoid patients are more significant when compared to the general population. Mathiowetz et al. (1985) have produced normative data for adults using the Jamar Dynamometer and found a high correlation between grip strength and age. Helliwell et al. (1987) compared normative results with rheumatoid patients using the Torsion Dynamometer and found that rheumatoid patients have 25% of the normal maximum grip strength with a reduction in pinch strength of approximately 40%. Time to maximum grip strength was also significantly reduced and the patient group showed considerably more fatigue.

Oedema Measurements

Measuring around the proximal interphalangeal joints (PIPJs) can be done with either a tape measure marked in centimetres, a finger circumference gauge marked in centimetres (McKnight & Kwoh, 1992), or ring sizers used in jewellery shops.

Total hand oedema can be measured using the Volumetrics test. This measures the whole hand to the wrist by measuring the amount of water displaced from a graduated volumeter (Fess & Moran, 1980).

Joint Deformity Score (Sharma et al., 1994)

All finger joints are scored according to the scale:
0 no deformity/instability.
1 ligamentous instability, lateral band or intrinsic shortening.
2 actively reducible deformity.
3 fixed or only passively reducible deformity.

The thumb and metacarpophalangeal joint (MCPJ) ulnar drift are scored as follows:
0 no deformity.
1 presence of deformity.

An overall deformity score is produced by adding together all scores for each hand.

Activities of Daily Living Score

The most widely used is the Stanford Health Assessment Questionnaire (HAQ) (Fries et al., 1980). This has since been modified by Kirwan & Reeback (1986). The 15 questions concerning activities specific to hand function can be administered using the 0–3 grading scale:
0 without any difficulty.
1 with some difficulty.
2 with much difficulty.
3 unable to perform.

The overall score is the sum of all the individual scores divided by the total number of tasks. This gives an indication of the patient's level of function, but it does not look at the underlying reasons for any difficulties. In order to do this, a functional assessment is required.

Functional Assessments

There are two main types of assessment:
• Quantitative—counts number of tasks performed in a set time.
• Qualitative—looks at the way the task is performed.

Within these groups there are many types of hand function assessments available (Dent et al., 1985), ranging from standardised to non-standardised. Only two examples of standardised tests will be described here.

Jebson Hand Function Test (Jebson et al., 1969)

This is one of the most widely used tests in general research, consisting of the timed performance by either hand of seven tasks:
• Writing a short sentence.
• Turning over 3 × 5" cards.
• Picking up small objects and placing them in a container.
• Stacking draughts.
• Simulated eating.
• Moving empty large cans.
• Moving weighted large cans.

The O'Neill Hand Function Test (O'Neill, 1995)

A more recent test which looks at the speed in which a task is performed (using any method) and also the manner in which it is performed using strict guidelines. There is also a non-prehension section looking at tasks which are essential to ADL but do not involve gripping. It consists of eight tasks:
• Picking up coins.
• Picking up pins.
• Lifting up plates.

- Picking up and turning piping.
- Picking up a tennis ball.
- Lifting blocks and handles.
- Bringing hand to mouth.
- Tapping keyboard.

This chapter will now consider various rheumatological conditions, describing briefly the development of deformities and possible surgical options for correction, before looking at the role of pre-operative assessment of the hand and outlining some outcomes of common surgical procedures.

HAND INVOLVEMENT IN RHEUMATOID ARTHRITIS

Rheumatoid arthritis in the hands primarily affects the synovium which is found in all the joints and around the flexor and extensor tendons and their sheaths. It can affect six anatomical structures in the hand leading to deformity: skin, muscle, nerves, tendons, joints and blood vessels.

In the early stages deformities could be reversible and this is where hand therapy can be most effective, particularly splinting and exercise. See Chapter 6 for more details.

Rheumatoid nodules may be found in the hand, particularly over bony prominences exposed to pressure. Common sites include the ulnar side of the hand and wrist, the dorsum of the fingers, any bony prominences created by a subluxed joint and, less commonly, on the palmar surface of the hand.

JOINT INVOLVEMENT
In the early stages the inflammation affects the synovium of the wrist, MCPJs, PIPJs and thumb interphalangeal joints (IPJs) (Figure 17.1). The resulting synovitis can lead to joint instability due to stretching and weakening of the ligaments and joint capsule. In the later stages joints may sublux and lose ROM due to soft tissue contractures, adverse tendon biomechanics, joint instability and muscle weakness.

MUSCLE INVOLVEMENT
The first dorsal interosseous often shows marked atrophy as a result of disuse, evidenced by the deep concavity on the dorsal aspect of the first webspace and the prominence of the second metacarpal head. If this muscle has wasted, it can be assumed the other interossei are affected.

Intrinsic muscle tightness may be the result of a protective reflex muscle spasm due to pain and swelling in the MCPJs which can cause contracture if prolonged or secondary to fixed flexion deformity of the MCPJs.

Muscle tightness contributes to joint deformities such as swan neck, ulnar drift and MCP flexion deformities. It also weakens power grip and reduces dexterity.

TENDON INVOLVEMENT
Tenosynovitis is common in RA and can have a marked impact upon function. The gliding of tendons within their sheaths is impeded and pain, swelling, crepitus and loss of function will be evident (Chandani, 1986). The end result can be rupture of the weakened tendon. Pain from flexor tenosynovitis is often severe and worse than that in joints. Morning stiffness is common (Towheed & Anastassiades, 1994).

Flexor Tenosynovitis
Tenosynovitis may occur at the wrist, palm or fingers. In the wrist it presents as a smooth, contoured swelling proximal to the volar wrist crease which can be seen to move proximally as the fingers flex. Symptoms which may be present are pain throughout the hand, and carpal tunnel syndrome. Loss of flexor tendon excursion leads to loss of active finger flexion and passive extension. Tenosynovitis in the palm and fingers can result in volar swelling over the proximal phalanges and possibly loss of flexor tendon excursion.

Trigger Finger
This is a snapping or catching of a finger during active flexion or extension resulting from a nodule, tenosynovium or thickened tendon becoming trapped at either the proximal, middle or distal flexor pulley. It presents in one of the following ways:
- A slight catch or snap during movement.
- Inconsistency in the degree of active movement.
- Palpable crepitus with tendon motion.
- An inability actively to extend or flex a finger completely.

In the early stages it is usually annoying rather than painful. As the lump grows bigger though, the catching can become painful and the finger can become locked in a flexed position so that extension involves a painful click, or may be impossible without assistance from the other hand. Triggering can occur in more than one finger at a time and is most common at the MCPJs.

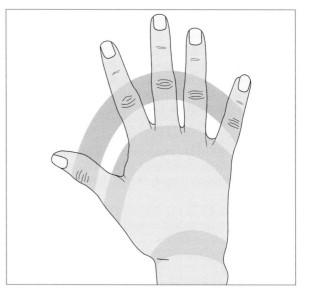

Figure 17.1 Common areas of synovitis.

Dorsal Wrist Tenosynovitis

The extensor tendons pass beneath their retinaculum in six compartments, any of which may be affected by tenosynovitis (Towheed & Anastassiades, 1994). The condition presents as a soft, non-tender mass either side of the extensor retinaculum which moves during active finger motion, so differentiating itself from wrist synovitis. Most commonly affected are the compartments of extensor carpi ulnari and extensor digitorum communis (EDC). Tenosynovitis in the compartment containing extensor carpi ulnaris may cause its supporting ligaments to stretch and allow volar displacement of the tendon which then becomes a major force in volar subluxation of the wrist (Figure 17.2).

DeQuervain's Disease

Inflammation of the first compartment containing extensor pollicis brevis and abductor pollicis brevis is usually painful. It is particularly important to detect as it causes severe discomfort and is easily treated. Pain can be demonstrated using Frinklestein's test—fully flex and adduct the thumb, then place the wrist into ulnar deviation to reproduce the pain. Splintage can be effective in reducing pain and swelling; however, immobilisation can increase stiffness and swelling. A local corticosteroid injection is also usually beneficial.

Tendon Rupture

There are two methods by which tendons rupture:
- Attrition or fraying of the tendon over diseased bone, e.g. extensor pollicis longus over Lister's tubercle on the dorsum of the radius.
- Intrinsic disease—rheumatoid pannus infiltrates the tendon causing it to weaken and eventually rupture.

The extensor tendons rupture more frequently than the flexor tendons due to the way they run across the carpal bones. Listed below is the order of frequency for tendon rupture:
- Extensor digiti minimi (EDM).
- Extensor digitorium communis (EDC).
- Flexor pollicis longus (FPL).
- Flexor digitorium superficialis (FDS).

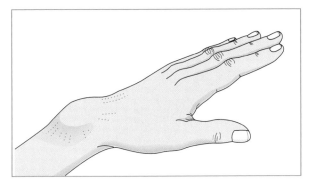

Figure 17.2 Volar subluxation of the wrist.

Extensor Tendon Ruptures

Tendon rupture presents as drooping of the affected finger at the MCP as the action of the intrinsics, which extend the IPJs and flex the MCPs, is unopposed by the extensors (Burke, 1995). It is most commonly seen in the little finger due to fraying of the extensor tendon over the ulnar styloid. Left untreated, the ring, middle and eventually index extensor tendons may all follow suit.

Flexor Tendon Ruptures

Usually seen at the wrist involving FPL, flexor digitorum profundus and FDS to the index finger. Flexor pollicis longus ruptures due to attrition from osteophytes on the scapho–trapezial joint whist the others rupture from pannus infiltration (Burke, 1995).

MANAGEMENT

Tenosynovectomy

Excision of diseased synovium can relieve the pain of soft tissue swelling, improve function and prevent tendon rupture (Wynn Parry & Stanley, 1993). Rehabilitation following tenosynovectomy is far simpler than following tendon rupture; therefore patients at risk of rupture should be referred for this safe and effective procedure as early as possible (Towheed & Anastassiades, 1994).

Chemical Synovectomy

Local corticosteroid injections into areas of persistent tenosynovitis are useful and can delay the need for surgery. The greatest risk is tendon rupture; therefore injections should be placed into the tenosynovium rather than the tendon.

Dorsal Wrist Tenosynovectomy

Dorsal wrist tenosynovectomy may be performed for failure of medical treatment after 3–6 months, tendon rupture(s), pain, combined with a Darrach's procedure or as a prophylactic measure to prevent tendon rupture.

Flexor Tenosynovectomy

May be performed for nerve compression, for example, combined with carpal tunnel decompression, triggering, rupture(s) or as prophylactic surgery to prevent tendon rupture if 3–6 months' medical treatment has failed to relieve the symptoms.

Trigger Finger

Particular attention must be paid to removal of the nodules causing triggering. The A1 pulley at the entrance to the flexor sheath must always be preserved as its excision can increase the ulnar movement of the flexor tendons on the MCPJs. Where synovectomy does not eliminate triggering, one slip of Flexor Digitorum Superficialis can be excised to allow more space within the sheath.

Tendon Grafting and Transfers

Often, with tendon ruptures, the proximal end retracts and it is not possible to perform an end-to-end repair, therefore tendon grafting or transfers may be considered. Tendon grafting is required when too much length has been destroyed to allow direct repair. Power remains in the motor unit of the muscle used for the donor tendon and therefore movements often have to be re-learnt.

Extensor Tendons
These include:
- Donor tendons—extensor indicis proprius.
- Flexor digitorium superficialis (FDS).
- Palmaris longus.

Common Transfers
These include:
- Extensor carpi radialis to extensor carpi ulnaris.
- Extensor indicis proprius to extensor pollicis longus.
- Extensor digiti minimi (EDM) to extensor indicis proprius.
- For extensor digitorium communis (EDC).

The little finger tendon is most commonly ruptured. The distal end of the tendon is sutured to adjacent extensor if undamaged—called side to side or piggy back transfer (Osterman & Hood, 1991). A single motor can act effectively for two fingers but not for three (Burke, 1995); therefore if there are also ruptures to the ring, middle or index fingers then more complex surgery is required often using extensor indicis proprius for a transfer or a tendon graft.

Flexor Tendons
Ruptures within the digital sheath cause problems because of the risk of adhesions. Protocols depend upon which tendon has ruptured:
- Flexor digitorum profundus only—excise the tendon and fuse the distal interphalangeal joint (DIPJ).
- Flexor digitorium superficialis (FDS) only—excision of the tendon and a tenosynovectomy of flexor digitorum profundus. Repair of FDS may only serve to increase the risk of adhesions without improving function.
- Both FDS and flexor digitorum profundus—common in the index finger—fusion of both IPJs and strengthening of the intrinsics for MCPJ flexion can provide a stable post for pinch grip, writing, etc.
- Ruptures at the wrist:
  Graft.
  Side to side transfer.
  DIPJ fusion if only flexor digitorum profundus involved.
  Tenodesis.
- FPL rupture:
  Donor is either FDS to the ring finger or palmaris longus, both of which have the required excursion (Burke, 1995).
  IPJ arthrodesis if MCPJ mobile.

The complex and multi-factorial mechanisims for the development of deformities in RA will now be outlined briefly.

COMMON DEFORMITIES IN RA

These include:
- Volar subluxation of the wrist.
- Radial deviation of the wrist.
- Ulnar deviation of the MCPJs.
- Volar subluxation of the MCPJs.
- Swan neck deformity of the fingers or thumb.
- Boutonnière deformity of the fingers or thumb.
- Lateral deviation of any IPJ.
- Prominent ulnar styloid.

The Z Collapse Principle
This principle underlies the development of many hand deformities (Osterman & Hood, 1991). When a deformity develops at one joint, the adjacent joints will adopt the opposite position, e.g. radial deviation at the wrist and ulnar deviation of the MCPJs (Figure 17.3). This is caused by the changes in the mechanical advantages of the tendons acting upon joints and the increased loading on the adjacent joints.

WRIST DEFORMITIES
The wrist is the key joint involved in hand function—a painful wrist can prevent the hand from functioning.

Wrist Joint Synovitis
Wrist joint synovitis causes pressure within the carpal spaces destroying ligaments, tendons and articular cartilage (Towheed & Anastassiades, 1994). Erosion of the ulnar styloid is common in RA. Integrity of the distal radio–ulnar joint (DRUJ) is destroyed by synovitis which also stretches the distal radio–ulnar ligament and ulnar collateral ligament (UCL) leading to rupture (Osterman & Hood, 1991). The ulnar head springs up dorsally where it 'floats' and can be easily depressed only to spring back up again ('piano key' sign). This is called a prominent ulnar

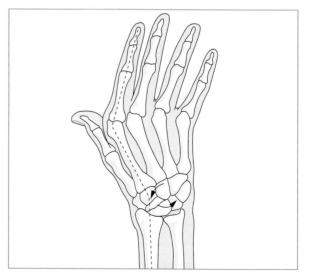

Figure 17.3 Z collapse principle.

styloid. Pronation and supination are painful and there is imminent danger of extensor tendon rupture.

Volar Subluxation/Dislocation of the Carpus on the Radius

As a result of ligament stretching due to chronic synovitis, and possibly also volar subluxation of extensor carpi ulnaris, the proximal row of carpal bones sublux in a volar direction. In severe cases, the carpus may dislocate completely beneath the radius.

Radial Deviation

There are three main mechanisms causing radial deviation:
- Chronic synovitis weakens the triangular fibrocartilage on the ulna side of the wrist allowing the carpus to slide down the distal radius which has a natural incline towards the ulna. The proximal row of carpal bones sublux in an ulnar direction, hence the term 'ulnar translocation of the carpus' and the distal row react by rotating radially. If erosive synovitis continues, the radio–carpal joint can dislocate at a marked 90° angle.
- Scapho-lunate dissociation caused by stretching of the ligament between the two carpal bones allowing a gap to appear. This instability results in the lunate and the rest of the carpus migrating in an ulnar direction and the scaphoid in a radial direction.
- Dislocation of extensor carpi ulnaris in a volar direction resulting in an over pull by extensor carpi radialis and extensor carpi radialis brevis.

Spontaneous Fusion

Progressive disease causes loss of joint space and bone, resulting in a shortened, fused carpus.

WRIST SURGERY

Some of the more common procedures will be described here.

Synovectomy

Surgical synovectomy is difficult due to the large area and complexity of the wrist joint (Burke, 1995). Chemical synovectomy is often the preferred option.

Ulnar Head Excision (Darrach Procedure)

Indications for this are a prominent ulnar styloid, painful forearm rotation or an unstable DRUJ.

Radio-Lunate Fusion (Chamay Fusion)

Removes all movement from the radio–lunate joint but permits mid-carpal motion of approximately 40°. Indications for a Chamay fusion are ulnar translocation of the carpus, radio–carpal deterioration being more pronounced than mid-carpal disease with useful movement remaining in the wrist joint.

Arthroplasty

The Swanson silastic flexible spacer was introduced in 1970 and is a cementless prosthesis. It is still one of the most frequently used wrist replacements (Burke, 1995) as it is easily revised to a fusion if required.

Indications

These include:
- Chronic wrist synovitis with subluxation/dislocation.
- Stiffness or fusion in a non-functional position.
- More movement required for function.

Good candidates for this procedure (Osterman & Hood, 1991) are:
- Those who no longer do heavy manual work.
- Those with bilateral wrist disease:
  non-dominant wrist—fuse for increased power and stability.
  dominant wrist—replace for improved movement and precision.

It is a non-weightbearing joint so careful patient selection is vital. The maximum recommended movement post-operatively is (Burke, 1995):
- 30° flexion.
- 30° extension.
- 15° ulnar deviation.
- 5° radial deviation.

Arthrodesis

Wrist fusion is a time-honoured, predictable and functional procedure. It is strong, stable and quick. The relief of pain and improved stability gained often result in better hand function and grip strength. Arthrodesis is preferable to arthroplasty:
- Where carpal bones cannot accept the implant.
- Where extensor tendons have ruptured.
- According to the surgeon's preference.
- According to the patient's physical status and functional needs.

Indications

These include (Burke, 1995):
- Severe pain.
- Restricted ROM or a stiff wrist in flexion.
- Rupture of the wrist extensors.
- Marked instability.
- Failure of replacement.
- Requirement for long-term walking aid use.
- Progressive disease.

Position of Fusion

This should be agreed between the patient, therapist and surgeon and tailored to ADL, occupational and hobby requirements. Whether it is to be a unilateral or bilateral fusion is relevant, along with hand dominance issues. The neutral is the best position for overall function but dorsi-flexion may be used to improve power. Palmar flexion is the worst overall functional position and can only be recommended if the hand's sole use is to reach the perineum.

ULNAR DEVIATION OF THE MCPJs
Predisposing Factors for Ulnar Drift
There are five predisposing factors for ulnar drift:
- The anatomy of the metacarpal head is such that the radial condyle is larger so creating a slope towards the ulnar side and the ulnar collateral ligament is stronger than the radial collateral ligament.
- The hand has a natural tendency towards ulnar drift as the hypothenar muscles rotate the little finger into ulnar deviation in order to produce a strong power grip. The ulnar interossei are stronger than the radial interossei. The ring and little finger flexor tendons cross the MCPJs from an ulnar angle helping to create an oblique power grip.
- There is an imbalance between the strength of the radial and ulnar intrinsic muscles as the radial side of the hand is constructed for precision activities and the ulnar side for power.
- All functional activities which include MCPJ flexion increase the ulnar forces over the joints.
- Radial deviation of the wrist results in a Z deformity as the hand attempts to keep the index finger in line with the radius.

Pathology of Ulnar Drift
Synovitis at the MCPJs causes stretching of the joint capsule, volar plate and collateral ligaments. The ligaments maintaining the location of the extensor tendons over the dorsum of the MCPJs are destroyed, allowing the extensor tendons to slip in the direction of the ulna and eventually displace into the webspace. This begins with the little finger extensor tendon and can result in these tendons becoming weak flexors if they pass the fulcrum of the joint (Figure 17.4).

Annular ligaments hold the flexor tendons in place at the MCPJs. If these are weakened by synovitis the tendon can slip in an ulnar direction, creating a strong deviating force. Later, the unopposed flexor tendons can pull the fingers in a volar direction, shortening the intrinsics and further stretching the extensor tendons.

Volar subluxation is caused by the resulting imbalance of the soft tissues and can progress to dislocation with the joints becoming completely flail. This is seen as a palpable 'step' over the dorsum of the joints (Figure 17.5).

Pain and stretch on the joint capsule can cause reflex muscle spasm of the intrinsics which contract; therefore even passive extension is impossible. The first dorsal interosseous weakens due to disuse and is unable to abduct and supinate the index finger to the thumb. Therefore, lateral pinch grip is often the only remaining effective grip.

The unbalanced hypothenar muscles frequently pull the proximal phalanx of the little finger into 90° of ulnar deviation and so into complete dislocation.

MCPJ SURGERY
Synovectomy
Indications
- Persistent pain and swelling, despite adequate medical treatment.
- Early erosions seen on X-ray.
- Near normal ROM.
- Displacement of the extensor tendons with synovitis—the radial extensor hood can be tightened (reefed) following synovectomy.

Soft Tissue Reconstruction
Where there is little bony damage this procedure may slow down the progression of the condition in patients with less active or well controlled disease. Prognosis is related to disease activity—progressive disease will overtake surgery in approximately 2 years.

Procedure
- Synovectomy.
- Relocation of dislocated extensor tendons.
- Reefing of extensor tendons.
- Reefing of radial collateral ligament (RCL) and removal of UCL.

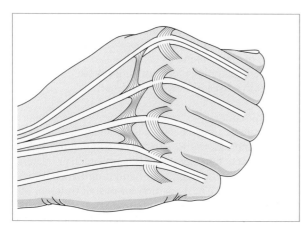

Figure 17.4 Extensor tendons over dorsum of metacarpophalangeal joints.

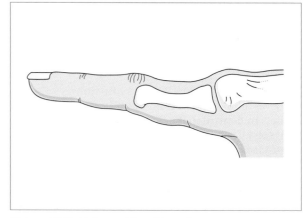

Figure 17.5 Volar subluxation of metacarpophalangeal joints.

- Sometimes also includes division or cross intrinsic transfer of abductor digiti minimi—move to become little finger adductor.
- Relocation of insertion of first dorsal interosseous distally may also be performed to provide more leverage for index finger abduction.

Prosthetic Arthroplasty

Indications
- Pain.
- Ulnar drift not amenable to soft tissue repair alone.
- Subluxation/dislocation of MCPJs severely limiting function.
- Stiff MCPJs in a non-functional position.

Before surgery can be performed there must be an intact neurovascular supply, intact flexor and extensor tendons, adequate bone density to accept implant and no infection.

Aims of Surgery
- Mid-line correction with stability.
- ROM of approximately 40–60°. Ideally 60–65° at the index finger and middle finger, whilst the ring finger and little finger require 70° to form an oblique power grip.
- Pain relief.
- Improved cosmesis—very important to patients.

Patient Selection
Patients must be able to understand the expectations of surgery. They will have a different ROM post-operatively. Ideally, the post-operative ROM or slightly less would still give functional improvement. For example, if a patient only has a range of 60–90° MCPJ flexion pre-operatively, changing this to 10–60° will take time for adjustment and may not produce the same degree of grip strength, thus preventing the patient from being able to flex the MCPJs fully. Good PIPJ movement can compensate for loss of full MCPJ flexion and therefore produce better results. However, the ability to open the hand will allow the patient to grasp many more objects than pre-operatively. Patients must also be able to comply with the detailed and lengthy post-operative regime as 50% of the result is dependent upon therapy (Souter, 1979).

Consideration must also be given to the limited lifespan of the prosthesis—very active patients will place greater strain on the implants and so require revision or salvage.

MCPJ Implants
There are two main designs:
- Swanson.
- Niebaur, also known as 'Sutter'.

Encapsulation Process
The joint capsule will completely re-grow around the implant within 6–8 weeks. The aim of therapy is to influence the collagen to form strong, straight fibres as it matures in order to produce stability and suppleness.

Post-operative Rehabilitation
Night splintage in extension and a dynamic outrigger for day use will usually be used for at least 6 weeks. The night splint is often maintained for between 3 and 6 months. These splints maintain the correct alignment of the joints at all times, whilst the encapsulation process takes place to ensure ligaments and the reforming capsule strengthen in the correct manner. Exercises are performed within the outrigger to strengthen the extensors and flexors, whilst exercises to strengthen the intrinsics are performed out of the splint.

Patient Education
Patients must be advised that there must be no active, functional use of their hand, other than for personal care and eating, for 6 weeks. They must not perform a lateral pinch as this can dislocate the implant. They should be given joint protection advice and be taught how to retrain the functional use of their hand once the outrigger is removed.

BOUTONNIÈRE DEFORMITY
The lateral bands of EDC separate like a buttonhole (Boutonnière) to allow the PIPJ to protrude between them (Figure 17.6).

Pathology
Synovitis weakens the extensor hood allowing the lateral bands to dislocate in a volar direction, crossing the axis of the joint so becoming PIPJ flexors. They are shortened by this displacement, and therefore increased pull is exerted on their distal insertion which hyperextends the DIPJ. As FDS is unopposed, the collateral ligaments quickly contract and a fixed flexion deformity develops.

Boutonnière deformity may also be caused by lengthening or rupture of the central slip. This forces EDC to transmit all of its power into the lateral bands which hyperextend the DIPJ. Later, the MCPJ hyperextends in an attempt to open the hand to improve grasp of objects. Nalebuff et al. (1988) classified Boutonnière deformities as:
- Mild—flexible and actively correctable.
- Moderate—intact joint space and passively correctable extension.
- Severe—joint destruction or fixed flexion deformity.

BOUTONNIÈRE CORRECTIONS
(Nalebuff et al. 1975a, Osterman & Hood, 1991)

Mild Deformity
- Synovectomy.
- Extensor tendon reefing and release of the terminal tendon proximal to the DIPJ.

Moderate Deformity
Tightening of the central slip and relocating the lateral bands dorsally to restore PIPJ extension. This can be combined with an extensor tenotomy at the DIPJ to correct hyperextension.

Severe Deformity

Options include:

- Extensor mechanism reconstruction and tenotomy.
- PIPJ arthroplasty and extensor mechanism reconstruction.
- Arthrodesis in a functional position for fixed flexion deformities greater than 70–80° and ruptured tendons. PIPJ arthroplasty is more appropriate for the ring finger and little finger, whilst index finger function is improved by the stability of a fusion.

SWAN NECK DEFORMITIES

Swan neck deformities—flexion of the DIPJ and MCPJ with hyperextension of the PIPJ—are present in 28% of rheumatoid hands and represent significant grip and functional loss, particularly if in conjunction with a thumb deformity (Nalebuff *et al.*, 1988). The deformity can occur as a result of synovitis in any of the joints (Figure 17.7).

Metacarpophalangeal Joint

The most common cause of swan necking, where chronic synovitis results in reflex intrinsic muscle spasm. This leads to shortening of these muscles causing MCPJ flexion to persist during attempted extension, thus increasing the tension on the dorsal extensor hood forcing the lateral bands to slip dorsally and hyperextend the PIPJ. This is exacerbated by any PIPJ disease which may stretch the volar plate or small ligaments maintaining the position of the lateral bands.

Interphalangeal Joint

Synovitis of the PIPJ is the least likely cause of swan necking since this usually results in a Boutonnière deformity as the synovium herniates dorsally and stretches the central slip. However, chronic synovitis can cause stretching of the volar plate and rupture of the insertion of FDS predisposing the PIPJ to hyperextension as the extensors are unopposed.

Chronic synovitis can cause rupture of the insertion of EDC into the distal phalanx resulting in a mallet finger deformity. The PIPJ becomes hyperextended due to the subsequent imbalance between the long flexors and extensors. In the late stages, intrinsic contracture, stretching of the PIPJ volar plate and capsule, collateral ligament shortening, tight skin and tension in flexor digitorum profundus lead to a fixed deformity.

Nalebuff *et al.* (1988) divided swan neck deformities into four categories based on joint mobility and X-ray appearance:

- Type I—flexible deformity; actively and passively correctable.
- Type II—as Type I but with intrinsic tightness.
- Type III—stiff joints but without destruction.
- Type IV—stiffness and joint destruction.

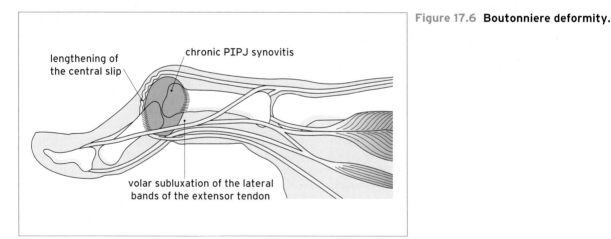

Figure 17.6 Boutonniere deformity.

lengthening of the central slip

chronic PIPJ synovitis

volar subluxation of the lateral bands of the extensor tendon

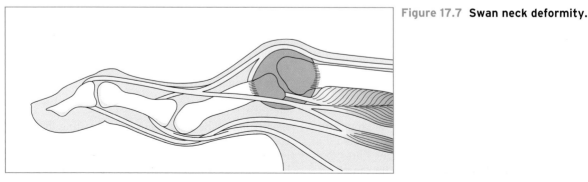

Figure 17.7 Swan neck deformity.

SWAN NECK CORRECTIONS
(Nalebuff & Millender, 1975b)

Type I—Swan Neck with Full PIPJ Flexion
- Chemical synovectomy.
- Dermadesis—removal of volar wedge of skin at the PIPJ to prevent hyperextension.
- Flexor tenodesis—slip of FDS relocated to hold the PIPJ in 20° flexion.
- Retinacular ligament reconstruction to restore DIPJ extension and prevent PIPJ hyperextension.
- DIPJ fusion in 5–10° flexion.

Type II—Flexible Deformity with Intrinsic Tightness
As for Type I, plus intrinsic release in order to eliminate lateral band tightness.

Type III—PIPJ Contracture and Intact Cartilage
- Manipulation under anaesthetic (MUA) and Kirschner wiring (K-wire) for 3 weeks performed if the flexor tendons are intact. 80–90° of flexion can be achieved. If gentle manipulation is impossible, soft tissue release of the collateral ligaments, central slip and skin may also be carried out.
- Flexor tenosynovectomy or tenolysis if the tendons are adherent.
- Lateral band release—relocation of the dorsally migrated lateral bands with release of the collateral ligaments and, possibly, central slip lengthening. Post-operatively, rehabilitation may be delayed for 2 weeks if a K-wire is used; then active and passive exercises to restore ROM, strength and dexterity.

Type IV—PIPJ Contracture and Damaged Cartilage
- Arthroplasty: a 40° arc of movement can be expected (Swanson *et al*. 1985).
- Arthrodesis.

THUMB DEFORMITIES
The thumb represents 50% of hand function and the rheumatoid thumb can cause significant disability (Osterman & Hood, 1991). Nalebuff (1984) has developed a useful classification of rheumatoid thumbs.

Type I - Boutonnière
This is most common thumb deformity. The MCPJ flexes, the IPJ hyperextends and there is compensatory carpo-metacarpal joint (CMCJ) abduction (Figure 17.8). MCPJ synovitis causes stretching of the joint capsule, collateral ligaments and dorsal hood mechanism, reducing the effectiveness of extensor pollicis brevis in extending the MCPJ. Extensor pollicis longus displaces in an ulnar direction and crosses the axis of the joint causing MCPJ flexion and IPJ hyperextension. There is no CMCJ limitation but it is held in an abducted posture in an attempt to form a pinch grip with the fingers. In severe cases, this pathology can result in subluxation of the MCPJ in 90° flexion and the IPJ in 90° hyperextension—called a '90/90 thumb'.

Type II – Swan Neck
The second most common deformity with CMCJ subluxation in adduction, MCPJ hyperextension and IPJ flexion (Figure 17.9). Subluxation or dislocation of the CMCJ into adduction leads to shortening of adductor pollicis causing a webspace contracture. Hyperextension of the MCPJ results due to the Z principle in an attempt to grasp objects. The IPJ flexes due to increased tension in FPL.

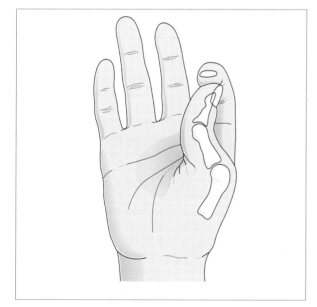

Figure 17.8 Boutonniere deformity of the thumb.

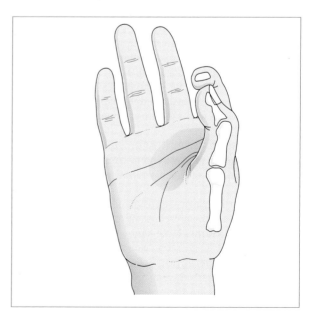

Figure 17.9 Swan neck deformity of the thumb.

Type III—Gamekeeper's Thumb

The third most common type with CMCJ adduction and MCPJ lateral deviation. MCPJ synovitis stretches the joint capsule and UCL causing lateral instability. The first metacarpal is drawn into adduction resulting in shortening of the first dorsal interosseous and a webspace contracture. The CMCJ is adducted due to the position of the first metacarpal; there is no CMCJ limitation.

Type IV—Swan Neck

MCPJ hyperextension and IPJ flexion; however, unlike Type II, the CMCJ is unaffected. MCPJ synovitis causes stretching of the volar capsule leading to MCPJ hyperextension. The IPJ flexes and the CMCJ may be held adducted in a compensatory posture, but there is no joint limitation.

Type V—Mutilans

Resorption of the bone at the MCPJ or IPJ causes shortening of the metacarpal or phalanges resulting in total instability of the affected joints and a short thumb. Mutilans deformity may also cause IPJ instability where the distal phalanx angles laterally away from the palm resulting from synovitis, erosive bony changes and the deforming forces applied by pinch grips.

THUMB SURGERY

Arthroplasty or arthrodesis is applicable to any joint; however, if one joint is to be fused there must be good movement at the other two to preserve function, otherwise an arthroplasty should be considered. Options include:
- IPJ fusion in slight flexion restores stability and overall function.
- MCPJ fusion in about 10–15° flexion, for isolated MCPJ problems, provides painfree stability for function (Stanley *et al.*, 1989).
- MCPJ arthroplasty—most useful when the CMCJ and IPJ are stiff and the ligamentous support to the MCPJ is intact. Patients who require MCPJ movement to perform ADL are ideal candidates. The average ROM is 25°. Patients with higher demands may be better treated with arthrodesis (Figgie *et al.*, 1990).
- CMCJ fusion—rare due to the success of CMCJ arthroplasty, but may be considered for patients with isolated CMCJ problems or those with strenuous occupations.

Carpometacarpal Joint Arthroplasty

For those who do not respond to conservative measures such as splintage or corticosteroid injections. Options include:
- Resection arthroplasty—excision of the trapezium.
- Silastic trapezium—preserves the anatomical CMCJ after arthroplasty (Kvarnes & Reikeras, 1985).

Boutonnière Correction

If the joints are passively reducible, laterally stable and the articular surfaces are adequate on X-ray, synovectomy of the MCPJ with insertion of extensor pollicis longus into the base of the proximal phalanx to improve MCPJ extension and reduce IPJ hyperextension may be carried out. Otherwise, MCPJ fusion is the only other option (Millender & Terreno, 1989).

Swan Neck Deformity
- To correct adduction of the first metacarpal—release adductor pollicis, or either the first dorsal interosseous or the overlying fascia, or all three procedures at the same time.
- To maintain correction, synovectomy and ligament reconstruction may be performed. If the articular surfaces are not adequate CMCJ arthroplasty is recommended.
- Once the adduction contracture has been overcome the hyperextension deformity can be treated by a tenodesis of extensor pollicis brevis to the MCPJ volar plate, achieving 30–40° flexion maintained with a K-wire for 3 weeks.

Table 17.1 is a summary of rheumatoid deformities and surgical options.

HAND INVOLVEMENT IN OTHER RHEUMATOLOGICAL CONDITIONS

JUVENILE RA

The deformities in the upper limb are different from the adult form:
- Shortening of the ulna.
- Flexion and ULNAR deviation of the wrist, often progressing to ankylosis.
- RADIAL deviation and loss of flexion of the MCPJs.
- Boutonnière deformities common, swan necks rare.
- Altered bone growth due to premature epiphyseal fusion.
- Tendon rupture and nerve compression are rare.

See Chapter 19 for further details of the pathology.

PSORIATIC ARTHRITIS

There is a difference between hand involvement in psoriatic arthritis (PsA) and RA (Moll & Wright, 1973):
- Digital swelling is firm and hard on palpation throughout the entire digit, not isolated to the volar aspect as with flexor tenosynovitis in RA.
- Smaller rather than large peripheral joints are affected asymmetrically:
  DIPJ involvement can be severe, causing asymmetrical mallet finger deformities (Figure 17.10).
  PIPJ and MCPJ involvement is random or asymmetric.
- There is a higher incidence of bony ankylosis in the digits and wrist.
- Extensor tendon tenosynovitis and ruptures are rare.
- Ulnar drift is less common.
- Swan neck and Boutonnière deformities can occur, but PIPJ flexion contractures are more common.
- Synovial hypertrophy is less severe.
- Contractures commonly occur due to peri-articular swelling and generalised capsular fibrosis.
- Absence of rheumatoid nodules.

PsA is described in Chapter 12.

Table 17.1 **Summary of rheumatoid deformities and surgical options.**

Summary of rheumatoid deformities and surgical options	
Deformity	Surgical Options
1. Nodules	Corticosteroid injection Surgical excision of nodule
2. Tenosynovitis	Tenosynovectomy
3. Trigger finger	Corticosteroid injection Tenosynovectomy/excision nodule
4. DeQuervain's disease	Corticosteroid injection
5. Tendon rupture	Tendon graft/transfer
6. Prominent ulnar styloid	Darrach (excision ulnar styloid)
7. Radial deviation of wrist	Charnay (Radio-lunate) fusion
8. Volar subluxation of wrist	Wrist arthroplasty/arthrodesis
9. Spontaneous fusion	Wrist arthroplasty/arthrodesis
10. Metacarpophalangeal joint ulnar deviation	Synovectomy Soft tissue reconstruction Metacarpophalangeal joint arthroplasty
11. Boutonniere deformity	Synovectomy Extensor tendon reconstruction Proximal interphalangeal joint arthroplasty/arthrodesis
12. Swan neck deformity	Synovectomy Dermadesis/tenodesis Distal interphalangeal joint fusion Intrinsic release Lateral band release Temporary K-wiring Proximal interphalangeal joint arthroplasty/arthrodesis
13. Thumb Boutonniere deformity	Interphalangeal joint fusion Metacarpophalangeal joint arthrodesis/arthroplasty Carpometacarpal joint arthrodesis/arthroplasty Soft tissue reconstruction
14. Thumb Swan neck deformity	Synovectomy/Tenodesis Intrinsic release Ligament reconstruction Carpometacarpal joint arthroplasty Temporary K wiring of metacarpophalangeal joint

Figure 17.10 **Mallet finger deformity.**

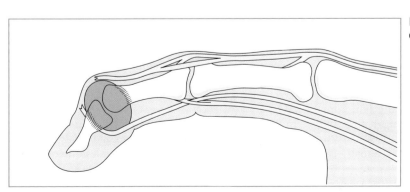

MUTILANS DEFORMITY (OPERA GLASS HAND)

Severe resorption of the bone ends leads to shortening and partially dislocated, unstable joints. It is associated with PsA and the end stage of RA, most commonly affecting the MCPJs, DIPJs, radio–carpal and radio–ulnar joints. The fingers are short and the skin becomes loose and overlaps, giving the characteristic telescoping appearance. The fingers feel soft, fleshy and floppy. The only treatment is surgery—arthrodesis arrests the resorption process and preserves the length of the finger if performed early enough.

OSTEOARTHRITIS

The pathology of osteoarthritis (OA) is described in Chapter 9. A common feature of OA is osteophyte formation. At the DIPJ they are known as Heberden's nodes and at the PIPJ, Bouchard's nodes. They can also occur at the thumb CMCJ, but are rare at the MCPJs. OA of the first CMCJ can occur in isolation. There is tenderness on palpation, stiffness and pain with crepitus on movement. Grip is impaired as a result of painful abduction of the thumb and weakness due to atrophy of the thenar muscles. It is typically bilateral and more common in women.

Management

- Rest by splinting continually for a short time, e.g. 2 weeks, or during painful activities.
- Active assisted exercises if joint ROM is becoming limited.
- Intra-articular injection to reduce pain and inflammation.
- Surgery if conservative measures have failed:
  Excision of the trapezium—shortens the thumb, decreasing its strength.
  Silastic trapezium—retains movement.
  Fusion of the CMCJ—may result in secondary stiffness and disuse atrophy in adjacent joints.

SCLERODERMA

The hand is commonly involved in scleroderma (Idler *et al.*, 1991) with taut, 'hidebound', scarred, atrophic skin causing limitation in joint motion. True inflammatory synovitis is rare. Early manifestations include Raynaud's phenomenon, digital swelling and arthralgias. Periarticular osteoporosis and erosions are rare but may result in a gradual loss of joint space and increased collagen formation leading to joint stiffness. Later, PIPJ flexion contractures may result in a stiff, claw hand deformity. Vascular compromise can cause painful, ischaemic ulcers in the fingers. Calcification of the soft tissues may produce chronic, painful, draining wounds.

The term 'sclerodactyly' is used to describe digits that are stiff, thin and covered in waxy appearing skin, commonly associated with atrophy of the finger pulp and resorption of the distal phalanx (Idler *et al.*, 1991).

For further discussion of systemic sclerosis, see Chapter 13.

SYSTEMIC LUPUS ERYTHEMATOSUS

Hand involvement is generally more benign than with RA or OA as the articular cartilage is not involved unless there are secondary degenerative changes resulting from the ligamentous laxity caused by systemic lupus erythematosus (SLE). However, due to this laxity, some of the most severe, unstable digital deformities are seen, and therefore early reconstructive surgery is recommended prior to dislocation or fixed deformity.

Wrist

- Ligamentous laxity leads to dorsal subluxation of the distal ulna which can be painful and limit pronation and supination.
- Ulnar translocation of the carpus is common and scapho–lunate dissociation can cause rotation of the lunate.

MCPJs

Subluxation of the extensor tendons can result in flexion deformities; however, unlike RA, ulnar drift is not common.

PIPJs

Swan neck deformities are usually seen, but Boutonnière and lateral deformities can occur. These may become fixed with secondary joint changes. If this happens, surgical fusion is a better option than soft tissue correction.

Thumb

In the early stages the most commonly seen deformity is extension lag at the MCPJ with hyperextension at the IPJ and laxity at the CMCJ. If this laxity increases, the CMCJ may dislocate changing the deformity to adduction of the first metacarpal with hyperextension of the MCPJ and flexion of the IPJ.

See Chapter 13 for further details of connective tissue disorders.

VASCULITIS

Involvement of small and medium-sized arteries results in:
- Nailfold infarcts—present as small, necrotic areas.
- Splinter haemorrhages.
- Poor capillary refill following local pressure.
- Digital sensory neuropathy.

Arterial lesions may be present in various stages of inflammation and healing and are important to report as they are an indication to cancel surgery due to the increased infection and healing risks. Digital infarctions can lead to gangrene and spontaneous amputation.

See Chapter 14 for further details of vasculitis.

GOUT

In the chronic stages, tophi can be seen in or about the joints and other tissues of the fingers and hands. Although the tophi themselves are relatively painless, there is often progressive stiffness and persistent aching of the affected joints. Eventually, extensive destruction of the joint occurs and large subcutaneous tophi can cause grotesque deformities in the hands. Progressive disability can result from marked limitation of range of movement by direct involvement of the joint structure or of the tendons. See Chapter 15 for further details of gout.

Table 17.2 is a summary of associated rheumatological conditions and common deformities.

PRE-OPERATIVE ASSESSMENT

Wynn Parry & Stanley (1993) state that a careful, detailed, pre-operative functional assessment by hand therapists is vital to indicate what needs doing and in what order. Stanley (1988) argues for a high level of influence for therapists in surgical choice and timing on the basis that they are most closely associated with the pre- and post-operative

Summary of associated rheumatological conditions and common deformities	
Condition	**Common deformities**
Juvenile rheumatoid arthritis	Shortening of ulna Flexion and ulnar deviation of wrist Radial deviation of metacarpophalangeal joints Boutonniere deformities
Psoriatic arthritis	Digital swelling Asymmetrical mallet finger deformities Joint stiffness Proximal interphalangeal joint flexion contractures
Mutilans	Shortened bones Subluxed/dislocated joints Telescoping fingers – short and flail
Osteoarthritis	Heberden's nodes (distal interphalangeal joint) Bouchard's nodes (proximal interphalangeal joint) First carpometacarpal joint affected
Scleroderma	Taut, scarred, atrophic skin Limited range of movement/joint stiffness Raynaud's phenomenon Digital swelling Arthralgia Proximal interphalangeal joint flexion contractures Ischaemic ulcers Atrophy of finger pulp Resorption of distal phalanx
Systemic lupus erythematosus	Dorsal subluxation of distal ulna Ulnar translocation of carpus Metacarpophalangeal joint flexion contractures Swan neck deformities Thumb abduction, metacarpophalangeal joint hyperextension Interphalangeal joint flexion
Vasculitis	Nailfold infarcts Splinter haemorrhages Poor capillary refill Sensory neuropathy
Gout	Tophi Joint stiffness Joint destruction and deformity

Table 17.2 **Summary of associated rheumatological conditions and common deformities.**

treatment. Key questions to consider include:
- How does the deformity affect function?
- Will surgery risk existing function?
- How much pain is there?
- Will surgery just exchange one set of problems for another?

Surgery represents a sudden change in a patient's functional ability. Rheumatoid patients adapt slowly to developing deformities, therefore a sudden change can leave patients unsure of the result for a considerable time until they have adapted to the new situation. What to assess?
- Function.
- Anatomy—deformities present?
- X-ray—how much bone is left? This is important when considering whether an arthroplasty or an arthrodesis is the best option.
- Medically—are they fit for surgery?
- What implications will surgery have upon other joints and muscle strength?
- Psychological factors—motivation, comprehension, compliance?
- Are the patients' expectations in line with the possible results of surgery?
- Are there any alternatives, e.g. adaptive devices?
- Any contra-indications, e.g. vasculitis, flare-ups?

Surgery aims to improve overall function by (Souter, 1979):
- Reducing pain.
- Improving mobility, providing stability or both.
- Preventing further damage.
- Correcting deformity.
- Improving power.
- Improving cosmesis.

SURGICAL PRIORITIES

Any damage to nerves which affects innervation must be corrected first before tendon ruptures can be repaired. Once ruptured, flexor tendons are more difficult to repair than extensors, and so usually take priority. The general rule is to work proximally to distally thereby producing stability throughout the limb and the ability to place the limb before considering the functional requirements of the hand. Therefore the shoulder will be operated on before the elbow, the elbow will come before the wrist, the wrist before the MCPJ or thumb and the MCPJ before the PIPJ. This is, however, only a general rule and there are times when the severity of the disease in one joint makes it take precedent over all others.

Lower limbs should be operated upon before upper limbs for weightbearing purposes, except for wrist arthrodesis which provides a solid, stable, pain free joint to assist with lower limb rehabilitation.

COMPLEX HAND PROBLEMS

Each component should be analysed individually looking at how it affects the whole upper limb. The functional needs of each joint should be considered. Stability for gripping is required in the wrist, MCPJ and IPJ of the thumb and DIPJs of the fingers, so therefore arthrodesis could most suitable.

Mobility is required in one elbow to reach out to objects and reach to the mouth, CMCJ of thumb for opposition and MCPJ of fingers to accomplish a grip on various sized objects, therefore arthroplasty could be the preferred option.

Where the PIPJs are concerned, arthrodesis of the index finger and others if the MCPJs have good movement will provide stability for gripping, otherwise arthroplasty if the MCPJs are stiff.

Grip Strength

Many patients asking for improved function actually require improved grip strength. Surgery can only alter the position of grip patterns in an attempt to improve strength. This must be discussed and explained fully to patients pre-operatively to ensure that their expectations are realistic.

TIMING OF SURGERY

Timing depends upon:
- Degree of urgency, e.g. nerve compression, tendon rupture will be treated as soon as possible.
- Stage of disease—surgery is best avoided during acute phases of the disease.
- Degree of disability—deformities do not always cause disability so therefore it is important to ascertain the severity of any problems pre-operatively.
- Priority order—see above description.
- Convenience in normal work and social schedule.

A programme should be worked out with the patient (Souter, 1979), working proximal to distal, and combining complimentary procedures which serve to remove mutually deforming disorders, e.g. the Z collapse principle of radial wrist deviation and MCPJ ulnar deviation (Millender & Phillips, 1978). Table 17.3 lists some possible combinations of surgery.

SURGICAL OUTCOMES

Souter (1979) has graded the range of surgical options according to how well they achieve the goals of surgery (described earlier). Expressed as an average percentage score:
- Thumb MCPJ fusion 85%.
- Extensor synovectomy with Darrach's 83%.
- Wrist fusion 73%.
- Flexor tenosynovectomy 68%.
- PIPJ fusion 68%.
- MCPJ arthroplasty 65%.
- Soft tissue correction of Swan neck 65%.
- IPJ thumb fusion 65%.
- MCPJ or PIPJ synovectomy 53%.
- PIPJ arthroplasty 43%.
- Soft tissue Boutonnière correction 35%.

Possible combinations of surgery	
Complementary: one from each group	
Group 1. Fingers	Tenosynovectomy OR Tendon transfers OR Swan neck/Boutonniere corrections OR Metacarpophalangeal joint arthroplasties
Group 2. Thumb	Tendon transfers/rebalancing OR Swan neck/Boutonniere corrections OR Interphalangeal joint fusion OR Metacarpophalangeal fusion/arthroplasty OR Trapezectomy/silastic trapezium
Group 3. Wrist	Formal wrist fusion OR Radio-lunate fusion OR Darrach's with tenosynovectomy
Contra-indicated combinations	
Metacarpophalangeal arthroplasties with proximal interphalangeal joint surgery: Swan neck/Boutonnière/soft tissue corrections/arthroplasty/arthrodesis	

Table 17.3 **Possible combinations of surgery.**

CONCLUSION

The therapist has an important role to play in the management of rheumatological conditions affecting the hand. This involves the identification and assessment of deformities whilst maintaining a holistic approach to the patient's condition and situation, and providing detailed information and opinions regarding the timing and needs of surgery for the patient and hand surgeon to discuss.

To this end Wynn Parry & Stanley (1993) have identified five factors which determine the results of surgery to the hand and wrist:

• The degree of damage suffered by the joints and soft tissues.
• The repertoire of the surgeon.
• The type of disease.
• The motivation and expectations of the patient.
• The quality of the therapy services. The quality of any surgical result is heavily dependent upon the initial assessment and identification of functional problems translated into anatomical terms and the quality of postoperative care.

REFERENCES

Burke FD. Surgery to the wrist joint. *Br J Rheum* 1995, **34**:274-282.

Chandani A. Tenosynovitis of the hand and wrist: A literature review. *Br J Occupat Ther* 1986:288-292.

Dellhag B, Wollersjo I, Bjelle A. Effect of active exercise and wax bath treatment in rheumatoid arthritis patients. *Arthritis Care Res* 1992, **5**:87-92.

Dent JA, Smith M, Caspers J. Assessment of hand function: a review of some tests in common use. *Br J Occup Ther* 1985:360-362.

Fess EE, Moran CA. Clinical assessment recommendations. *Am Soc Hand Ther* 1980.

Figgie MP, Inglis AE, Sorbel M, Bohn WW, Fisher DA. Metacarpophalangeal arthroplasty of the rheumatoid thumb. *J Hand Surg* 1990,**15A**:210-216.

Fries JF, Spitz P, Kraines RG, Holman HR. Measurement of patient outcome in arthritis. *Arthritis Rheum* 1980, **2**:137-145.

Helliwell P, Howe A, Wright V. Functional assessment of the hand: reproducibility, acceptability and utility of a new system for measuring strength. *Ann Rheum Dis* 1987, **46**:203-208.

Idler RS, Strickland JW, Creighton JJ. Scleroderma and its manifestations in the hand. *Indiana Med* 1991, **84(10)**:702-703.

Jebson RH, Taylor N, Trieschmann RB, Trotter M, Howard LA. An objective and standardized test of hand function. *Arch Phys Med Rehabil* 1969, **50(6)**:311-319.

Jones E, Hanly JG, Mooney R, Rand LL, Spurway PM, Eastwood BG, Jones JV. Strength and function in the normal and rheumatoid hand. *J Rheum* 1991, **18**:1313-1318.

Kirwan J, Reeback J. Stanford Health Assessment Questionnaire modified to assess disability in British patients with rheumatoid arthritis. *Br J Rheum* 1986, **25**:206-209.

Kraft GH, Detels PE. Position of function of the wrist. *Arch Phys Med Rehabil* 1972, **53**:272-275.

Kvarnes L, Reikeras O. Rheumatoid arthritis at the base of the thumb treated by trapezial resection or implant arthroplasty. *J Hand Surg* 1985, **10**:195-196.

Mathiowetz V, Kashman N, Volland G, Weber K, Dowe M, Rogers S. Grip and pinch strength: Normative data for adults. *Arch Phys Med Rehabil* 1985, **66**:69-74.

Millender LH, Philips C. Combined wrist arthrodesis and metacarpophalangeal arthroplasty in rheumatoid arthritis. *Orthopaedics* 1978, **1**:43-48.

Millender LH, Terreno A. Surgical treatment of the Boutonniere rheumatoid thumb deformity. *Hand Clin* 1989, **5**:239-248.

Moll JMH, Wright V. Psoriatic arthritis. *Sem Arthritis Rheum* 1973, **3(1)**:55-78.

McKnight PT, Kwoh CK. Randomized, controlled trial of compression gloves in rheumatoid arthritis. *Arthritis Care Res* 1992, **5**:223-227.

Nalebuff EA, Millender LH. Surgical treatment of the boutonniere deformity in rheumatoid arthritis. *Orthop Clin North Am* 1975a, **6(3)**:753-763.

Nalebuff MD, Millender LH. Surgical treatment of the swan neck deformity in rheumatoid arthritis. *Orthop Clin North Am* 1975b, **6**:733-752.

Nalebuff EA. The rheumatoid thumb. *Clin Rheum Dis* 1984, **10**:589-608.

Nalebuff EA, Felden D, Millender LH. In Green, ed. *Operative hand surgery.* New York:Churchill Livingstone;1988:1665-1759.

Nordenskiold UM, Grimby G. Grip force in patients with rheumatoid arthritis and fibromyalgia and in healthy subjects: a study with the Grippit instrument. *Scand J Rheumatol* 1993, **22**:14-19.

O'Neill G. The development of a standardized assessment of hand function. *Br J Occupational Therapy* 1995, **58**:477-480.

Osterman AL, Hood J. Synovectomy, arthroplasty and arthrodesis in the reconstruction of the rheumatoid wrist and hand. *Curr Opin Rheumatol* 1991, **3**:102-108.

Scott J, Huskisson EC. Vertical or horizontal visual analogue scales. *Ann Rheum Dis* 1979, **38(6)**:560.

Sharma S, Schumacher HR, McLellan T. Evaluation of the Jebson Hand Function Test for use with patients with rheumatoid arthritis. *Arthritis Care Res* 1994, **7**:16-19.

Souter WA. Planning treatment of the rheumatoid hand. *Hand* 1979, **11**:3-16.

Stanley JK. The surgical management of the rheumatoid wrist and hand. In: Howard Beddow F, ed. *Surgical management of rheumatoid arthritis.* London: Wright; 1988.

Stanley JK, Smith JE, Muirhead AG. Arthrodesis of the metacarpophalangeal joint of the thumb: review of 42 cases. *J Hand Surg* 1989, **14B**:291-293.

Swanson A, Maupin B, Gajjar N, DeGroot Swanson G. Flexible implant arthroplasty in the proximal interphalangeal joint of the hand. *J Hand Surg* 1985, **10**:796-805.

Towheed TE, Anastassiades TP. Rheumatoid hand: practical approach to assessment and management. *Can Family Physician* 1994, **40**:1303-1309.

Wynn Parry CB, Stanley JK. Synovectomy of the hand. *Br J Rheumatol* 1993, **32**:1089-1095.

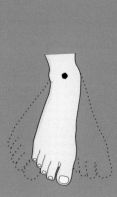

18 J Stewart & M Monoghan

THE FOOT IN RHEUMATOLOGY

CHAPTER OUTLINE

- Anatomy
- Gait
- Assessment

- Rheumatological conditions and the foot
- Management of the foot

INTRODUCTION

Rheumatological conditions present a varied clinical picture in the foot. Problems range from discomfort in the first metatarsal head to complete destruction of the structural complex of the foot; from ridging of the nail to absorption of the distal tissues and bone. This chapter is designed to give an overview of the various pathologies which may affect the foot in rheumatological conditions and describes how these effects are clinically manifested and managed. There have been few studies other than those focusing on rheumatoid arthritis (RA) investigating foot pathology and therefore, as yet, some of the suggested management remains unsubstantiated.

ANATOMY

The foot is a complex multi-jointed structure comprising of 26 bones. It may be divided into three areas: the hindfoot (calcaneum and talus), midfoot (navicular, cuboid and three cuneiforms) and the forefoot (metatarsals and phalanges) (Figure 18.1). The foot is an arched structure with the calcaneum acting as the posterior pillar for both the medial longitudinal arch and the lateral longitudinal arch. The medial longitudinal arch comprises of the calcaneum, talus, navicular, three cuneiforms and the metatarsals 1 to 3. The lateral longitudinal arch is made up of the calcaneum, cuboid and metatarsals 4 and 5. The

transverse arch is situated at the tarso-metatarsal joints but has little functional significance.

The arches of the foot are maintained by the various muscles and ligaments which insert or pass through the area. These include the spring ligament (plantar calcaneo navicular ligament), long plantar ligament (calcaneo cuboid ligament) and the plantar aponeurosis. Muscles which have a major influence in supporting the arches are tibialis anterior, tibialis posterior, the long flexors and extensors and the intrinsic muscles of the foot.

The foot contains four layers of intrinsic muscles. Layer 1, the most superficial layer, comprises abductor hallucis, abductor digiti minimi and flexor digitorum brevis. Layer 2 comprises flexor digitorum accessorius and the lumbrical muscles. Layer 3 is made up of flexor hallucis brevis, adductor hallucis (oblique and transverse parts) and flexor digiti minimi brevis. Layer 4 contains the four dorsal interossei and the three plantar interossei. The main weightbearing areas at the heel and forefoot are protected by fat pads (Figure 18.2). At the forefoot these are situated between the metatarsal heads and the base of the proximal phalanges. Their main function is to offer protection to the blood vessels and digital nerves which may be at risk from weightbearing pressure.

Before considering how the foot is affected by rheumatological conditions, it is useful to examine the component parts of the gait cycle, the principles and concepts regarding foot function and to define terms.

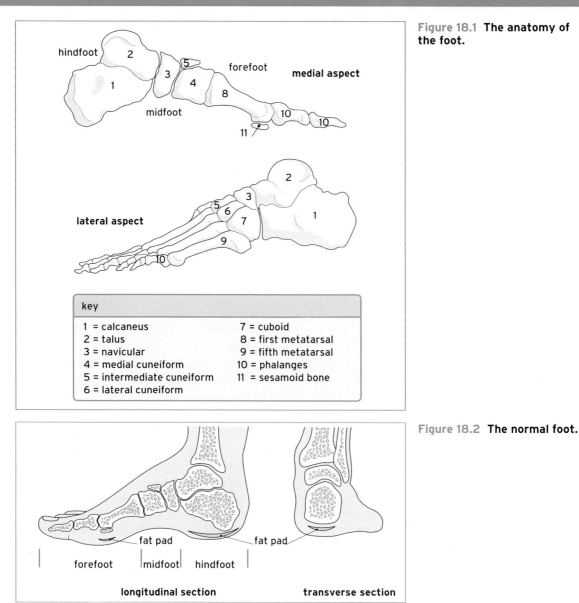

Figure 18.1 **The anatomy of the foot.**

key

1 = calcaneus	7 = cuboid
2 = talus	8 = first metatarsal
3 = navicular	9 = fifth metatarsal
4 = medial cuneiform	10 = phalanges
5 = intermediate cuneiform	11 = sesamoid bone
6 = lateral cuneiform	

Figure 18.2 **The normal foot.**

DEFINITION OF TERMS

Figure 18.3 illustrates foot movement, where the following can be noted:

- Abduction—a transverse plane motion where the forefoot is directed towards the midline of the body.
- Adduction—a transverse plane motion where the forefoot is directed away the midline of the body.
- Angle of Gait—the angle which the foot makes to the sagittal plane during forward propulsion.
- Pronation—a complex triplane motion consisting of eversion, abduction and dorsiflexion of the foot on the leg.
- Supination—a complex triplane motion consisting of inversion, adduction and plantarflexion of the foot on the leg.
- Varus—a fixed frontal plane position in which the foot is inverted.
- Valgus—a fixed frontal plane position in which the foot is everted.

THE FOOT AS A DYNAMIC STRUCTURE

The foot has two basic functions: to act as a platform on which the body is supported and to aid in propelling the body forward during gait. This is possible due to kinetic chain motion, which is an important feature of gait (Boyd & Rendall, 1993). The lower limb is seen as comprising a number of units which have the ability either to move on each other or to become fixed as a stable column for weightbearing.

Open kinetic chain motion occurs when the end unit (the non-weightbearing foot) is free to move on the leg when assisting in ground clearance (see 'swing phase').

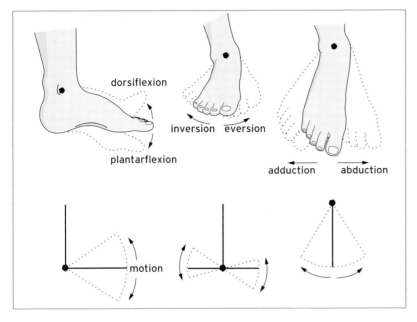

Figure 18.3 **Foot movement.**

Closed kinetic chain motion occurs when the end unit (the weightbearing foot) is fixed by body weight allowing the leg to move over the top of the foot (see 'stance phase').

The subtalar (talocalcaneal) joint exhibits a complex triplane motion consisting of pronation and supination. The component movements are dorsiflexion/plantarflexion, inversion/eversion and adduction/abduction. The midtarsal joint displays similar triplanar motion but the amount of midtarsal joint motion is solely dependent on the position at the subtalar joint.

Through the relative positioning of these intrinsic joints, the foot has the ability to change from a mobile adaptor, necessary for accommodating to variances in terrain and for shock absorption, to a rigid lever required for propulsion.

GAIT

Human gait is a co-ordinated series of events which occur in a cyclical manner. One gait cycle is from the heel strike of one foot to the heel strike of the same foot, one stride on. The cycle is made up of a series of events, e.g. pronation and supination at the subtalar joint and midtarsal joints, dorsiflexion/plantarflexion at the ankle and flexion/extension at the first metatarsophalangeal joint (MTPJ). These events all happen at a specific time within the gait cycle. In clinical evaluation it is the timing of events within this cycle and not the events themselves which allows a comparison to be made. In dysfunction there is not necessarily a loss of function but the timing is altered. For example, with a pronated foot the ability to supinate is not necessarily lost but because pronation is increased the time in pronation is lengthened and therefore as a consequence of this supination is delayed. So when assessing the abnormal foot one compares the timings against known 'normal' timings.

The gait cycle may be divided into two separate functional phases: the non-weightbearing swing phase (40%) and the weightbearing stance phase (60%). The swing phase is functionally less important, occurring from toe off to heel strike, while the stance phase occurs from heel strike to toe off. It can be further divided into three sub-phases: contact, midstance and propulsive phase (Figure 18.4). A double support phase (10%) also exists when both feet are weightbearing. As cadence (walking speed) increases the double support phase is reduced until running speed is achieved when both feet will be airborne (float phase).

CONTACT PHASE

At heel strike the foot is in a supinated position thereby accounting for wear on shoes to the outside of centre at the heel. Immediately after heel strike, the foot pronates at the subtalar joint initiating the shock absorption facility. This in turn 'unlocks' the midtarsal joint and the smaller joints distal to it. With subtalar joint pronation the calcaneum everts and the talus plantarflexes and adducts. As it is 'locked' within the ankle mortise the talus takes on the role of torque convertor, allowing its movement to force the lower leg into internal rotation which in turn forces the knee and the hip to flex. The fat pad at the heel, the plantar aponeurosis and the long and short plantar ligaments all play a major part in shock attenuation.

MIDSTANCE

When the foot moves into the midstance phase the subtalar joint moves out of its pronated position and starts to supinate, moving through the subtalar neutral position. With supination comes calcaneal inversion whilst the talus abducts and dorsiflexes. In doing so torque conversion will force the lower leg to rotate externally enabling the knee and the hip to extend, passing the subtalar neutral position at the midpoint of midstance. With the centre of load

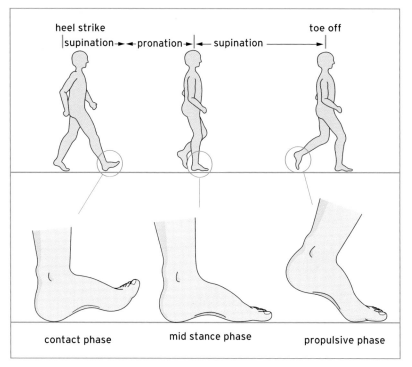

Figure 18.4 **Stance phase.**

passing over the foot, the heel lifts from the ground and the foot moves into its propulsive phase.

PROPULSION

At this point the subtalar joint is in a fully supinated position with the midtarsal and other joints in the foot locked in a rigid position. This then allows for propulsion of body weight from the weightbearing foot to the other foot which has now commenced its stance phase. Timing is of great importance in the gait cycle. Dysfunction occurs when the phases of gait are mistimed, resulting in the foot staying a mobile adaptor when it should be a rigid lever and vice versa.

When the subtalar joint is affected by disease, subjects will invariably adopt a pronated stance. They do so for a number of reasons. It may be that if the knee has adopted a valgus position then the forces acting on the foot will force the joint into a pronated position. When the subtalar joint is swollen the individual will pronate as this tends to be the most comfortable position to adopt.

The rheumatoid flatfoot may never move from a pronated position during the stance phase of gait. The consequences of this are that the leg will remain internally rotated with a reduction of knee and hip extension. The result of this will be a foot with a low arch profile producing an apropulsive and inefficient gait.

ASSESSMENT

The lower limb should be examined in static and if possible in dynamic stance; the foot may be too painful to walk on for any distance especially without shoes. The foot needs to be examined weightbearing and non-weightbearing and

particular attention given to joint movement and cutaneous changes. The symptoms which the patient reports may further facilitate an understanding of the individual's foot and the mobility problems.

ASSESSMENT OF THE WEIGHTBEARING FOOT

When studying the weightbearing foot, significant changes in the position of the foot in relation to the leg from a non-weightbearing stance should be noted.

The rearfoot (made up from the hindfoot and the midfoot)—the most common deformity is over pronation at the subtalar joint. Excessive pronation at the subtalar joint will result in a flattened medial longitudinal arch and if there is instability at this joint it can lead to complete collapse of the midfoot.

The forefoot—the most common deformity in this area is splaying at the MPJs which makes the foot difficult to accommodate. Rigidity and loss of fibro-fatty padding at the forefoot on weightbearing can cause high pressure areas leading potentially to tissue necrosis at these points. Understandably the forefoot is the area that causes individuals the most pain in rheumatological conditions.

The toes—different toe deformities will result in specific patterns of callus (Figure 18.5). An understanding of toe deformities will help when accommodating the feet in footwear and fitting orthotics.

ASSESSMENT OF THE NON-WEIGHTBEARING FOOT

Joint assessment of the rheumatic foot must be carried out with care as the foot is often very painful, either from skin

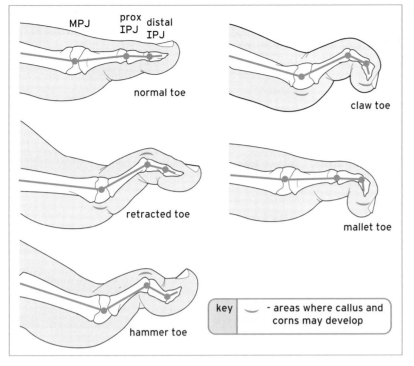

Figure 18.5 **Toe deformities.**

lesions at the joint site or from the joints themselves. The ankle, subtalar joint, midtarsal, MTPJs and interphalangeal joints should be carefully examined to assess the range of movement and quality of the movement. Patterns of joint involvement will differ depending on the specific disease process and also variations will occur from individual to individual. Therefore each joint should be assessed and compared with other joints and with the other foot.

The ankle should be tested for dorsiflexion and plantarflexion with the knee straight and flexed, to release the soft tissue structures. The subtalar joint is assessed by grasping and holding firm the talus whilst inverting and everting the calcaneum. With this movement there should be approximately two-thirds inversion to one-third eversion from a neutral position. The midtarsal joint is made up of a collection of joints, principally inverted and everted. The midtarsal joint motion is elicited by holding the calcaneum in one hand and grasping the foot proximal to the MTPJs with the other, gently inverting and everting the distal part of the foot to the tarsus.

In RA the patient often complains of 'walking on marbles' and experiences considerable discomfort if lateral pressure is applied at the MTPJs when the foot is squeezed, similar to its position in tight footwear. With this disorder there may also be 'day-light sign' where the enlargement of the MTPJs causes the toes to separate from one another causing spaces between the toes.

Callus, corns or bursae will indicate where the foot is subject to pressure. Callus indicates intermittent compressive stresses accompanied by some movement. With corns, the pressure is more localised and severe. Adventitious bursae are caused by sheering stresses within the tissues but as these structures are lined with synovial membrane the disease process may lead to bursitis without a mechanical cause.

Rheumatological conditions affect multiple systems so assessment of the foot must be holistic in its approach. Vascular and neurological assessment may also be indicated but examination should always be goal directed and dependent upon the needs of the individual and the disease process.

RHEUMATOLOGICAL CONDITIONS AND THE FOOT

RHEUMATOID ARTHRITIS

Although the cause of RA is still speculative, its pathology is undoubtedly related to an inflammatory process described as having two phases. The first is an acute synovitis with the classical signs of inflammation being present. The second is a severe anatomical deformity due to the destructive process in the joints which results in excessive loading of the metatarsal heads (among other areas) of the foot (Betts *et al.*, 1988). In the early stages of RA it is almost impossible to predict the outcome of the disease (Luukkainen *et al.*, 1983) or its progress (Reeback & Silman, 1984). However, it has been reported that onset involving the medial MTPJs is usually associated with a poorer prognosis or a more malignant disease course (Roth, 1993).

There is little doubt that the foot is affected in most patients who suffer from RA. It is the small joints of the feet, especially the MTPJs, which are affected early in the course of the disease with a common feature being complete destruction of these joints. Other major areas of involvement are the plantar aspect of the heel and the joints of the hindfoot. Little has been written about the ankle (Waugh, 1988) although Cracheola *et al.* (1992) report that it is commonly affected in RA, when it can cause major problems regarding patient mobility.

Valgus deformity of the hindfoot occurs for a number of reasons. When the subtalar joint is affected by the disease the patient will adopt a pronated stance. This in turn will cause the load line to be displaced laterally, relative to the line of action of bodyweight. This leads to a moment on the joint which increases the deformity (Foulston, 1987). When the subtalar joint is inflamed, the rheumatoid patient will pronate the foot causing more intra-articular space to be made available for the increased volume of joint fluid. This is the most comfortable position to adopt when weightbearing. Little is known about the pathogenesis of valgus deformity of the hindfoot. Keenan *et al.* (1991) have offered several hypotheses as to the cause of hindfoot deformity. These include cartilaginous and osseous changes in the subtalar and midtarsal joints, soft tissue problems including laxity of joint capsules due to inflammation and swelling, rupture and tenosynovitis of tibialis posterior tendon.

At heel strike the rheumatoid flatfoot will already be in a pronated position. This may be seen on the shoe as wear on the medial side of the heel. At midstance, when the foot is completely plantigrade, the subtalar joint will not be in the process of supination in readiness for propulsion; rather the joint will remain pronated. This will result in a low arch profile to the foot and will allow the midtarsal joint to remain unlocked, thereby rendering the foot hypermobile. As weightbearing load is transferred along the length of the foot the first and fifth rays will dorsiflex leaving the lesser metatarsal heads to receive the load. The instability of the hindfoot may subsequently lead to forefoot deformity (Dimonte & Light, 1982) and to hallux valgus (Schoenhaus & Cohen, 1992). It is generally accepted that metatarsal heads 3 and 4 will become overloaded with resultant lesion formation.

As a result of hallux valgus and the resultant joint malalignment, the weightbearing capacity of the first toe diminishes. The rheumatoid flatfoot will almost always present with an abducted angle of gait and this will result in medial roll-off at the interphalangeal joint. The forces acting on the medial side of the hallux will increase the lateral deviation of the hallux. Within the normal foot the loadbearing pattern is such that the load is shared equally between the heel and the forefoot with the lateral border of the foot also loadbearing. The toes are involved in loadbearing for about three-quarters of the stance phase (Hughes *et al.*, 1990) with the hallux taking the main thrust during propulsion.

The loadbearing pattern of the rheumatoid foot has been investigated by many researchers (e.g. Minns & Craxford, 1984, Samnegard *et al.*, 1990). It has been shown that the classic rheumatoid foot demonstrates a pattern where metatarsal heads 3 and 4 take most load during the stance phase of gait. This may be due to severe hallux abducto valgus inhibiting the function of the first MTPJ, thereby shifting the load to the lateral metatarsal heads. Dorsal subluxation of the lesser MTPJs results in the toes playing little or no part in toe-off. This leaves the metatarsal heads maintaining ground contact until load has been transferred to the other foot.

Such is the variable nature of the disease that any metatarsal head may become subject to excessive load. Indeed as the disease increases in chronicity so the load pattern may change as deformity becomes more evident.

See Chapter 8 for more information on rheumatoid arthritis.

OSTEOARTHRITIS

Osteoarthritis (OA) is a common, age-related change to joints characterised by the erosion of articular cartilage with hypertrophy of the subchondral bone at the joint margins (Dieppe, 1995). The joints of the foot are subjected to considerable stress from biomechanical anomalies and trauma. The resultant arthritic changes and limitation of movement will further alter the mechanics of gait. In the joint affected by arthritis there is often pain and stiffness on initial weightbearing until the individual 'gets going' but if the joint is overworked the pain will resume. It is also likely to be painful at the extreme parameters of its range of motion. All joints in the foot can be potentially affected by OA but in the foot the most commonly affected joint is the first MTPJ (Cawley & Smidt, 1993). When this joint is affected the subject is unable to dorsiflex the first MTPJ as this movement is often painful; to compensate the foot 'supinates' on forefoot loading allowing the interphalangeal joint of the first to 'toe-off'. This will eventually lead to problems at this joint and excessive pressure also on the second and fifth metatarsal heads. At the first MTPJ osteophytic growth is common and may result in dorsal and/or lateral enlargement of the joint, leading to further deformity and discomfort.

Management of OA in the foot is concerned with the control of painful motion and the progressive rigidity compensated for by shock absorbing materials. As with many rheumatic problems, the foot needs to be accommodated and therefore footwear is chosen to fulfil these roles. Training shoes will help deal with all of these issues although some people do not find them aesthetically acceptable.

See Chapter 9 for more information on osteoarthritis.

PSORIATIC ARTHRITIS

This seronegative arthritis presents several clinical pictures in the feet from a mild involvement of the joints to gross destruction. The clinical picture may vary but the involvement of the interphalangeal joints is most common in the foot (MacKie, 1993). This can give rise to dactylitis where the arthritic changes coupled with the flexor tenosynovitis make the digits shapeless and 'sausage like'. Arthritic changes are likely to be accompanied by nail changes, such as pitting of the nail and onycholysis (elevation of the nail plate from the nail bed) (Veale *et al.*, 1994). The more severe clinical pictures can resemble RA, where hallux valgus, retraction of the lesser digits, subtalar pronation and hence collapse of the mid-foot may all be present. Arthritis mutilans, although less common, will cause severe destruction of the feet, where the digits look as if they are telescoped into the adjacent bone resulting in very short and deformed digits. This manifestation of psoriatic arthritis is extremely difficult to accommodate as, although they are short, the digits may lie in varied positions relative to the metatarsals.

Pain does not occur only on weightbearing and consequently it is difficult to manage this foot topically. Management therefore will depend upon the clinical picture presented.

See Chapter 12 for more information on psoriatic arthritis.

REITER'S DISEASE

Reiter's disease is similar to psoriatic arthritis in its clinical manifestation in the feet (Toivanen, 1995). Foot pain is common and heel pain is the most common site for pain within the foot followed by pain in the MTPJ and then the interphalangeal joints (Calmels *et al.*, 1993). Enthesopathy is the most marked feature of this condition when it occurs early in the disease (Deesomchok & Tumrasvin, 1993). As with psoriatic arthritis, the digits can appear sausage shaped and keratoderma blennorrhagica can occur on the skin. This looks similar to pustular psoriasis and occurs on any part of the plantar aspect of the foot. Nail dystrophies such as pitting, onycholysis and paronychia, also common in psoriasis, occur in Reiter's.

Heel pain from the enthesopathy can be controlled by sorbothane heel cups placed into the shoe, or if the pain is located to one specific point on the plantar shock-absorbing material can be used with an aperture cut over the painful point. These measures are needed until the acute symptoms subside.

See Chapter 12 for more information on Reiter's disease.

ANKYLOSING SPONDYLITIS

Ankylosing spondylitis can result in bony spurs in the feet especially around the calcaneum. Achilles peritendinitis and retrocalcaneal bursitis may also be seen. Bony spurs are most common at the insertion of the tendo achilles and origin of the plantar fascia (West & Woodburn, 1995). These are a result of enthesopathy and are painful.

Drug intervention or steroid injections are more successful at treating this condition than palliative care, although similar interventions to those used in Reiter's disease may alleviate some discomfort. For calcaneal spurs, heel lifts in shoes reduce the stress on the tendo achilles and medial longitudinal arch support will reduce stress on the plantar fascia.

See Chapter 10 for more information on ankylosing spondylitis.

COLLAGEN-VASCULAR DISEASES

This group includes systemic lupus erythematosus, systemic sclerosis or scleroderma and polyarteritis nodosa. They are problematic to the feet due to changes in the small- and medium-sized blood vessels (Cawley & Smidt, 1993). The clinical features are dependent upon the underlying pathology but Raynaud's phenomenon, vasculitis, fibrosis and calcinotic nodules will have the most devastating effect on the feet. The peripheries are prone to anything from small areas of necrosis, splinter haemorrhage under the nail and nail fold infarctions to large areas of necrosis or gangrene. Over time there is a loss of the soft tissues at the apex (end) of the toes and fibrous tissue is laid down in its place. The soft tissue at the pulp of the digits is slowly lost and the nail becomes thin and friable and in some instances lost altogether. In extreme cases there is also bone absorption of the distal phalanx and as a result the digits look as if they have been whittled away at the distal margins. The skin under these circumstances is thin, shiny and devitalised. These changes can also cause atrophy of the fibro-fatty padding on the plantar aspect of the foot causing pain on weightbearing and reduced capacity to deal with stress.

The main aim in the management of these foot problems is to maintain the integrity of the tissues. Therefore any high pressure areas must be reduced by redistributing weight evenly over the plantar aspect of the foot with accommodative orthoses. Thermoplastics are useful in the management of these conditions either as insoles or covering materials for insoles which help maintain a consistent temperature within the footwear. Tissue contraction, especially in scleroderma, will result in retraction of the digits, making the dorsal surface prominent and subject to pressure from the footwear. Thus as with all of the above conditions, footwear is of major importance in the management and protection of the feet.

GOUT

The foot is a common site to be affected by this condition, especially the first MTPJ, being reported to occur in 90% of cases (Cohen & Emmerson, 1995). In acute gout the affected joint will be inflamed and exquisitely painful. The pain is so severe the patient may not be able to tolerate even the slightest amount of pressure on the area. Chronic gout can lead to severe destruction of the articular cartilage and gross osteoarthritic changes. Tophi deposits in the foot are frequently noted (Kerman *et al.*, 1993). Deposits around the nail plate will result in the nail becoming brittle, split and 'reeded' with longitudinal ridges (Fenton & Wilkinson, 1984).

The pain in acute gout needs to be controlled by drugs as strapping will only add to the pain the patient is already experiencing. When the initial symptoms have subsided, semi-immobilising strapping with padding to prevent movement of the joint will help to keep the patient ambulant. Rigid orthoses will also prevent painful movement. A 2 mm thick and approximately 4 cm wide piece of sprung steel placed along the length of the medial border of a shoe will prevent any movement of painful first MTPJs and help reduce pain. This is also an appropriate management for OA in this joint.

See Chapter 15 for more information on gout.

MANAGEMENT OF THE FOOT

The management of the foot in rheumatological conditions is arguably as complex as that of the 'diabetic foot'. Management is dependent upon the severity of the systemic disease, the specific clinical picture, the pharmacological status (especially with long-term corticosteroids) and the patients' attitude towards their illness. Prevention of deformity in the foot is not well researched due to incomplete understanding of the 'normal' dynamic foot and the lack of valid and reliable tools for measuring this phenomenum. The aims of foot-care for this group are therefore:

• To maintain tissue integrity.
• To minimise pain.
• To maximise existing foot function and in doing so:
• facilitate ambulation.

This can be done in several ways but principally by the use of orthoses and footwear.

ORTHOSES

There is no single commonly accepted definition for a podiatric orthosis. Jahss (1991) described an orthosis as 'a mechanical device made for the foot or toes that is used to either stabilise the foot or hold it in an optimal position, increase function, limit motion of a painful joint, decrease weightbearing on painful areas, or protect the foot or toes from pressure or excess friction against each other or the shoe'. This definition amply sets out the role of an orthosis but it would be useful to offer more specific operational definitions for the two main categories of orthosis.

A functional orthosis corrects or attempts to correct a pathological state within the foot. It has been defined as a device that aligns an improperly balanced foot by controlling subtalar motion (D'Ambrosia, 1985) and as a device which controls excessive and potentially harmful subtalar and midtarsal movement (Donatelli & Wooden, 1990). An accommodative orthosis allows for relief of pressure or friction without attempting to correct dysfunction or deformity.

The decision to prescribe one or other must be made after diagnosis and formulation of a planned management. As a general rule, functional orthoses may be prescribed before joint deformity has become established but are contra-indicated where fixed non-reducible deformity is present. In these cases accommodative orthoses would be the preferred option. The rheumatoid foot may be divided into several component parts where podiatric orthoses may be considered for use. These are: the heel, the plantar metatarsal head area, the medial eminence of the first metatarsal head in hallux abducto valgus (bunion), the lateral eminence of the fifth metatarsal head in 'Tailor's' bunion and the lesser toes.

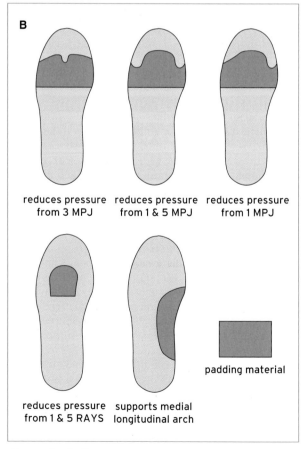

reduces pressure from 3 MPJ   reduces pressure from 1 & 5 MPJ   reduces pressure from 1 MPJ

reduces pressure from 1 & 5 RAYS   supports medial longitudinal arch

padding material

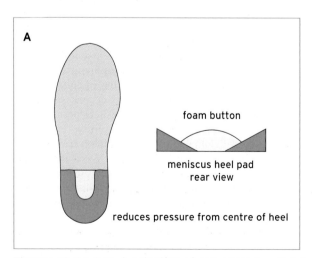

foam button

meniscus heel pad
rear view

reduces pressure from centre of heel

Figures 18.6A & B **A selection of non-casted podiatric orthoses including a rear view of menicus heel pad.**

The Heel

The heel may be affected by calcaneal erosions or enthesopathy or by atrophy of the plantar fat pad. The preferred accommodative orthosis used in this area is a meniscus heel pad which may include a foam button placed centrally (Figure 18.6A).

The Metatarsal Head Area (Plantar)

The main objective in managing pain is to attempt to relocate load from painful metatarsal heads to unaffected areas. (Figure 18.6B). This may be achieved by the use of non-casted insoles which are fitted into the footwear or by the use of prescription orthoses which are manufactured to previously taken casts of the patients' feet. Prescription orthoses tend to offer more protection as the padding can be approximated very closely to the presenting foot lesions.

The Metatarsophalangeal Joint Area (Lateral) and Lesser Toes

These areas invariably suffer from frictional forces from the shoe and have traditionally been protected by the use of latex rubber shields which are manufactured onto a plaster cast of the patient's foot. These incorporate oval aperture or crescent-shaped pads made from open or closed cell foam rubber. Although the basic shape of the padding has not changed the need for casting the foot prior to the manufacture of latex orthodigita is no longer necessary, as silicone devices may now be manufactured directly onto the patient's foot.

MATERIALS USED IN THE MANUFACTURE OF PODIATRIC ORTHOSES

Non Cellular Polyurethane Foam

This material is manufactured from shock-absorbing polyurethane elastomers. The material deforms on impact and the shock waves are spread over a greater area of contact between the foot and the ground.

Cellular Polyurethane Foam

This material is a frothed cellular urethane which is soft, resilient and protective. Both types of foam are useful in reducing shock, especially at heel strike.

Sponge Rubbers

These have been used for many years in the manufacture of insoles. Structurally there are two types of sponge rubber: open cell and closed cell sponge rubbers. They vary widely in structure and function.

Open Cell Rubber (OCR)

These consist of a mass of rubber honeycombed with interconnected cells communicating with the atmosphere at the surfaces of the material. When a force is placed upon unsealed OCR it collapses instantly leaving only the thickness of the rubber material between the force and the structure supporting the material. When the force is removed the cells refill with air and the material springs back resuming its former dimensions. Repeated and intermittent force will cause the material to 'bottom out' retaining less than 50% of its original thickness. Useful for applying cushioning to an area.

Closed Cell Rubber

These consist of a mass of rubber or synthetic rubber containing many small isolated pockets of nitrogen gas, blown evenly throughout the material. This material will retain 70% of its original thickness when compressed. It will return to shape after the deforming force is removed. This material feels harder to the touch than OCR.

Silicone elastomers

Silicone orthodigita (removable pads manufactured from silicone elastomers, which are also used in dentistry for casting impressions of teeth and gums) have largely superseded the latex rubber techniques.

Crosslinked Polyethylene Foam (Plastazote)

Plastazote is a closed cell crosslinked polyethylene. It is a lightweight material and in soft and medium densities is very cushioning. It is very popular with rheumatoid patients because of these properties. One major drawback is that it 'bottoms out' very rapidly and does require regular renewal.

Most materials used in the manufacture of podiatric insoles are available in thicknesses ranging from 1 to 10 mm.

FOOTWEAR

The most taxing of all tasks in the management of the 'rheumatic foot' is its encasement in a shoe which will accommodate both constantly changing deformities and orthotic devices and will meet the wearer's aesthetic needs.

Constant compressional pressure on tissues from footwear causes necrotic breakdown, whilst intermittent pressure can cause hyperkeratotic lesions to develop. Footwear which allows the foot to be subjected to shearing stresses can cause nail disorders, apical callus, blisters and/or adventitious bursae. The deviation of the digits predisposes the inter-digital spaces to maceration and ulceration. As healing is often compromised, the ill-fitted shoe or boot has serious implications. Correct initial fitting does not guarantee a trouble free foot. Changes in foot shape can mean that footwear becomes obsolete very quickly and is then no longer comfortable or fitted.

Hip and knee deformities will also influence the correctness and continuing fit of the footwear. The destruction of the hip and knee will change stance and gait. Valgus knee deformities are likely to put increased pressure on the medial border of the foot and hence the shoe. Hip involvement may prevent adequate ground clearance during the swing phase of the walking cycle.

Footwear selection depends on the needs of patients and their disease process. For example, deformity of the joints means that the foot must be accommodated, whilst a vascularly impaired foot requires materials which protect the foot from changes in temperature and external factors without causing added pressure to the foot. There are currently three alternatives: shop bought footwear which has been adapted, stock footwear bought from specialist retailers made on modified lasts, and bespoke or made-to-measure footwear.

Shop bought footwear with adaptations is the cheapest alternative, although less favoured today because of the improved quality of stock shoes. Examples of modifications include heel raises (to take the strain of the tendo achilles) and balloon patches (to accommodate single prominent joints). Rocker bars and metatarsal bars can be externally fixed to boots or shoes by orthotists but care must be taken with any adaptation which requires individuals to alter their already compromised gait.

Stock footwear, designed for forefoot deformities, is becoming increasingly utilised (Kaye, 1994). It is considerably cheaper than bespoke footwear and is designed with extra-depth or extra-width toe box or both (Figure 18.7) This footwear will accommodate marked digital deformity and also extra padding and orthoses. Some examples are designed to be opened up so that rigid feet, which cannot move to allow a shoe to be slipped on, can be placed onto the sole and the shoe wrapped around it.

Bespoke footwear is an expensive option which does not guarantee comfort and fit (Stewart, 1996). Its appearance has improved considerably over the last few years, but the materials used and the prescribed designs make it often inappropriate for indoor and summer use.

All footwear should be selected on the basis of individual need but generally the footwear should be light in weight, have soft and malleable uppers with some form of adaptable fixation. Velcro is especially helpful for those with hand problems. If the individual is house-bound, shoes designed for out-door use may be too warm, heavy and difficult to walk on carpeted areas. Alternatives need to be sought.

Training shoes are helpful for people with rheumatological conditions, being light and warm, with shock-absorbing properties and in some instances Velcro fastenings. They are usually broad across the MTPJs and have a high toe-box which accommodates toe deformities. With 'rheumatoid flatfoot', care must be taken to ensure that the shoes of choice have a strong heel counter in order that it may withstand the forces of pronation.

Decisions about what footwear is best for people is governed by the presenting clinical picture. If the individual is experiencing pain and excessive pronation from the subtalar joint, a shoe with a strong medial heel counter and shank is necessary. Dorsal, medial or lateral deformities can usually be accommodated if not too severe by stretching soft leather uppers, although designs with stitching on the uppers of the shoes will be damaged in this process.

SUMMARY

Understanding the foot dynamically can give insight into the resultant changes in rheumatological conditions and therefore the management of the foot. As mechanical forces are not the only cause of deformity and pain in the feet, an appreciation of the pathological process will ensure a more complete understanding of the foot within specific disease processes and the management necessary to promote ambulation.

There is little research to suggest what is the best way to manage the foot in rheumatic disease. Therefore clinicians must base their therapeutic management upon the clinical manifestations with which the patient presents and review the aims of care with each episode of change.

ACKNOWLEDGEMENTS
Mr Peter Ball, Department of Podiatric Medicine, New College Durham.
Media Services Department at New College Durham.
David Price, Cosy Feet.

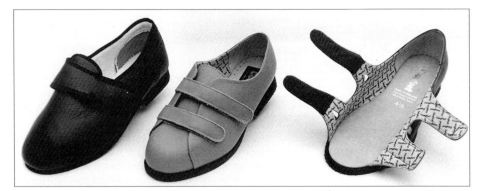

Figure 18.7 Stock footwear.

REFERENCES

Betts RP, Stockley I, Getty CJM *et al.* Foot pressure studies in the assessment of forefoot arthroplasty in the rheumatoid foot. *Foot Ankle* 1988, **8**:315-325.

Boyd PM, Rendall G. Structure and function. In: Lorimer DL, ed. *Neale's common foot disorders, 4th edition*. Edinburgh: Churchill Livingstone; 1993:7-18.

Calmels C, Eulry F, Lechevalier D *et al.* Involvement of the foot in reactive arthritis. A retrospective study of 105 cases. *Rev Rheumatisme Edition Francaise* 1993, **60**:324-329.

Cawley MID, Smidt LA. Rheumatic disorders. In: Lorimer DL, ed. *Neale's common foot disorders, 4th edition*. Edinburgh: Churchill Livingstone; 1993:367-376.

Cohen MG, Emmerson BT. Gout. In: Klippel JH, Dieppe PA, eds. *Practical rheumatology*. London: Mosby; 1995:255-276.

Cracheola A, Cimino WR, Lian G. Arthrodesis of the ankle in patients who have rheumatoid arthritis. *J Bone Jt Surg* 1992, **74A**:903-909.

D'Ambrosia RD. Orthotic devices in running injuries. *Clin Sports Med* 1985, **4**:611-618.

Deesomchok U, Tumrasvin T. Clinical comparison of patients with ankylosing spondylitis, Reiter's syndrome and psoriatic arthritis. *J Med Assoc Thailand* 1993, **76**:61-70.

Dieppe PA. Clinical features and diagnostic problems in osteoarthritis. In : Klippel JH, Dieppe PA, eds. *Practical rheumatology*. London: Mosby; 1995:141-156.

Dimonte P, Light H. Pathomechanics, gait deviations and treatment of the rheumatoid foot. *Phys Ther* 1982, **62**:1148-1156.

Donatelli R, Wooden M. Biomechanical orthotics. In: Donatelli M, ed. *The biomechanics of the foot and ankle*. Philadelphia: Davis; 1990:193-216.

Fenton DA, Wilkinson JD. The nail in systemic disease and drug induced changes. In: Baran R, Dawber RPR eds. *Diseases of the nail and their management*. Oxford: Blackwell Scientific Publications; 1984:205-266.

Foulston J. Biomechanics of the foot. In: Jayson MIV, Smidt LA, eds. *Clinical rheumatology*. London: Ballière and Tindall; 1987.

Hughes J, Clark P, Klenerman L. The importance of the toes in walking. *J Bone Jt Surg* 1990, **72B**:245-251.

Jahss M. Arch Supports Shielding and Orthodigita. In: Jahss M, ed. *Disorders of the foot and ankle*. Philadelphia: Saunders; 1991:2857-2865.

Kaye RA. The extra-depth toe box: a rational approach. *Foot Ankle* 1994, **3**:146-150.

Keenan MAE, Peabody TD, Gronley JK *et al.* Valgus deformities of the feet and characteristics of gait in patients who have rheumatoid arthritis. *J Bone Jt Surg* 1991, **73A**:237-247.

Kerman BL, Mack G, Moshirfar MM. Tophaceous gout of the foot: an unusual presentation of severe chronic gout in undiagnosed patient. *J Foot Ankle Surg* 1993, **32**:167-170.

Luukkainen R, Kaarela K, Isomaki H *et al.* The prediction of radiological destruction during the early stage of rheumatoid arthritis. *Clin Expl Rheumatol* 1983, **1**:295-298.

MacKie RA. Psoriatic and other papulo-squamous disease. In: *Clinical dermatology: an illustrated textbook, 3rd edition*. Oxford: Oxford University Press; 1993:38-70.

Minns RJ, Craxford AD. Pressure under the forefoot in rheumatoid arthritis: a comparison of static and dynamic methods of assessment. *Clin Orthop* 1984, **187**:235-242.

Reeback J, Silman A. Predictors of outcome at two years in patients with rheumatoid arthritis. *J Roy Soc Med* 1984, **77**:1002-1005.

Roth RD. Joint diseases associated with aging. *Clin Podiatric Med Surg* 1993, **10**:137-159.

Samnegard E, Turan I, Lanshammar H. Post operative pressure under the rheumatoid foot. *J Foot Surg* 1990, **29**:593-594.

Schoenhaus HD, Cohen RS. Etiology of the bunion. *J Foot Surg* 1992, **31**:25-29.

Stewart J. Patient satisfaction with bespoke footwear in people with rheumatoid arthritis. *J Br Podiatric Med* 1996, **51**:21-23.

Toivanen A. Reactive arthritis. In: Klippel JH, Dieppe PA, eds. *Practical Rheumatology*. London: Mosby; 1995:287-294.

Veale D, Roger S, Fitzgerald O. Classification of clinical subjects in psoriatic arthritis. *Br J Rheumatol* 1994, **33**:133-138.

Waugh W. Ankle disorders. In: Helal B, Wilson D, eds. *The foot*. Edinburgh: Churchill Livingstone; 1988:550-566.

West SG, Woodburn J. Pain in the foot. *BMJ* 1995, **310**:860-864.

GENERAL READING

Alexander IJ. *The foot: examination and diagnosis*. New York: Churchill Livingstone; 1990.

Helal B, Wilson D, eds. *The foot*. Edinburgh: Churchill Livingstone; 1988.

Janisse DJ. The art and science of fitting shoes. *Foot Ankle* 1992, **13**:257-262.

Merriman LM, Tollafield DR. *Assessment of the lower limb*. Edinburgh: Churchill Livingstone; 1995.

Valmassy RL. *Clinical biomechanics of the lower extremities*. St. Louis: Mosby; 1996.

Whittle MW. *Gait analysis - an introduction*. Oxford: Butterworth-Heinemann; 1996.

SECTION 5

PAEDIATRICS

rheumatology (roo·mat·ol·o·je). Branch of medicine which is concerned with the diagnosis and treatment of rheumatic disorders.

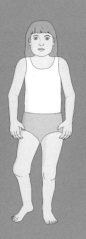

19 E Hall

ARTHRITIS IN CHILDREN

CHAPTER OUTLINE

- Juvenile chronic arthritis
- Juvenile ankylosing spondylitis
- Juvenile psoriatic arthritis
- Juvenile systemic lupus erythematosus
- Juvenile dermatomyositis
- Management of juvenile chronic arthritis

INTRODUCTION

Children of all ages complain from time to time about aches and pains in their joints and muscles. Fortunately most of these conditions are short-lived and have no long-term complications for the children and their families. Some diseases, however, may present with musculoskeletal aches and pains but can have serious consequences. These include leukaemia, neoplasia, trauma (accidental and non-accidental), rheumatic fever and chronic arthritis. It is therefore important to take the child's complaint seriously until such time that no cause is found. Even if there are no organic reasons for the child's symptoms it is always important to bear in mind the possibilities of sexual and /or mental abuse, as these can present with physical signs and symptoms.

This chapter aims to address some of the more common rheumatic diseases of childhood, many of which have similarities to the disease in adults whereas others are unique to the young person. At present there are two sets of criteria for the classification of chronic childhood arthritis—those of the American College of Rheumatology (ACR) and those of the European League Against Rheumatology (EULAR) (Table 19.1).

INCIDENCE

1 in 5000 children develop chronic arthritis, and 1 in 1000 will develop significant joint inflammation following an episode of viral illness. However, the frequency of rheumatic disease in childhood and adolescence is thought to be rare, thus inappropriately delaying diagnosis. Approximately 80% of children will have complete remission of their arthritis while still in childhood. There is, however, a small but significant number who will continue to have problems in adulthood. These are more likely to be children with seropositive polyarthritis and juvenile ankylosing spondylitis (JAS). The most commonly recognised of the childhood rheumatic diseases is juvenile chronic arthritis (JCA) of pauci-articular onset accounting for 40–50% of children.

JUVENILE CHRONIC ARTHRITIS

This, the most common group can be subdivided into three distinct types depending on mode of onset:
- Systemic.
- Polyarticular.
- Pauci-articular.

Table 19.1 **Criteria for classification of childhood arthritis.**

Criteria for classification of childhood arthritis		
	American College of Rheumatology Criteria	**European League against Rheumatology Criteria**
Age at onset	Under 16 years	Under 16 years
Duration	6 weeks or more	3 months or more
Onset types	Juvenile rheumatoid arthritis (JRA): Pauci-articular (<5 joints) Polyarticular (>4 joints) Systemic arthritis with characteristic fever	Still's Disease Pauci-articular (<5 joints) Polyarticular (>4 joints seronegative) Systemic arthritis with characteristic fever
Other groups	None	JRA – seropositive polyarthritis Ankylosing spondylitis Psoriatic arthritis
Exclusions	Other forms of arthritis	

Some other types of childhood arthritis, though less common, include:
- JAS.
- Juvenile psoriatic arthritis (JPsA).
- Systemic lupus erythematosus (SLE).
- Dermatomyositis.

Systemic

George Fredric Still was the first person to record the classic symptoms of systemic-onset JCA (Still, 1897). In the US this tends to be known as juvenile rheumatoid arthritis (JRA). It is also known as Still's disease; this is more old fashioned but is still in current use. This group is defined by:
- The majority having the onset before 5 years old.
- There being an equal sex incidence.

The characteristic features of JCA include:
- Swinging fever which can be 40°C at night and subnormal by the morning.
- A macular rash which is associated with the high fever.
- Lymphadenopathy, splenomegaly and pericarditis.
- Acute-phase proteins will be elevated indicating high levels of inflammation. These include C-reactive protein (CRP) and serum complement.
- Erythrocyte sedimentation rate (ESR) will be raised and may be as high as 100 mm/hour.
- White cell count may be as high as $50 \times 10^9/l$ and platelet count as high as $600 \times 10^9/l$.
- Moderate anaemia.

At the time of presentation the child, who is often very ill, may have had bouts of arthritis or arthralgia affecting many joints, but not yet have developed persistent joint symptoms. However, all children will go on to develop persistent arthritis, and it is often only then that a definite diagnosis of systemic-onset JCA will be made (Figure 19.1).

Once developed, it tends to have a symmetrical distribution. The most commonly affected joints are the knees, wrists and ankles closely followed by the cervical spine, hips and the temporomandibular joints. The hips and wrists are most frequent sites for progressive and destructive changes; these may be seen as early as 1 year after onset and indicate a poor prognosis in terms of functional outcome (Schneider et al., 1992).

Delayed growth is another common feature. The delayed growth is said to be related to disease activity, inadequate calorie intake and the use of corticosteroids to treat the disease. Bacon et al. (1990) indicated that the link between nutritional state and growth could be due to alterations in the requirements, absorption and use of circulating nutrients in the presence of chronic inflammation. Bernstein et al. (1974) noted that a third of those with arthritis in his study group were below the 3rd centile for height at disease diagnosis, perhaps reflecting unrecognised early disease.

Course and Prognosis

This is very difficult to predict and consequently it is very difficult to give parents and the child any clear indication as to what the future holds. Systemic-onset JCA may follow a monocyclic course that will lead to full remission in about 2 years. Other children follow a polycyclic course that is characterised by exacerbations and remissions of disease activity. A few will have persistent, active polyarthritis. A study by Calabro et al. (1976) reported that the average period of active disease duration is 5–6 years; however, as stated earlier, approximately 5% of children will have persistent disease activity well into their adult life.

The amount and severity of joint involvement cannot be predicted; however, the longer the duration of disease activity, the greater the number of involved joints. Progressive destructive arthritis occurs in approximately one third of all patients. The majority of these children have significant disability at long-term follow up. It is also within this group that most of the systemic complications occur.

Mortality

It needs to be remembered that children who fall into this sub-group of JCA have systemic as well as joint disease and as a consequence have a higher mortality rate when compared with the other groups. Several large European studies report the death rate to be about 14% (Ansell & Wood, 1976, Stroeber, 1981, Häfner & Truckenbrodt, 1986). The major causes of death are:
• Amyloidosis with renal failure.
• Infection.
• Hepatic failure.

• Myopericarditis.
• Haematological disorders.

Polyarticular

This subset of JCA is identical to rheumatoid arthritis (RA) in adults both clinically and genetically. The group is defined as:
• Onset under 15 years (around 10 being the most common).
• More than five joints involved within 6 months.
• Active synovitis present for 3 months.
• Sex ratio F>M 3:1.

Characteristic features of polyarticular JCA (Figure 19.2) are:
• A symmetrical polyarthritis affecting large joints (i.e. knees) and the small joint of the hands and feet.
• Approximately 10% will be rheumatoid factor (RF) positive.
• The inflammatory indices are usually raised.

The subtype of children who are RF negative tend to be younger girls and generally have a better prognosis. The older, RF positive children will on the whole not do so well,

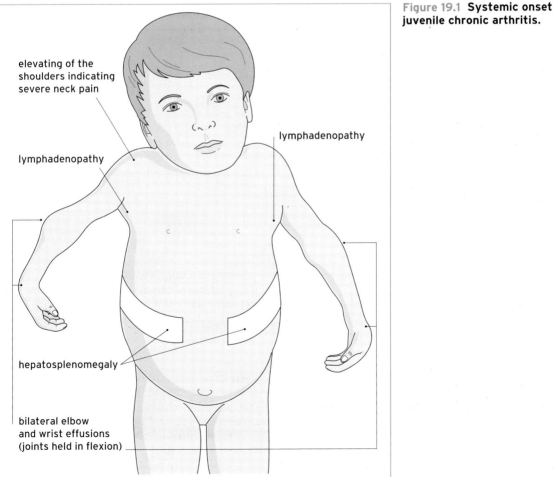

Figure 19.1 Systemic onset juvenile chronic arthritis.

elevating of the shoulders indicating severe neck pain

lymphadenopathy

lymphadenopathy

hepatosplenomegaly

bilateral elbow and wrist effusions (joints held in flexion) especially with the presence of rheumatoid nodules and signs of early erosions on X-ray. It is these children who are most likely to continue having active disease into adulthood and consequently a poor functional outcome (Cassidy *et al.*, 1989).

Course and Prognosis

The disease pattern tends to be one of progressive, destructive polyarthritis affecting many joints including knees, ankles, neck and hips. The involvement of the hips at an early stage in the disease is a poor prognostic indicator. Controlling the severity of inflammation will help to reduce the destruction of the joints. However, in long-term follow-up studies about 30% of children had severe functional difficulties (Ansell & Wood, 1976). This results in loss of independence as help is required to perform various activities of daily living (David *et al.*, 1994).

Pauci-articular

This sub-group is the most common among all the childhood arthritides, accounting for approximately 50% of all the children with JCA. This group is defined as:
• Onset under 16 years.
• Less than four joints involved in the first 6 months.
• Active synovitis in at least one joint for 3 months.

The characteristic features include:
• A high incidence among pre-school-age girls.
• Large joint involvement, usually the knees, elbows and ankles and rarely the hip or shoulder.
• Frequent occurrence of chronic anterior uveitis.
• High incidence of positive anti-nuclear antibody (ANA).
• Inflammatory indices are usually normal.

The classic clinical picture is one of a normal healthy toddler, usually female, who develops a monoarthritis or an asymmetrical arthritis in a few joints (Figure 19.3). The joints most commonly affected are the knee, ankle and the elbow (in order of frequency) (Ansell, 1977). The child may not complain of pain but the parents notice that the joints are swollen, and the child may start limping or want to be carried more often. Even at this early stage there may be a noticeable flexion deformity of the knee and associated muscle wasting. Despite the obvious clinical signs the child may not be incapacitated and his or her activities may be only modestly limited.

There is, however, another subset within pauci-articular JCA. These children tend to be older boys often with lower limb arthritis. They are frequently human leukocyte antigen (HLA)-B27 positive and present with enthesitis. The pattern of disease has more resemblance

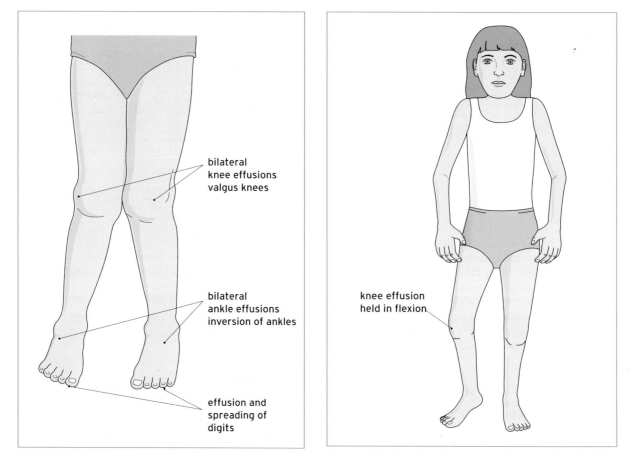

Figure 19.2 Polyarticular juvenile chronic arthritis.

bilateral knee effusions valgus knees

bilateral ankle effusions inversion of ankles

effusion and spreading of digits

knee effusion held in flexion

Figure 19.3 Pauci-articular juvenile chronic arthritis.

to a spondyloarthropathy than JCA. This group will be discussed later.

Course and Prognosis

Most children with pauci-articular onset remain within this group. The total number of joints involved will remain at less than five, and the typical length of time for active disease is 2–5 years (Sherry *et al.*, 1993). Joint destruction is rare except in those children who progress to a poly-articular course. Most children will have little if any disability once the disease has run its course.

Children with pauci-articular JCA are at risk of developing severe muscle wasting and bony enlargement of a joint as well as inequality of leg length with knee involvement. If the disease develops before the age of 3 the affected leg is longer due to the inflammation, which increases the blood flow thus stimulating growth (Vostrejs & Hollister, 1988). If, however, the disease starts after the age of 9, there is a tendency for premature closure of the epiphyses which will result in the affected leg being shorter (Simon *et al.*, 1981).

There may also be one-sided closure of the epiphysis thus leading to a valgus or varus deformity. In the hands and feet there may be odd length digits. Controlling the inflammation can help to reduce these effects but will not necessarily eliminate them altogether.

The potentially most disabling consequence of pauci-articular JCA is chronic iridocyclitis or anterior uveitis. It is suggested that approximately 20% of children with this type of arthritis develop chronic iridocyclitis (Sherry *et al.*, 1991). Kanski (1990) stated that 10% will be blind at the 10-year follow-up, 50% will have decreased visual acuity and 25% will have cataracts or glaucoma. Chronic iridocyclitis is described as inflammation of the anterior part of the eye and the reason it is a serious complication is that it usually remains asymptomatic until significant damage has been done. Children who are ANA positive and RF negative are at most risk. It is essential, though, that all children have regular ophthalmic (slit lamp) examinations. If the uveitis is missed there is a high risk of severe damage which can result in blindness. Thus the child may not have any significant disability as a result of the arthritis but may be disabled due to lack of vision (David *et al.*, 1994).

The arthritis and uveitis usually develop at different times, with arthritis often the first to develop; however, asymptomatic and consequently undetected uveitis may already be present at diagnosis. The uveitis can last for many years after remission of joint symptoms. The relative severity of joint and eye disease can differ widely; severe joint disease does not necessarily mean that the eyes will be similarly affected.

JUVENILE ANKYLOSING SPONDYLITIS

In children the diagnosis of JAS is often delayed. For a definite diagnosis the sacroiliac joints must be involved and this involvement usually follows the development of peripheral arthritis. The classic clinical features of AS are described in Chapter 10. Briefly, AS primarily involves the axial and peripheral skeleton and is accompanied by enthesitis (inflammation at the teno–osseous junction) and iritis (inflammation of the eye). The common features of JAS are:

- Asymmetrical, pauci-articular arthritis.
- Weightbearing joints, especially the knee, are most commonly involved.
- Sex ratio M:F, 8:1.
- Common age at onset is 8–10 years.
- Strong family history of spondyloarthropathies.
- Approximately 75% are HLA B27 positive.

It is important to observe for sacroiliac involvement in boys who are HLA B27 positive (see Chapter 10 for the importance of this marker) and have a large joint arthropathy.

In contrast to adults, children rarely complain of pain relating to the axial skeleton. This probably explains why many children are initially diagnosed as having pauci-articular JCA, as the presenting feature is often persistent swelling of a lower limb joint, e.g. the knee. Treatment of these children is the same as for adults with AS and is therefore discussed in Chapter 10.

JUVENILE PSORIATIC ARTHRITIS

This arthropathy is defined as being arthritis commencing before the age of 16 years and associated with psoriasis either preceding the arthritis or following it within 15 years. In the majority of children the arthritis precedes the psoriasis (this is opposite to adults) and the clinical arthritic picture is similar to that found in adults. Southwood *et al.* (1989) revised the diagnostic criteria and consequently stated that the number of all childhood arthritides attributed to juvenile psoriatic arthritis (JPsA) could be as high as 19%.

DIAGNOSTIC CRITERIA FOR JUVENILE PSORIATIC ARTHRITIS

Southwood *et al.* (1989) documented the Vancouver criteria for the diagnosis of JPsA as:

Definite JPsA:
- Arthritis with typical psoriatic rash.
- Arthritis with three of the four following minor criteria:
    Dactylitis.
    Nail pitting or onycholysis.
    Psoriasis-like rash.
    Family history (first or second degree relative) of psoriasis.

Probable JPsA:
- Arthritis with two of the four minor criteria listed above.

Southwood *et al.* (1989) and Cassidy & Petty (1990) stated that the clinical manifestations need not be present simultaneously. The management of these children is similar to that of JCA and will be discussed later in this chapter.

JUVENILE SYSTEMIC LUPUS ERYTHEMATOSUS

This type of arthritis in childhood and adolescence closely resembles the adult type. Silverman & Eddy (1993) documented the common clinical features, the prevalence of which were taken from a range of studies from 1956 to 1990 (Table 19.2). In children arthritis and arthralgia occur in more than 90%; this is usually episodic, affecting large and small joints alike. This arthritis does not usually lead to any deformity and is treated symptomatically by physiotherapists and the medical profession.

The classical malar rash, in the butterfly distribution, is said to occur in 80% of children during the course of the disease and may be the first sign of a disease flare-up (Silverman & Eddy 1993). The more complex manifestations of the disease include widespread inflammation of the blood vessels (vasculitis), involvement of the central nervous system (psychiatric disorders, headaches and neuropathies), cardiac involvement (pericarditis), and renal disease (nephritis). If these complications of the disease are not adequately controlled then there is a high mortality risk, especially if the renal involvement is severe. Lacks & White (1990) reported an 85% survival rate at 5 years for those children with renal disease. These figures are similar to the survival rates in the adult population.

The treatment of SLE is dependent on the prevalence and severity of symptoms. For mild disease, usually arthralgia and myalgia with no evidence of multi-system involvement, the treatment of choice would be non-steroidal anti-inflammatory drugs (NSAIDs) and an antimalarial drug (e.g.

hydroxychloroquine). The presence of vasculitis, renal involvement and other systemic features requires steroids and immunosuppressant drugs as the outcome of uncontrolled severe disease in these children is not good.

JUVENILE DERMATOMYOSITIS

This is a chronic and progressive weakness usually affecting proximal muscles, namely the hip and shoulder girdle, with associated vascular and skin manifestations. Some children, usually those with more severe disease, develop soft tissue calcifications (calcinosis). Pachman *et al.* (1985) indicated that the figure for this was approximately 30% but as more intensive therapy was being instituted they felt that numbers would reduce. The calcinosis can vary from a few calcific lumps which can resolve spontaneously to more extensive lesions which can severely inhibit function. This calcinosis is rare in adult onset dermatomyositis but can present in adults when their disease onset occurred in childhood (Cohen *et al.*, 1986).

The weakness presents itself as difficulty in functional activities, for instance climbing stairs and getting up off the floor, and the child may push off its legs with its hands in an attempt to stand up. Pain is not a common complaint among these children.

Due to the weakness there is a tendency to develop early flexion contractures. In the early inflammatory stage gentle passive stretching, splinting and functional positioning of the joints are all that should be done as any active exercising can exacerbate the condition. It must also be remembered that the weakness is due to the inflammatory process and not lack of use. Once the acute stage is over then gentle graded exercise regimes can be started. Close monitoring of inflammatory parameters is necessary to ensure that the exercise programmes do not induce a flare-up.

MANAGEMENT OF JUVENILE CHRONIC ARTHRITIS

The management of these children is a potentially long and sometimes difficult task. It often involves many years of routine exercises, splinting and medication. For some children it also includes major orthopaedic surgery.

Each type of arthritis has distinct features which can influence the overall outcome for the child. As physiotherapists, it is important to take these distinctions into account when planning and implementing treatment.

A team approach is essential to obtain the best outcome in terms of physical and psychosocial well-being. The team members must communicate with each other to enable a consistent and co-ordinated care plan to be developed and followed. This plan will need to be adapted because circumstances will change due to progression of the disease and the fact that children grow up! Children have different physical and psychosocial needs at the various stages of development, i.e. childhood, adolescence and young adult.

The main team is highlighted in Figure 19.4. Ideally the consultant should be a paediatric rheumatologist.

Features of juvenile systemic lupus erythematosus	
Clinical features that can occur at any time during the disease course	
Feature	**%**
Fever	80-100
Arthritis	60-90
Skin rash (any)	60-90
Malar rash	30-80
Renal	48-100
Cardiovascular	25-60
Pulmonary	18-81
Central nervous system	26-44
Gastrointestinal	24-40
Hepatosplenomegaly	19-43
Lymphadenopathy	13-45

Table 19.2 **Features of juvenile systemic lupus erythematosus.**

However, in many hospitals an adult rheumatology consultant and a paediatrician work closely together to provide the medical support. Other members of the team who may be needed in the management of these children are:
- Chiropodists/Podiatrists.
- Orthotists.
- Orthopaedic surgeons.
- Ophthalmologists.
- Medical social workers.
- Clinical psychologists.

Management of arthritis can be divided into many different elements. Each element needs the involvement and co-operation of the others if the outcome for the child, in terms of functional ability, is to be as favourable as possible. The term management encompasses many facets and includes:
- Drug therapy.
- Physiotherapy/Hydrotherapy.
- Occupational therapy.
- Splinting.
- Surgery.
- Schooling.

DRUG THERAPY

Drug therapy is an important treatment modality and the aims of treatment are two-fold:
- To control inflammation and provide analgesia.
- To control disease activity.

The drugs used in the treatment of children are the same as those used in adults. They will produce the same effect as well as having the same side effects. For further information, see Chapter 3.

The inflammation is controlled by NSAIDs, i.e. ibuprofen, naproxen, diclofenac, etc. These can be in tablet, suppository or liquid form. There are currently only six NSAIDs licensed for use in paediatrics. For persistent disease activity NSAIDs will usually be taken as a regular dose (i.e. three times a day); however, in less severe disease the drugs can be used as required (i.e. if the child has a

increase in joint symptoms then the NSAIDs can be used for a few days to get the child over an acute episode).

Reducing the level of inflammation may have a good analgesic effect but should more pain relief be required then paracetamol may be used as well; for very small children and babies there are liquid forms. Aspirin is not recommended because of its association with Reye's syndrome.

In children whose arthritis cannot be controlled with simple NSAIDs the next step is to use slow-acting anti-rheumatic drugs (SAARDs). Their action is to try to control the disease process itself and not just alleviate the signs and symptoms. The drugs used are:
- Hydroxychloroquine.
- D-penicillamine.
- Gold (oral or intramuscular).
- Sulphasalazine.
- Methotrexate.

In very severe disease or cases of vasculitis, cyclophosphamide and azathioprine may be needed.

Oral corticosteroids for the treatment of rheumatological conditions, especially in children, are used with caution due to the long-term complications. However, as inflammation decreases skeletal growth they may be used as a first choice. Complications can include osteoporosis with subsequent vertebral collapse, delayed growth and, in the short-term, weight gain and cushingoid features. An alternate day dose regime reduces these side effects. In cases of severe life-threatening manifestations of juvenile rheumatoid disease, oral or intravenous steroids will be administered to reduce the inflammation rapidly. Steroids quickly reduce the signs and symptoms of rheumatoid disease (i.e. inflammation) and may play a part in controlling the underlying disease process

The use of intra-articular steroids, however, has an important role to play in the management of these children. In cases where one or two joints are a persistent problem despite continued or increased medication, an injection, normally under general anaesthetic, will usually settle the symptoms and allow for effective physiotherapy. In children with polyarticular disease a treatment plan of multiple joint injections and physiotherapy has been shown to be beneficial in re-mobilisation.

PHYSIOTHERAPY

Physiotherapy is an extremely important aspect in the management of JCA. The physiotherapist requires an understanding of the particular aspects of the disease, together with an ability to communicate and build up a rapport with the children and their families. A great deal of energy and enthusiasm is needed as treatment is often prolonged (i.e. years) and unwelcome, especially if the child is in a lot of pain.

As children approach their teenage years they begin to develop a certain amount of independence in thought and deed that can often lead to conflict. To maintain the rapport therapists may need to 'back off' from formal treatment to allow children to make certain decisions themselves. This can often be frustrating as one can visualise these children

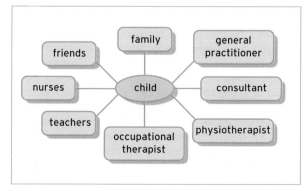

Figure 19.4 Members of the team involved in the management of children with juvenile chronic arthritis.

achieving more in terms of functional independence if only they would participate more with their exercises. Unless children are willing to be in partnership with the therapist in planning their treatment programme they may rebel and possibly do nothing in terms of exercise, wearing splints, etc. However, gentle persuasion with discussion and the development of achievable targets will often work. Working together with the child to set goals that are relevant to them at that time is essential to retain their confidence. The aims of physiotherapy are:

• To maintain and/or improve joint range.
• Increase muscle power.
• Reduce pain.
• Prevent deformity.
• Maximise functional potential.
• Provide support and encouragement.

Physiotherapy should be started as soon as a diagnosis is made. The severity of the arthritis as well as the particular type of onset will indicate the amount of involvement by physiotherapists.

Assessment

The assessment of children is not always straightforward. A subjective assessment should include a history from both the child and the parents. This way the therapist can get a good overall picture of the problems being experienced by both parties (as these may differ). Inclusion of children indicates to them that they are believed in respect to the problems they are having, especially if the arthritis is mild. This provides a good platform for the development of the professional relationship. During the subjective assessment it is also important to ascertain a child's hobbies and interests as this knowledge will often be useful when planning treatment goals. It will also demonstrate an interest in the child as a person and not just his or her arthritis.

Objective Assessment

The objective assessment should include observations and measurements on the following:

• General appearance.
• Pain.
• Swelling.
• Muscle power.
• Joint range.
• Deformity and posture.
• Extra-articular manifestation, i.e. nodules.
• Functional ability.
• Gait analysis.

When assessing functional ability it is important to take into account children's ages, especially those under 5 years, as they may not yet be able to achieve a functional activity even without arthritis. Following the assessment the therapist should be able to:

• Determine the best treatment plan for that particular child.

• Monitor the effect of subsequent treatment against base line data.
• Provide information to assist other members of the team.

The physical management of all types of juvenile arthritis can involve a variety of treatment modalities which may include:

• Daily exercise regimes.
• Hot/cold therapy.
• Electrical therapy.
• Hydrotherapy.
• Splinting.

The exercise regimes not only maintain joint range and muscle power but also help to stimulate skeletal growth. The children are encouraged to perform the exercises daily because inflamed joints have a tendency to stiffen quickly and develop flexion deformities. Specific passive stretches to all affected joints should be done twice daily. A routine to include all joints is the ideal but acceptance of other family pressures needs to be taken in to account. It is better that the child concentrates on problem areas, especially if time is limited due to the hectic family schedule.

Older children can be taught specific routines and be expected to carry them out. In the young child, age-appropriate activities need to be taught to the parents or guardians as well as the child. The specific aims of the activities need to be fully explained. The parents or guardians need to be shown the correct way the child has to perform these activities as well as how to handle and perform the soft tissue stretches to the joint. Normal play cannot be substituted for direct physiotherapy as the child will automatically use the unaffected limb or use the affected limb in the position of most comfort—usually a degree of flexion. This does not mean that play is ruled out but that play has to be supervised and directed to ensure that the muscles and joints are used correctly.

In the systemically ill child with high levels of inflammation, rest in a good functional position is important; however, the joints need to be exercised passively to ensure joint mobility is not lost. Vigorous exercise at this stage will not only be too painful but can increase the levels of inflammation within a joint potentially leading to more joint damage in terms of cartilage and bone loss. Hydrotherapy is the most effective treatment modality at this stage. Progression to active-assisted and then active exercises can be implemented when the child is able.

Exercise regimes need to ensure that all joints are fully stretched and all muscle groups are strengthened. There should be a daily routine and the numbers of each exercise performed will depend on the severity of symptoms. Older children need to be encouraged to take responsibility for their own exercise programme. If the child has a flare-up it is important to concentrate on maintenance of joint range rather than strengthening.

Hot and Cold Therapy

The use of hot and cold therapy in children is as important as in the adult. It is important to bear in mind the age of the child as the very young will not be able to sit still long enough to comply with some of the treatment modalities, e.g. ice, hot packs and wax.

Moist heat in the form of hot packs or a hot bath helps to reduce pain and muscle spasm as well as aid relaxation. Heat prior to exercises will enable the joints and muscles to work more effectively. If serial splints need to be applied, heat used prior to the application of the splint will allow for a greater stretch to the joint, thus obtaining a better result.

Wax therapy is also very useful prior to hand exercises. The child can also use the wax to make shapes and objects using the different actions of the hand, i.e. pinch grip, full fist, metacarpophalangeal, proximal and distal interphalangeal flexion. This modality is not suitable for younger children as they tend to find the wax too hot.

A hot bath in the mornings will often help to reduce the early morning stiffness. This is important to enable the child to get to school. In the very small child, bathtime can be an important time for exercising as well as having fun. In very swollen joints ice therapy is preferable but some children may not tolerate this treatment modality well.

Electrical Therapy

Electrotherapy modalities are not often used when treating children due to the problems of compliance as mentioned earlier. They can be used in older children to reduce the pain and swelling. Another important reason for avoiding electrotherapy is that the treatment cannot be done at home thus requiring more frequent visits to the hospital, which is not conducive to education or to promoting a sense of independence. The modalities that may be used are ultrasound, pulsed shortwave and interferential.

Hydrotherapy

Hydrotherapy is an ideal medium for the treatment of JCA. The warm water not only helps to reduce pain and muscle spasm but the buoyancy will assist movement of painful limbs. Progression to buoyancy resisted exercises can be implemented when the child is able. Posture correction and gait re-education can be started early even in the very ill child, and as the child recovers then the good habits learnt in the water can be transferred to dry land.

The ability to swim or at least be comfortable in water is important for the psychosocial development of these children. It is a medium where they can compete with their peers and be part of a group and not left on the outside as can happen on dry land, if the children cannot keep up with other more boisterous play activities.

Above all hydrotherapy is fun. Most children do not realise that they are exercising when in water. It is important for the therapist to devise games and activities that exercise the joints correctly. The therapist has to be very inventive and prepared to get very wet!

Prone Lying

When joints are swollen the position of most comfort is in a degree of flexion (loose packed position). This tends to enlarge the joint space, reducing the pressure on the soft tissues and reducing pain. As a consequence of this, an arthritic child will adopt a posture of hip and knee flexion when standing and a curled up position when in bed. If this is prolonged then deformities will develop. To counteract this posture the children are encouraged to lie prone for at least 1 hour a day. This can be done watching television, reading, doing homework or playing games. Ideally prone lying should be done on the floor but if the child has severe neck involvement this may not be practical and supine lying on the bed may have to be an acceptable compromise. In some cases it may be necessary to use night traction to maintain good hip extension.

Splinting

Splinting of joints in arthritic children has a varied and valuable role. The main reasons for splinting are to:

- Rest a joint in a functional position, especially if active synovitis is present.
- Provide support and improve function if there is instability present.
- Correct and prevent deformity.

Compliance in children, especially the older ones, can be a problem. The main reasons for lack of compliance are discomfort and that the splints are not aesthetically pleasing. The discomfort factor can easily be addressed by either remaking the splint or remoulding it if thermoplastic materials are used. The image factor is not so easily sorted out. Children of all ages find it hard to be different, they tend to get picked on and left out of peer social groups. This can have a marked psychological effect on these children. A thorough explanation of the reasons for the splints is needed, and making the splints in flesh or currently fashionable coloured materials may help. Sometimes compromises have to be reached, i.e. wrist splints have to be worn when not in school (even though school is the best time to wear them). Eventually the child may realise that there is less pain by wearing them and so will comply.

Resting splints are used to maintain the joint in a good position (Figure 19.5) and are usually worn at night. The splints are in the forms of paddle splints for the hands and wrists and full leg gutters for the knees and ankles (Figure 19.6). The materials used are either plaster of Paris or thermoplastic. For the very young child giving the splint a name or drawing features on it may make the child less frightened. Having got the young child to accept the splint, compliance is not usually a problem.

Working splints are most commonly applied to the wrists to maintain extension as it is in this position that the grip is at its strongest and consequently most functional. Wrist extension is quickly lost in children with JCA and is very difficult to regain; therefore the saying 'prevention is better than cure' is very appropriate in this instance. The splints can be made of thermoplastic materials or leather and need to be adjusted as the child grows or as the swelling fluctuates. This ensures that they are a good fit, comfortable and functionally correct.

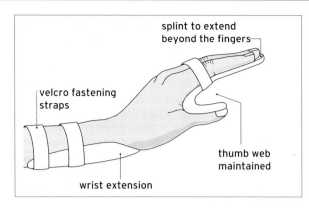

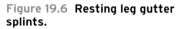

Figure 19.5 **Resting hand splints.**

splint to extend
beyond the fingers

velcro fastening
straps

thumb web
maintained

wrist extension

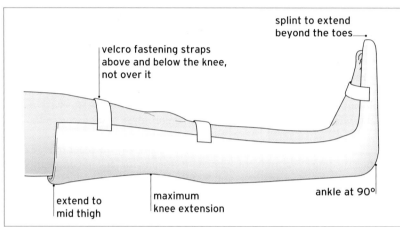

Figure 19.6 **Resting leg gutter splints.**

splint to extend
beyond the toes

velcro fastening straps
above and below the knee,
not over it

extend to
mid thigh

maximum
knee extension

ankle at 90°

Serial splints are used to correct severe flexion deformities, especially of the knees. The splints need to be used in conjunction with intensive physiotherapy. There is no point in straightening a leg which has inadequate muscle power to maintain the straight position; therefore the muscle imbalance has to be corrected. A good regime for serial splinting would be to wear the splint at weekends, followed by active exercises throughout the week with the leg in the bivalved splint when not exercising and during the night.

Collars are worn to reduce pain and maintain good head and neck posture. In cases of long-standing disease there may be some instability so the collar needs to be worn to prevent damage to the spinal cord prior to any surgical intervention.

Other splints that may be used in the management of JCA are foot orthoses in the form of moulded heel cups to maintain the calcaneus in a good position, or full length insoles to correct excessive forefoot pronation.

OCCUPATIONAL THERAPY

The occupational therapist (OT) is a valuable member of the team. There may be considerable overlap between OTs and physiotherapists depending on the facilities and personnel available. The major role of OTs is to assess functional skills and provide training in independence. They will also assess the needs of the child regarding aids and equipment adaptations to assist in independence. In some units the OTs are the main providers of made-to-measure splints.

The assessment should cover all aspects of activities of daily living including personal care, play, schooling, social activities and the child's ability to cope with its environment, as well as ensuring that developmental milestones are achieved.

SURGERY

There is an increasing awareness of the valuable role that surgery has to play in the management of these children. It is not now seen as a salvage procedure to fall back on when all else has failed but rather as an important part in the overall management of these children. Timely surgical intervention can prevent or at least delay the onset of severe musculoskeletal problems.

It is important that there is joint consultation between orthopaedic surgeons and rheumatologists at an early stage if there is an indication that surgery might be needed. The main surgical procedures are:

- Soft tissue release.
- Joint replacements, e.g. hip and knee.
- Arthrodesis, e.g. ankle and fingers (for function and stability).
- Femoral osteotomy (delays joint replacement surgery).

The main reason for surgery would be the restoration of function and then the reduction of pain. It is well recognised that there has to be active physiotherapy following any surgical procedure to obtain maximum benefit from the operation. It is therefore necessary to establish that the child and the parents or guardians can and will comply with the post-operative regime, otherwise surgery may not be considered.

An interesting note is that only 10% of children with JCA are seropositive (RF positive); however, of those who require surgical intervention about 50% are seropositive thus reflecting the aggressive nature of seropositivity in joint destruction.

SCHOOLING

This section is not at the end of the chapter because it is least important. In fact for many of these children it is very important because due to their joint problems they will have to make a living by 'brains and not brawn'.

The majority of children cope well in mainstream schools but it may be necessary to discuss the problems these children have with their teachers. The main problems they encounter are climbing stairs and carrying heavy bags. Communication between the relevant parties will usually overcome these problems.

Some children, due to the severity of their functional problems, will go to special schools where facilities are more suitable. These schools usually have a physiotherapy service available which will help to maintain the child's independence by providing possibly daily treatment. This treatment can be fitted in around lessons thus ensuring an adequate level of education which could not be achieved if the child had to be brought out of school so regularly for physiotherapy.

CONCLUSION

The treatment of JCA is a long and often difficult task involving many years of routine exercises, splinting and medication. It is therefore important to establish a good rapport with the children and their families at an early stage as this makes the task of the therapist easier. A positive approach from all members of the team is essential to ensure that the children grow up to lead as full a life as possible despite the constraints of their arthritis. The main philosophy of physiotherapy management for these children is to keep them active and set treatment goals that are relevant to the individual child at that moment.

REFERENCES

Ansell BM, Wood PHN. Prognosis in juvenile chronic polyarthritis. *Clin Rheum Dis* 1976, **2**:397-412.

Ansell BM. Joint manifestations in children with juvenile chronic polyarthritis. *Arthritis Rheum* 1977, **20**:204-206.

Bacon M, White PH, Raiten DJ *et al*. Nutritional status and growth in juvenile rheumatoid arthritis. *Sem Arthritis Rheum* 1990, **20**:1-11.

Bernstein BH, Stobie D, Singsen BH *et al*. Growth retardation in juvenile rheumatoid arthritis. *Arthritis Rheum* 1974, **20**:213-216.

Calabro JJ, Holgerson WB, Sonpal GM, Khoury MI. Juvenile rheumatoid arthritis: a general review and report on 100 patients observed for 15 years. *Sem Arthritis Rheum* 1976, **5**:257-298.

Cassidy JT, Levenson JE, Brewer EJ Jr. The development of classification criteria for children with juvenile rheumatoid arthritis. *Bull Rheum Dis* 1989, **38**:1-7.

Cassidy JT, Petty RE, eds. *Textbook of paediatric rheumatology, 2nd edition*. New York: Churchill Livingstone; 1990.

Cohen MG, Nash J, Webb J. Calcification is rare in adult onset dermatomyositis. *Clin Rheum* 1986, **5**:512-551.

David J, Cooper C, Hickey L *et al*. The functional and psychological outcomes of juvenile chronic arthritis in young adulthood. *J Rheum* 1994, **33**:876-881.

Hafner R, Truckenbrodt H. Course and prognosis of systemic juvenile chronic arthritis retrospective study of 187 patients. *Klinische Paediatrie* 1986, **198**:401-407.

Kanski JJ. Uveitis in juvenile chronic arthritis. *Clin Rheum* 1990, **8**:499-503.

Lacks S, White P. Morbidity associated with childhood systemic lupus erythematosis. *J Rheum* 1990, **17**:941-945.

Pachman LM, Friedman JM, Maryjowski-Sweeney ML *et al*. Immunogenetic studies of juvenile dermatomyositis III: study of antibody to organ-specific and nuclear antigens. *Arth Rheum* 1985, **28**:151-157.

Schneider R, Lang BA, Reilly BJ *et al*. Prognostic indicators of joint destruction in systemic-onset juvenile rheumatoid arthritis. *J Paeds* 1992, **120**:200-205.

Sherry DD, Mellins ED, Nepom B. Pauciarticular-onset juvenile chronic (rheumatoid) arthritis. In: Maddison PJ, Isenberg DA, Woo P, Glass DN, eds. *Oxford Textbook of Rheumatology*. Oxford: Oxford University Press; 1993, vol 2:710-722.

Sherry DD, Mellins ED, Wedgewood RJ. Decreasing severity of chronic uveitis in children with pauciarticular arthritis. *Am J Dis of Child* 1991, **145(9)**:1026-1028.

Silverman ED, Eddy A. Systemic lupus erythematosis in childhood and adolescence. In: Maddison PJ, Isenberg DA, Woo P, Glass DN, eds. *Oxford Textbook of Rheumatology*. Oxford: Oxford Univeristy Press; 1993: vol2:756-771.

Simon S, Whiffen J, Shapiro F. Leg length discrepancies in monarticular and pauciarticular juvenile rheumatoid arthritis. *J Bone & Joint Surg* 1981, **63A**:209-215.

SouthwoodTR, Petty RE, Malleson PN *et al*. Psoriatic arthritis in children. *Arthritis Rheum* 1989, **32**:1007-1013.

Still GF. On a form of chronic joint disease in children. *Medical-chirurgical Transactions* 1897, **80**:47-59.

Stroeber E. Prognosis in juvenile chronic arthritis. *Eur J Paeds* 1981, **135**:225-228.

Vostrejs M, Hollister JR. Muscle atrophy and leg length discrepancies in pauciarticular juvenile rheumatoid arthritis. *Am J Dis of Child* 1988, **145**:343-345.

GENERAL READING

Ansell B. *Colour Atlas of Peadiatric Rheumatology*. London: Wolfe Publications; 1991.

Arthritis Rheumatic Council. *When your Child has Arthritis*. ARC

Emery HM, Bowyer SL. Physical modalities of therapy in peadiatric rheumatic disease. *Rheum Dis Clin North Am* 1991, **17(4)**:1001-1014.

Holroyd J. *Arthritis at Your Age?* Ipswich: The Grindle Press; 1992

Varni JW. Evaluation and management of pain in children with juvenile rheumatoid arthritis. *Rheum* 1992, **19(33)**:32-35.

Wallace CA, Levison JE. Juvenile rheumatoid arthritis: outcome and treatment for the 1990s. *Rheum Dis Clin North Am* 1991, **17**:891-905.

Woo P. *Paediatric Rheumatology Update*. Oxford: Oxford University Press; 1990.

INDEX